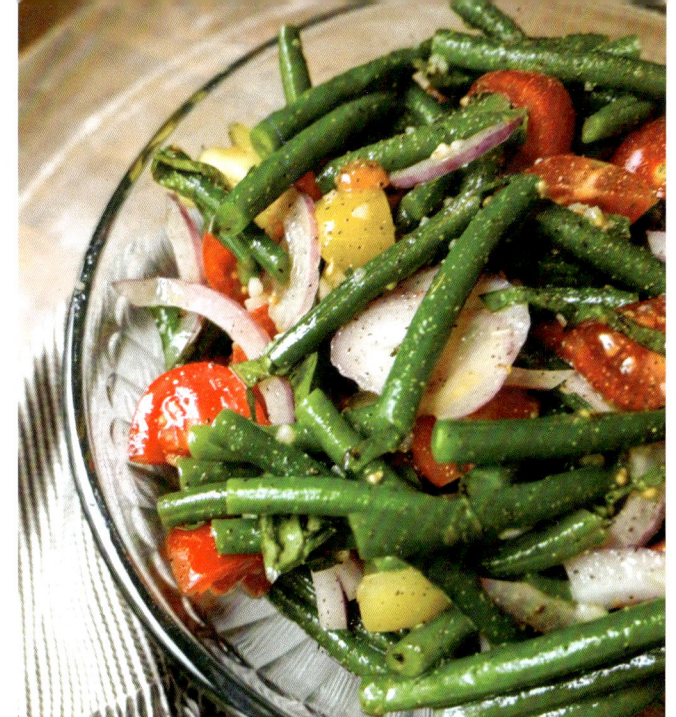

D1788354

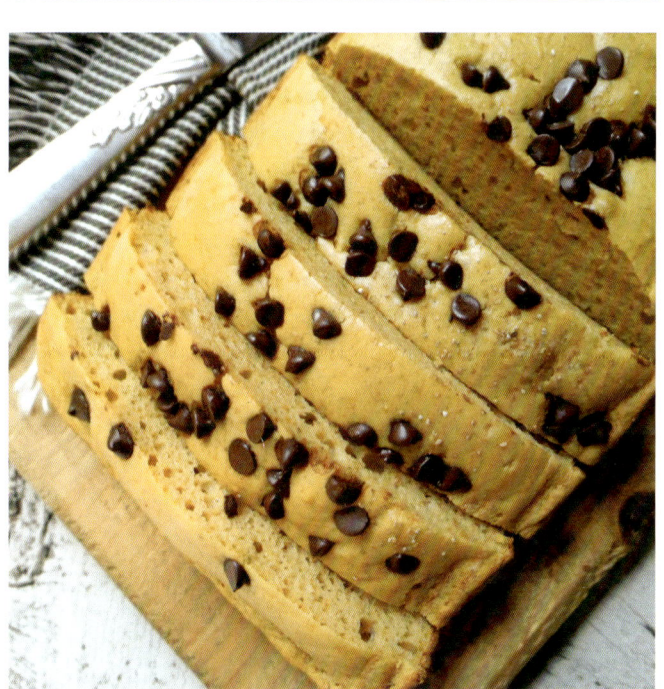

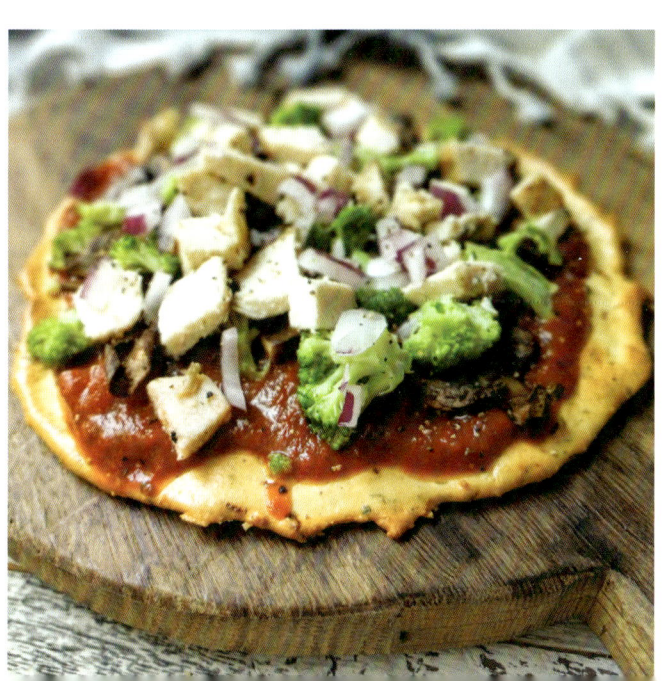

contents

how to use janeva's ideal recipe cookbook

The purpose of Janeva's Ideal Recipes cookbook is to provide a resourceful tool filled with a variety of phase 1 protocol recipes, taking you through your entire phase 1 journey. Have some fun in the kitchen while preparing your own meals, now and for a lifetime!

- Each recipe provides serving sizes for phase 1. The serving sizes include Ideal Protein packet counts (whether unrestricted or restricted), lean protein, veggie, oil, and dairy counts, as they pertain to each recipe. Any 'extras' such as syrups or condiments should be considered and are not included in the serving size counts. Consult your coach or clinic for supporting ingredients that qualify as an 'extra'.

- The 6 oz. lean protein US protocol has been used in these recipes throughout the cookbook. If you are using the 8 oz. lean protein protocol, it is very easy to add 2 oz. more lean protein to the recipes. The alternative option is to prepare the recipes as written (6 oz. lean protein) and fill the 8 oz. protein requirement with 2 oz. additional protein by eating hard boiled eggs as a snack or adding lean protein to a lunch meal. Consult your coach or clinic for further information.

janeva's baking tips

- When a recipe calls for shredded squash (zucchini or chayote), it may be used peeled or unpeeled unless otherwise specified.

- Always mix dry ingredients well to incorporate baking powder or baking soda into the mixture. This will ensure an even rise of the baked goods.

- After mixing batter and filling pan(s), bake immediately as the leaveners (rising ingredients) are activated by the liquid and need to be baked promptly before deactivation.

- Spray metal pans with cooking spray before adding batter - silicone pans/molds do not need cooking spray.

- If using baking liners for the muffin and cupcake recipes, be sure they are made of parchment paper; standard paper baking liners will cause the proteins to stick to the paper.

- Bake on center rack of oven for even baking.

- Remove baked goods from the pan immediately after baking - cool completely on a cooling rack before serving unless the recipe states otherwise. Baked goods moisten as they cool resulting in the best texture.

- To store, place baked goods in a plastic resealable bag; refrigerate up to 2 days. To freeze, remove as much air as possible from the bag and freeze.

meet janeva

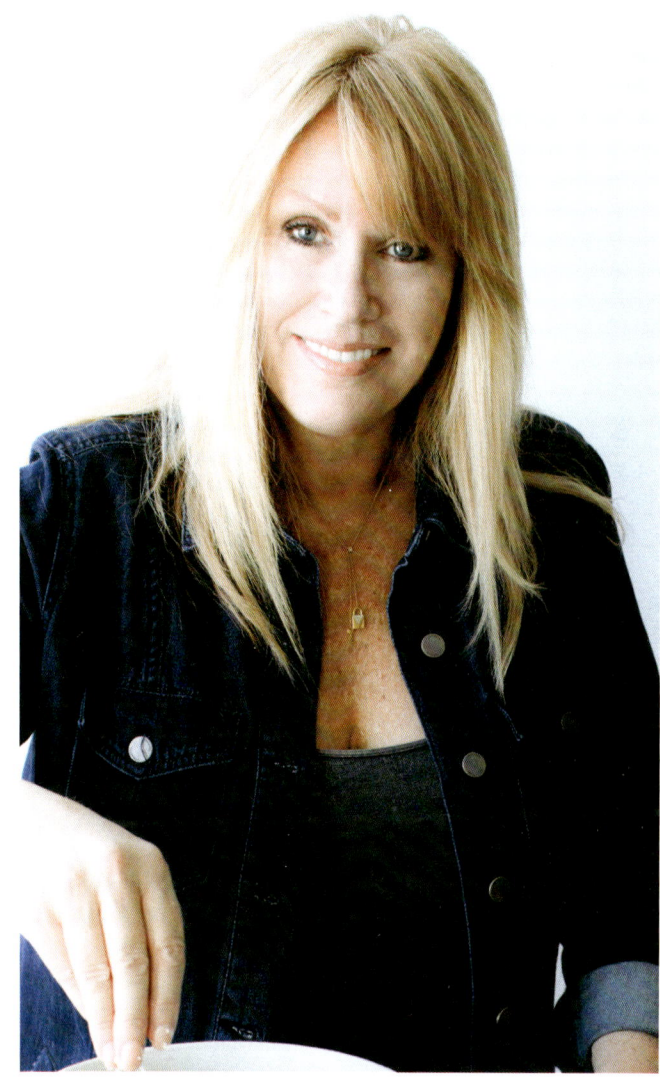

International cookbook author, Janeva Eickhoff, struggled with her weight as the years brought her into her 50's. In 2013 she began her weight loss journey with the Ideal Protein® weight loss program and found she still wanted the classic comfort dishes she was used to cooking and eating. While re-creating those homestyle classic comfort recipes using healthier ingredients, Janeva successfully lost 33 lbs. in just 10 weeks. Janeva began baking with Ideal Protein® food packets, thus pioneering over 80+ baked goods recipes. This gained the attention of fellow social media dieters, and soon they were asking for a cookbook. Janeva gathered 300+ of her original phase 1 recipes, and in June 2015, she published her first and very successful cookbook, Janeva's Ideal Recipes, a personal collection of recipes for the Ideal Protein® weight loss program. Janeva is passionate about helping others succeed with their own weight loss goals and interacts daily with her followers on her Facebook cookbook page. Since publishing her first cookbook, Janeva has gone on to create, write, and publish 6 cookbooks for a healthy and nutritional lifestyle; her current cookbooks are available online at her website.

After Janeva lost her only son in 2001, she began a charity in his name in 2015. A portion of the proceeds from her cookbook sales are donated to Samuel's House Foundation via Feed My Starving Children. Donations thus far have provided a meal for over 70K children worldwide.

Janeva lives in central Minnesota with her life love, Rory, and their lovable cat, Luey.

For daily support and recipe ideas for the Ideal Protein® phase 1 journey, join us at:

WWW.JANEVASKITCHEN.COM

Janeva's Ideal Recipes Cookbook – Phase 1

Instagram @janevasidealrecipes

beverages & smoothies

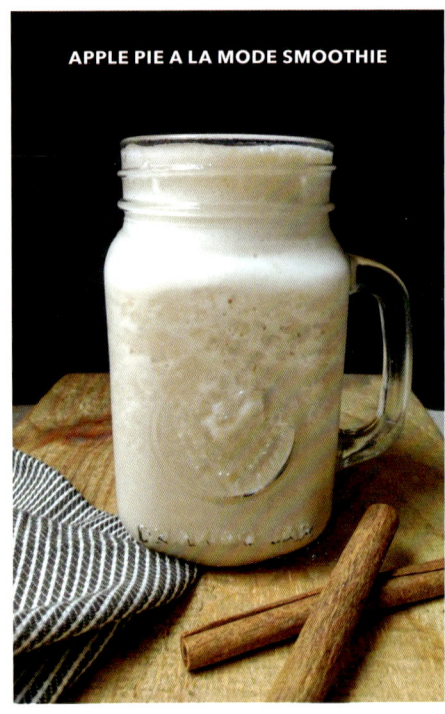

APPLE PIE A LA MODE SMOOTHIE

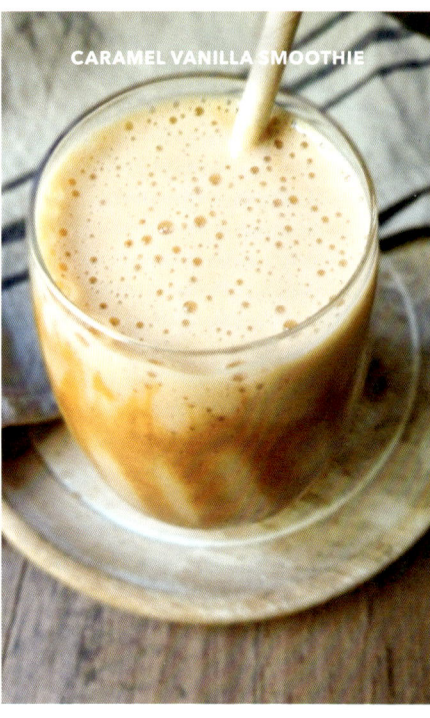

CARAMEL VANILLA SMOOTHIE

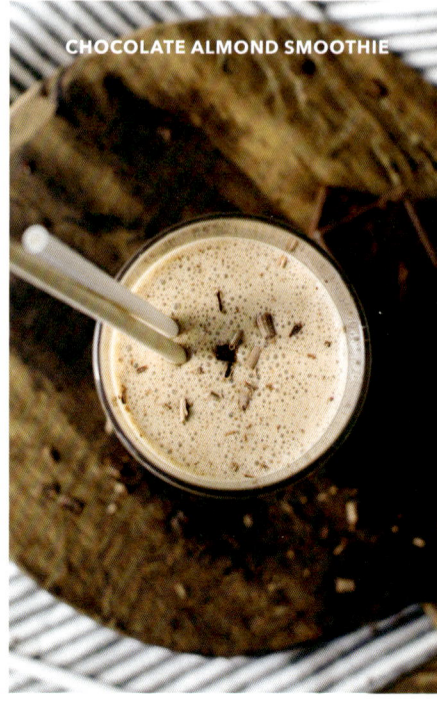

CHOCOLATE ALMOND SMOOTHIE

Apple Pie a la Mode Smoothie

INGREDIENTS
1 Ideal Protein vanilla shake (ready-to-drink)
1 C. ice
⅔ C. Caramel Fried Apples, pg. 127

DIRECTIONS
1. Blend ingredients in a 900+ watt blender until smooth and creamy.

SERVINGS
Entire recipe yield = 1 unrestricted + 1 C. veggies (⅔ C. cooked Caramel Fried Apples = 1 C. raw veggies)

Caramel Vanilla Smoothie

INGREDIENTS
1 Ideal Protein vanilla pudding mix
2 T. Walden Farms caramel syrup
1 tsp. vanilla extract
10 oz. water
1 C. ice (or more for desired consistency)

DIRECTIONS
1. Blend ingredients in a 900+ watt blender until smooth and creamy.

SERVINGS
Entire recipe yield = 1 unrestricted

Chocolate Almond Smoothie

INGREDIENTS
1 Ideal Protein dark chocolate pudding mix
10 oz. cold water
¼ tsp. almond extract
1 C. ice (or more for desired consistency)

DIRECTIONS
1. Blend ingredients in a 900+ watt blender until smooth and creamy.

SERVINGS
Entire recipe yield = 1 unrestricted

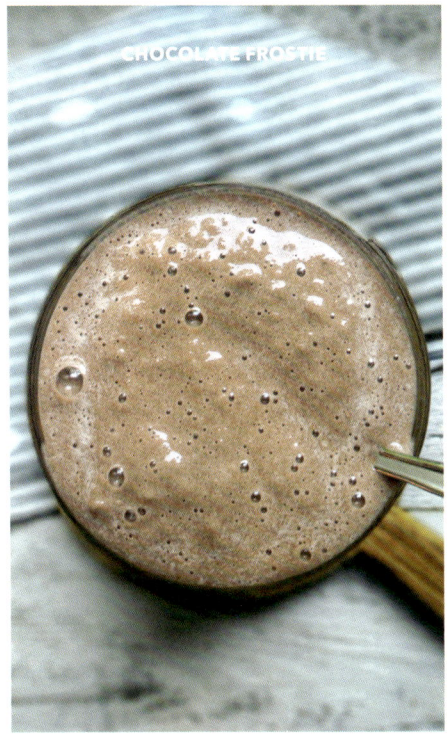
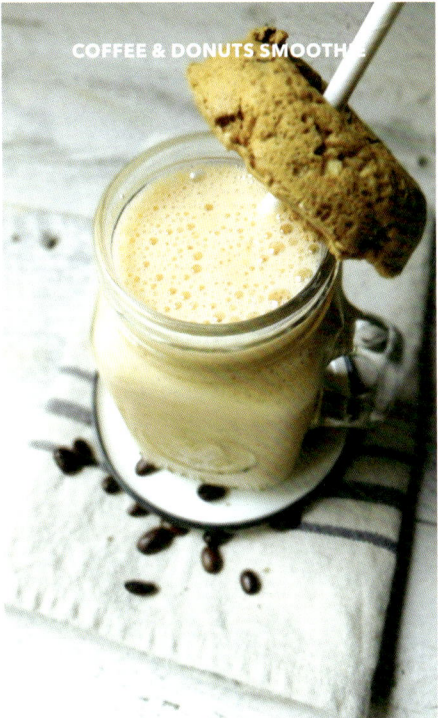
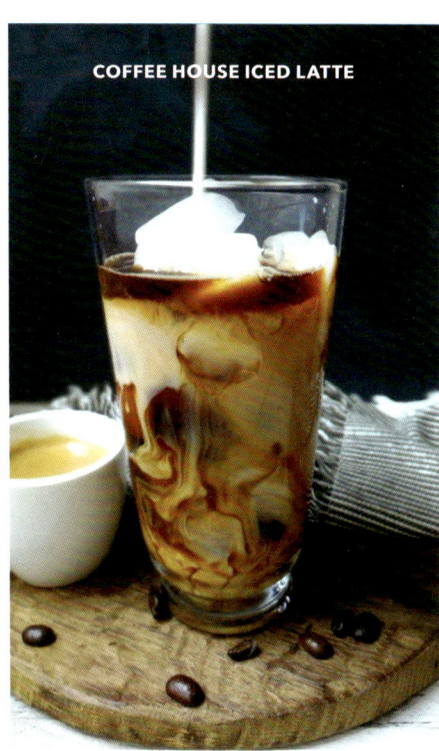

CHOCOLATE FROSTIE

COFFEE & DONUTS SMOOTHIE

COFFEE HOUSE ICED LATTE

Chocolate Frostie

Great way to get your veggies in—and you won't taste the cauliflower!

INGREDIENTS

5.25 oz. frozen cauliflower rice
1 Ideal Protein chocolate smoothie mix
⅓ C. (about 5) ice cubes
1 C. cold water

DIRECTIONS

1. In order listed, place ingredients in a blender. Blend on high until smooth and creamy.

SERVINGS

Entire recipe yield = 1 unrestricted + 1 ½ C. veggies

Coffee & Donuts Smoothie

INGREDIENTS

1 Ideal Protein vanilla pudding mix
½ tsp. butter extract
1 tsp. instant espresso or coffee granules
¼ tsp. cinnamon
10 oz. cold water
1 C. ice

DIRECTIONS

1. Blend ingredients in a 900+ watt blender until smooth and creamy.

SERVINGS

Entire recipe yield = 1 unrestricted

Coffee House Iced Latte

INGREDIENTS

Ice
1 Ideal Protein vanilla shake (ready-to-drink)
2 oz. (2 shots) espresso
1 pump sugar free coffee syrup, any flavor (optional)

DIRECTIONS

1. Fill a large cup or glass with ice. Add remaining ingredients; stir to mix.

SERVINGS

Entire recipe yield = 1 unrestricted

TIP: When ordering at a coffee house, ask for a doppio (2 shots espresso) over ice in a tall glass. Add one Ideal Protein vanilla shake and stir.

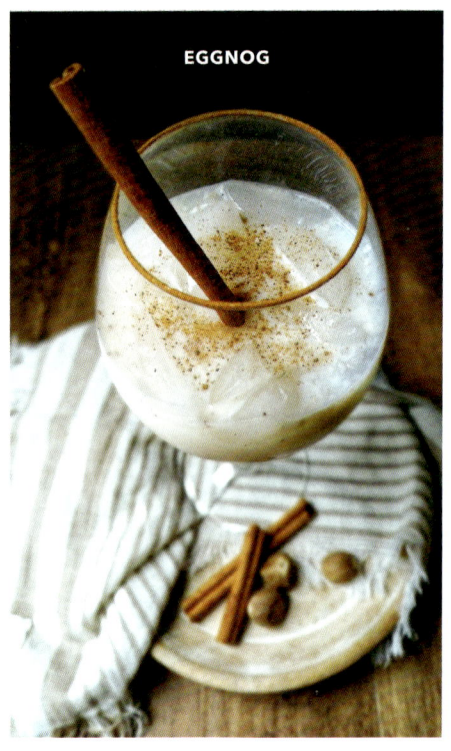

EGGNOG

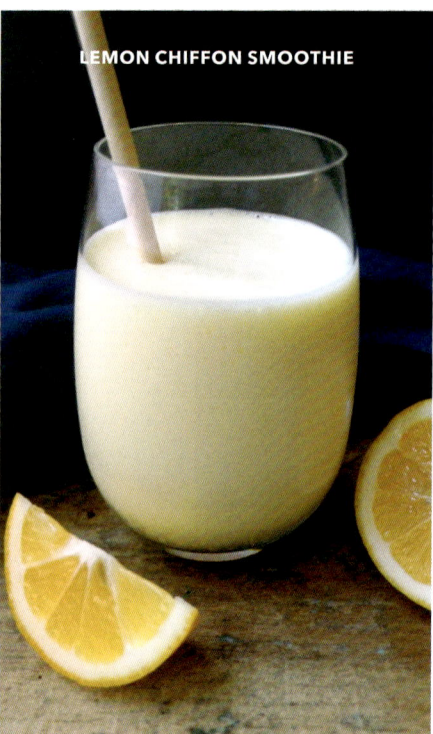

LEMON CHIFFON SMOOTHIE

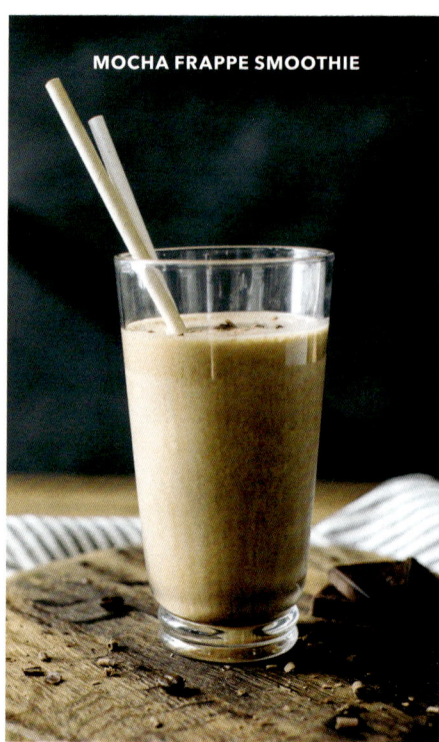

MOCHA FRAPPE SMOOTHIE

Eggnog

INGREDIENTS

1 Ideal Protein vanilla shake (ready-to-drink)
1 ½ tsp. Ideal Protein vanilla pudding mix
⅛ tsp. rum extract
¼ tsp. nutmeg

DIRECTIONS

1. Place ingredients in a blender; blend. Serve over ice.

SERVINGS

Entire recipe yield = 1 unrestricted

TIP: The 1 ½ tsp. vanilla pudding mix helps to thicken and flavor the eggnog. I reserve a pudding packet for recipes like this and store in fridge.

Lemon Chiffon Smoothie

INGREDIENTS

1 Ideal Protein vanilla pudding mix
9 oz. water
⅛ tsp. lemon extract
2 T. half and half cream
1 ½ C. ice

DIRECTIONS

1. Blend ingredients in a 900+ watt blender until smooth and creamy.

SERVINGS

Entire recipe yield = 1 unrestricted + 1 oz. half and half cream

TIP: Yellow food coloring may be added to enhance the lemon color.

Mocha Frappe Smoothie

INGREDIENTS

1 Ideal Protein dark chocolate pudding mix
4 oz. cold coffee
6 oz. cold water
½ tsp. instant espresso granules
½ tsp. vanilla extract
⅛ tsp. liquid stevia extract (optional)
2 C. ice

DIRECTIONS

1. Blend ingredients in a 900+ watt blender until smooth and creamy.

SERVINGS

Entire recipe yield = 1 unrestricted

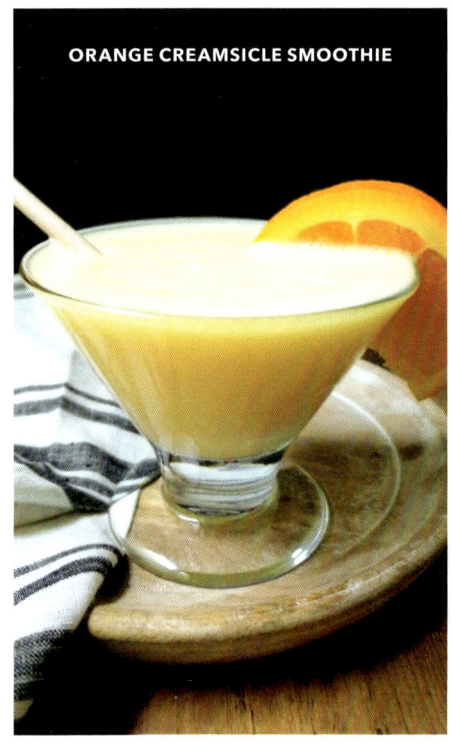

ORANGE CREAMSICLE SMOOTHIE

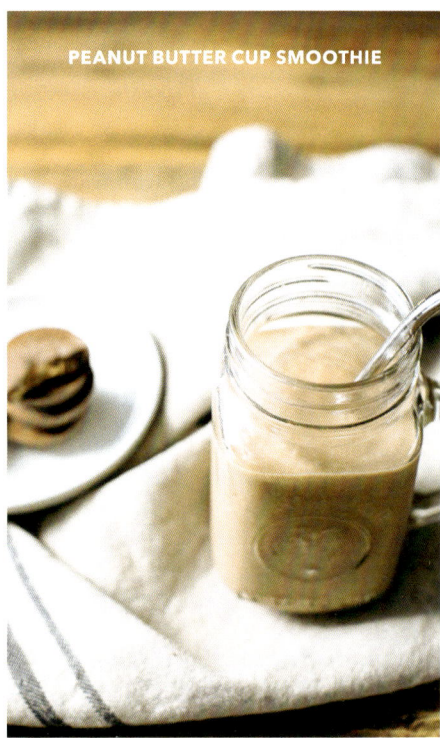

PEANUT BUTTER CUP SMOOTHIE

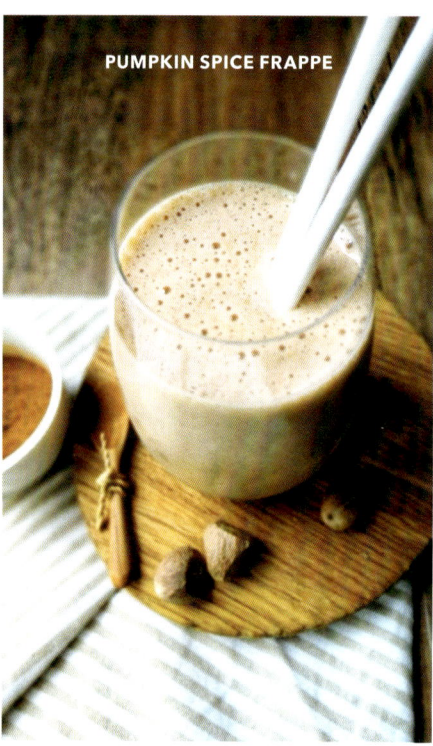

PUMPKIN SPICE FRAPPE

Orange Creamsicle Smoothie

INGREDIENTS
1 Ideal Protein vanilla smoothie mix
2 T. Walden Farms orange marmalade
1 tsp. vanilla extract
8 oz. cold water
1 C. ice

DIRECTIONS
1. Blend ingredients in a 900+ watt blender until smooth and creamy.

SERVINGS
Entire recipe yield = 1 unrestricted

Peanut Butter Cup Smoothie

INGREDIENTS
1 Ideal Protein dark chocolate pudding mix
1 T. Walden Farms peanut butter
10 oz. cold water
¼ tsp. vanilla extract
1 C. ice (or more for desired consistency)

DIRECTIONS
2. Blend ingredients in a 900+ watt blender until smooth and creamy.

SERVINGS
Entire recipe yield = 1 unrestricted

Pumpkin Spice Frappe

INGREDIENTS
1 Ideal Protein vanilla smoothie mix
6 oz. water
½ tsp. Pumpkin Pie Spice, pg. 145
1 T. Walden Farms caramel syrup
2 T. half and half cream
1 C. ice

DIRECTIONS
1. Blend ingredients in a 900+ watt blender until smooth and creamy.

SERVINGS
Entire recipe yield = 1 unrestricted + 1 oz. half and half cream

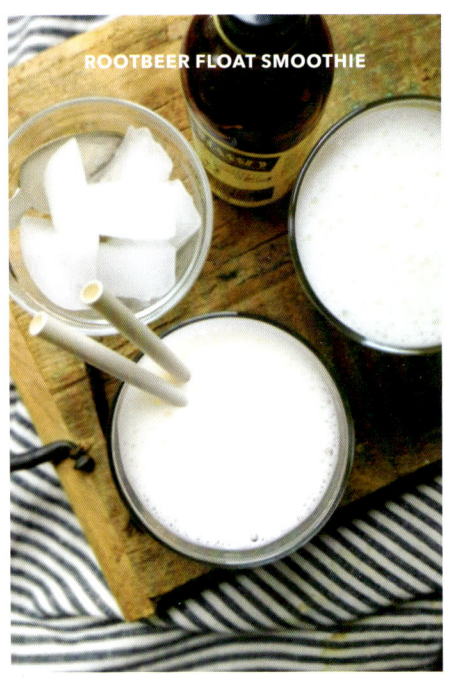
ROOTBEER FLOAT SMOOTHIE

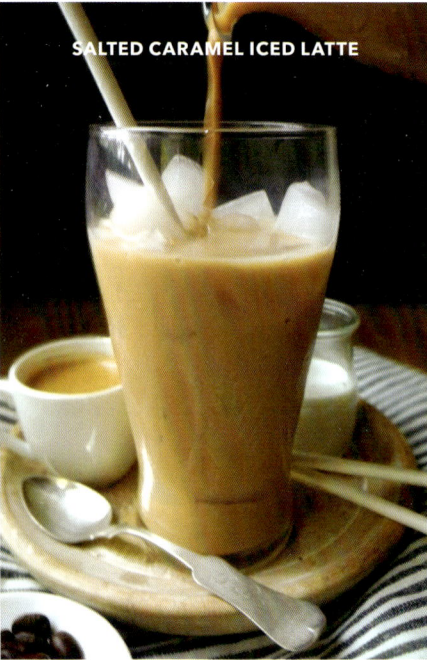
SALTED CARAMEL ICED LATTE

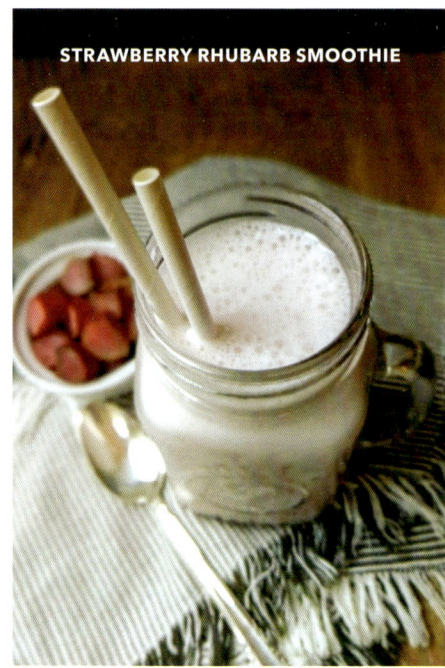
STRAWBERRY RHUBARB SMOOTHIE

Rootbeer Float Smoothie

INGREDIENTS

1 Ideal Protein vanilla smoothie mix
8 oz. cold water
¼ tsp. vanilla extract
¼ tsp. rootbeer extract
1 C. ice

DIRECTIONS

1. Blend ingredients in a 900+ watt blender until smooth and creamy.

SERVINGS

Entire recipe yield = 1 unrestricted

Salted Caramel Iced Latte

INGREDIENTS

1 Ideal Protein vanilla shake (ready-to-drink)
2 oz. (2 shots) espresso
2 T. Walden Farms caramel syrup
2 T. half and half cream
1 pinch sea salt

DIRECTIONS

1. Fill a large cup or glass with ice. Add remaining ingredients; stir to mix.

SERVINGS

Entire recipe yield = 1 unrestricted + 1 oz. half and half cream

Strawberry Rhubarb Smoothie

INGREDIENTS

1 Ideal Protein vanilla smoothie mix
⅔ C. Strawberry Rhubarb Compote, pg. 137
6 oz. cold water
1 C. ice (or more for desired consistency)

DIRECTIONS

1. Blend ingredients in a 900+ watt blender until smooth and creamy.

SERVINGS

Entire recipe yield = 1 unrestricted + 1 C. veggies (⅔ C. cooked rhubarb = 1 C. raw veggies)

TIP: The Ideal Protein chocolate smoothie mix may be subbed for the vanilla smoothie mix in this recipe.

Strawberry Shortcake Smoothie

INGREDIENTS
1 Ideal Protein vanilla smoothie mix
6 oz. cold water
1 T. Walden Farms strawberry syrup
½ tsp. strawberry or vanilla extract
¼ tsp. butter extract
1 C. ice

DIRECTIONS
1. Blend ingredients in a 900+ watt blender until smooth and creamy.

SERVINGS
Entire recipe yield = 1 unrestricted

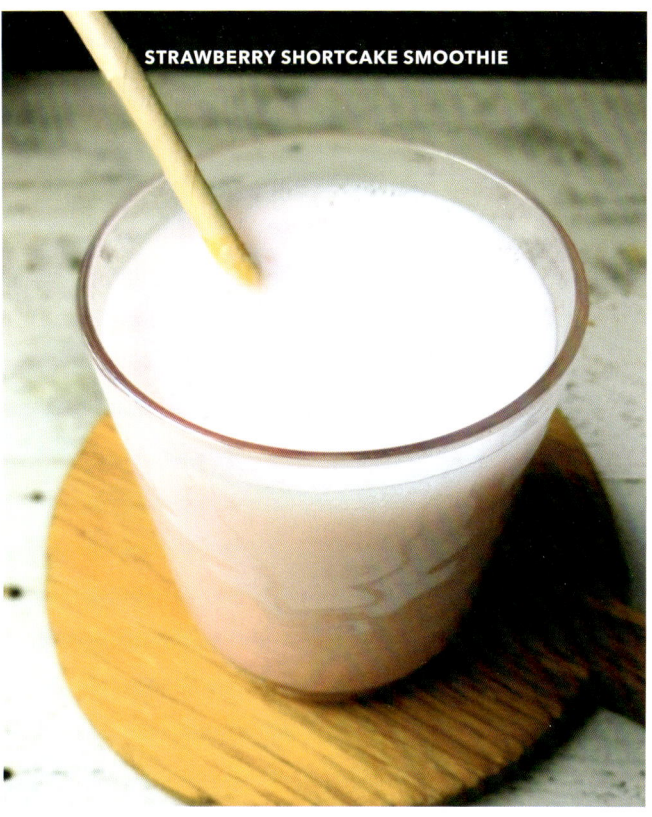

STRAWBERRY SHORTCAKE SMOOTHIE

Whipped Coffee
Also known as Dalgona coffee

INGREDIENTS
2 T. instant coffee granules
2 T. cold water
1 tsp. sugar free sweetener, granular
⅛ tsp. cinnamon, optional
1 Ideal Protein vanilla or chocolate shake (ready-to-drink)

DIRECTIONS
1. Place instant coffee granules, water, sweetener, and cinnamon in a small mixing bowl.
2. Using an electric hand mixer, beat on high speed until foamy and whipped. (This will take 1-2 minutes.)
3. Pour shake into a clear glass over ice. Spoon desired amount of whipped mixture over the top and admire for a few minutes. Give it a few stirs with a spoon; serve.

SERVINGS
Entire recipe yield = 1 unrestricted

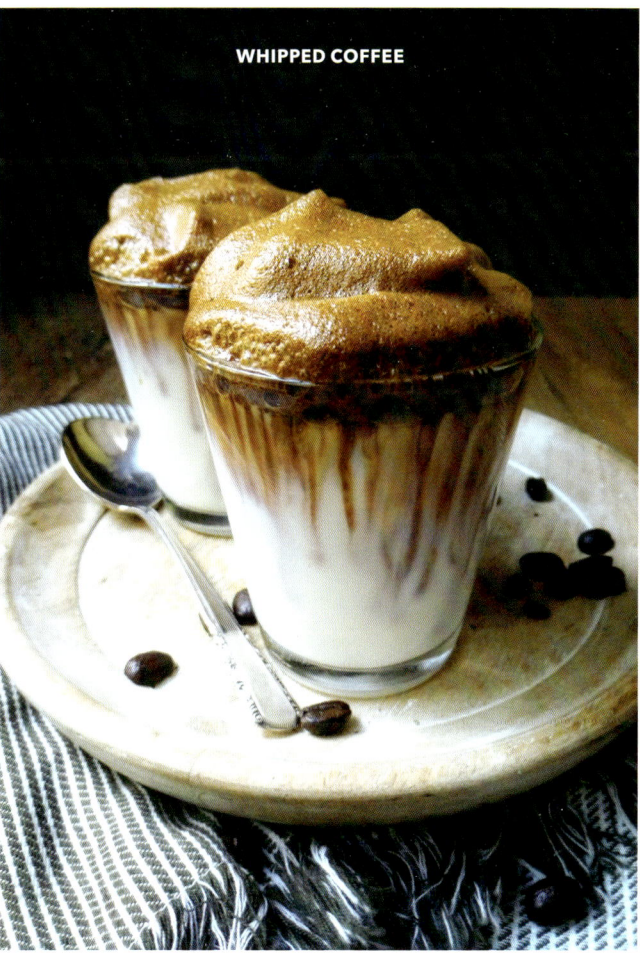

WHIPPED COFFEE

Apple Harvest Bread

Eggless recipe

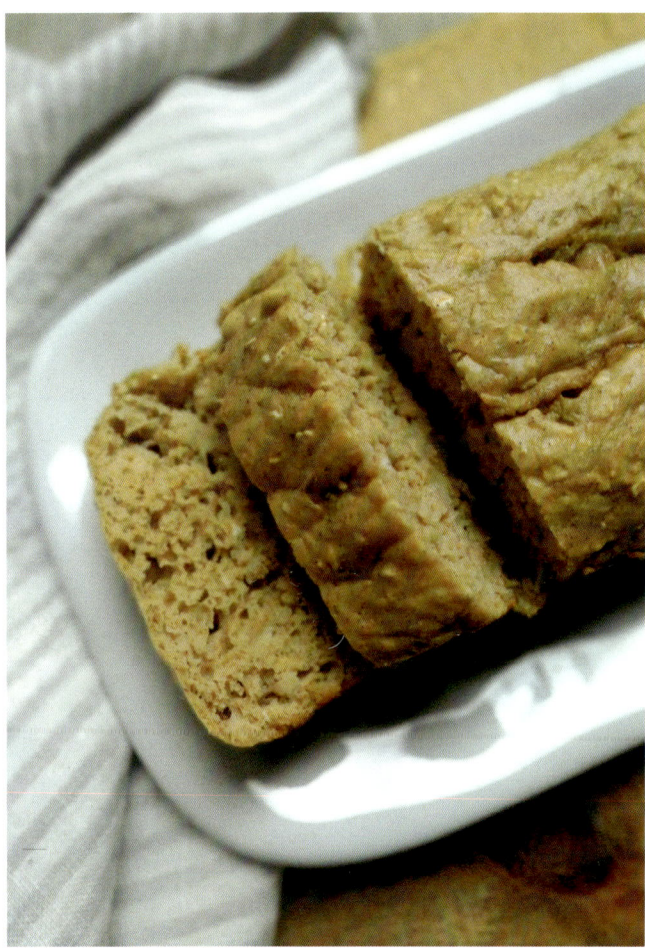

INGREDIENTS

½ C. shredded chayote or zucchini squash
1 Ideal Protein apple cinnamon oatmeal mix
1 Ideal Protein golden pancakes mix
¼ tsp. baking soda
½ tsp. cinnamon
¼ C. water
2 T. Ideal Protein maple syrup
2 tsp. olive oil
1 tsp. vanilla extract
1 tsp. apple cider vinegar
Cooking spray

DIRECTIONS

1. Preheat oven to 350°F degrees.
2. Place shredded squash between paper towels; squeeze to absorb excess moisture. Set aside.
3. Add dry ingredients to a mixing bowl; stir to mix.
4. Add liquid ingredients (including shredded squash) to a separate mixing bowl; whisk to mix. Stir into dry ingredients.
5. Pour batter into a sprayed (5 3/8 x 3 x 2 ⅛-inch) mini loaf pan; level batter.
6. Bake 15-17 minutes or until an inserted cake tester comes out clean.
7. For best texture, remove bread from pan and cool completely on a cooling rack before serving.

SERVINGS

Entire loaf = 2 unrestricted + ½ C. veggies + 2 tsp. oil
½ loaf = 1 unrestricted + ¼ C. veggies + 1 tsp. oil

Apple Pie Scones

INGREDIENTS (SCONES)
¼ C. shredded chayote or zucchini squash
1 pkg. Ideal Protein apple cinnamon puffs
1 Ideal Protein golden pancakes mix
1 tsp. baking powder
1 tsp. apple pie spice
1 large egg
1 T. Ideal Protein maple syrup
2 T. water
¼ tsp. butter extract
¼ tsp. vanilla extract
Cooking spray

INGREDIENTS (GLAZE, TOPPINGS)
1 T. Walden Farms marshmallow dip
2 tsp. Ideal Protein maple syrup
Pinch of apple pie spice
Chopped Caramel Fried Apples, pg. 127 (optional,
   for topping)

DIRECTIONS
1. Preheat oven to 350°F degrees.
2. Blot shredded squash with paper towels to absorb excess moisture; set aside.
3. Place the dry ingredients in a bullet blender or food processor; pulse to fine crumbs. Transfer to a mixing bowl.
4. Add liquid ingredients to a separate mixing bowl; whisk to mix. Stir into dry ingredients. Fold in zucchini.
5. Pour batter into a sprayed scone pan making 4 scones.
6. Bake 11-13 minutes or until an inserted cake tester comes out clean.
7. Remove scones from pan and cool completely on a cooling rack before glazing.
8. Combine glaze ingredients and drizzle over scones; top with chopped apples, if desired.

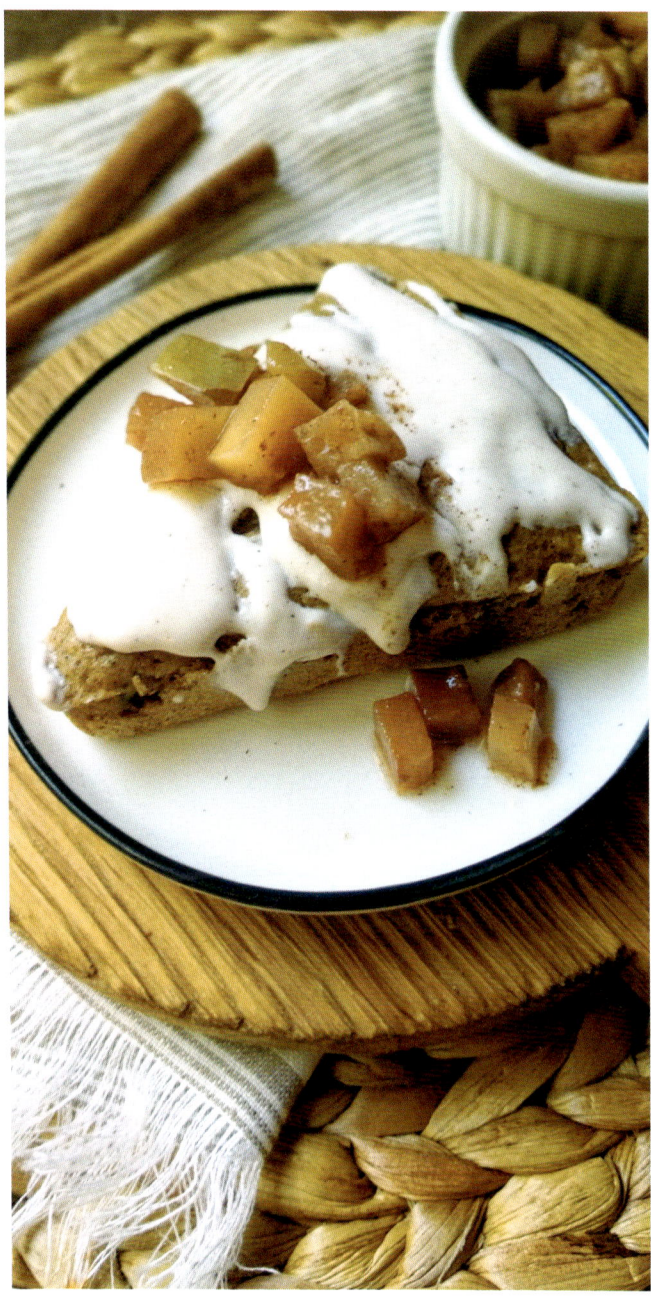

SERVINGS
4 scones = 1 unrestricted + 1 restricted + 1 oz. lean protein (egg) + ¼ C. veggies
2 scones = ½ unrestricted + ½ restricted + 0.5 oz. lean protein (egg) + 2 T. veggies

NOTE: Because this recipe includes a restricted packet, and 1 serving (2 scones) contains ½ restricted, I count it as 1 full restricted for the day. This ensures the carb or calorie count won't exceed protocol amounts. Servings do not include glaze.

Banana Nut Muffins

Eggless recipe

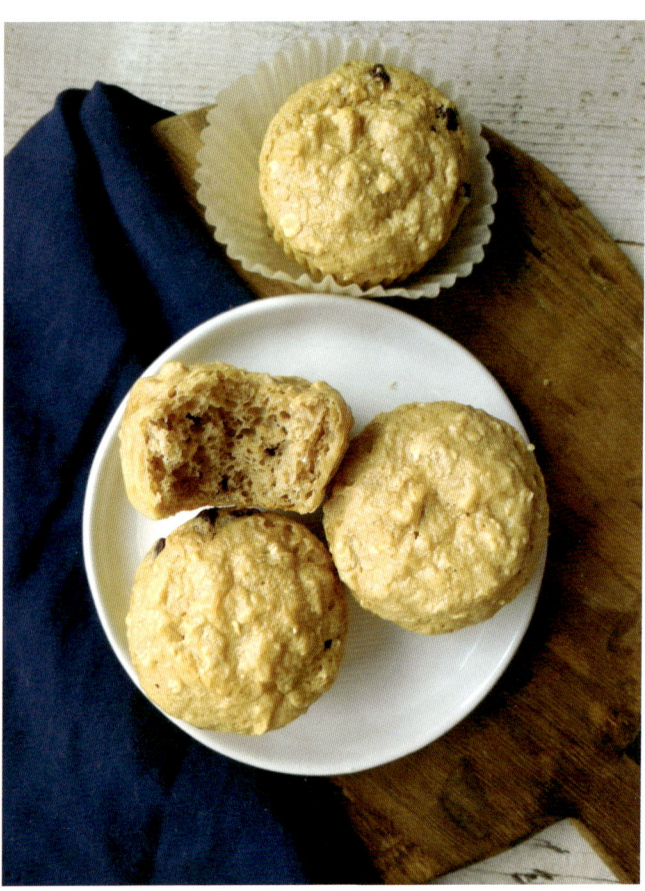

INGREDIENTS
¼ C. shredded zucchini
1 Ideal Protein golden or chocolate chip pancake mix
1 Ideal Protein maple oatmeal mix
¼ tsp. baking soda
¼ C. water
2 T. Ideal Protein maple syrup
1 T. walnut oil
1 tsp. apple cider vinegar
½ tsp. banana extract
Cooking spray

DIRECTIONS
1. Preheat oven to 350°F degrees.
2. Place shredded zucchini between paper towels; squeeze to absorb excess moisture. Set aside.
3. Add dry ingredients to a mixing bowl; stir to mix.
4. Add liquid ingredients to a separate mixing bowl; whisk to mix. Stir into dry ingredients; fold in zucchini.
5. Scoop batter into a sprayed standard size muffin tin making 4 muffins.
6. Bake 11-13 minutes or until an inserted cake tester comes out clean. Do not overbake.
7. For best texture, remove muffins from pan and cool completely on a cooling rack before serving.

SERVINGS
4 muffins = 2 unrestricted + ¼ C. veggies + 1 T. oil
2 muffins = 1 unrestricted + 2 T. veggies + 1 ½ tsp. oil

Breakfast Buzz Muffins

Jumbo size

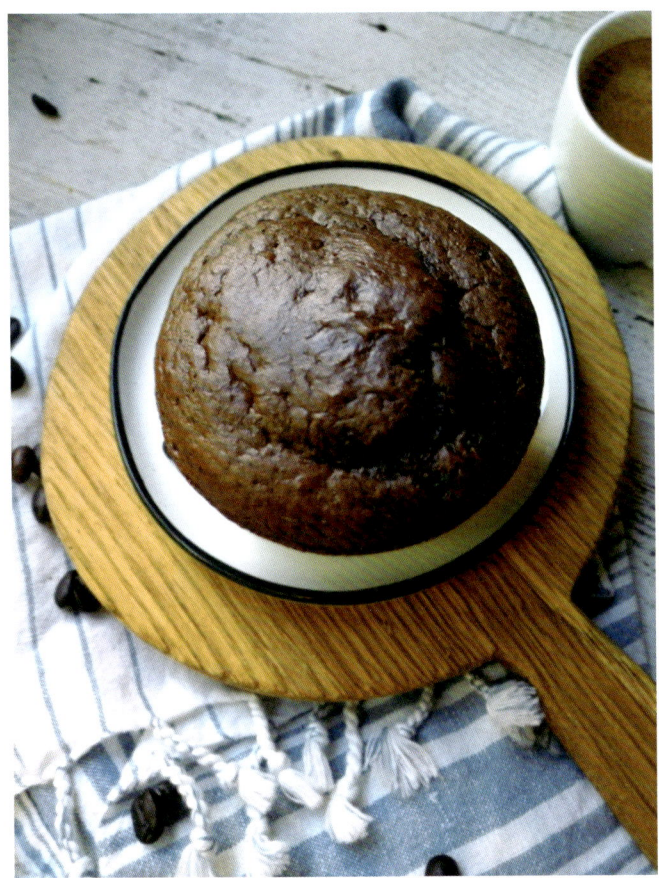

INGREDIENTS

¼ C. shredded zucchini
1 Ideal Protein chocolate caramel mug cake mix
1 Ideal Protein chocolate crispy square (broken in pieces)
2 tsp. instant coffee or espresso granules
1 tsp. baking powder
½ tsp. cinnamon
1 large egg
¼ C. cold coffee
1 T. Walden Farms chocolate syrup
½ tsp. vanilla extract
Cooking spray

DIRECTIONS

1. Preheat oven to 350°F degrees.
2. Blot zucchini with paper towels to absorb excess moisture; set aside.
3. Place the dry ingredients in a bullet blender or food processor; pulse to fine crumbs. Transfer to a mixing bowl.
4. Add liquid ingredients to a separate mixing bowl; whisk to mix. Stir into dry ingredients. Fold in zucchini.
5. Pour batter into a sprayed jumbo size muffin tin* making 2 muffins.
6. Bake 16-18 minutes or until an inserted cake tester comes out clean.
7. For best texture, remove muffins from pan and cool completely on a cooling rack before serving.

SERVINGS

2 jumbo muffins = 2 unrestricted + 1 oz. lean protein (egg) + ¼ C. veggies
1 jumbo muffin = 1 unrestricted + 0.5 oz. lean protein (egg) + 2 T. veggies

TIP: *If a jumbo muffin tin is not available, use a standard muffin tin making 4 muffins; bake approximately 11-13 minutes or until an inserted cake tester comes out clean.

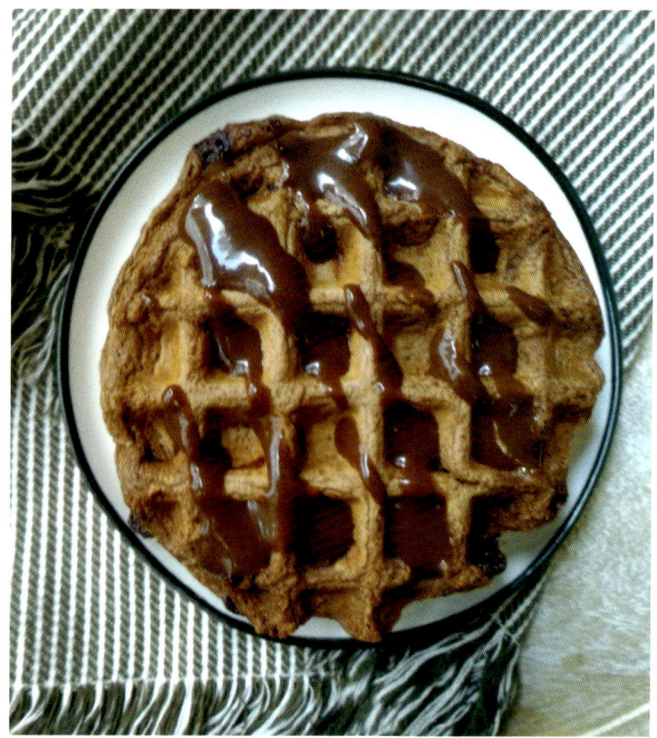

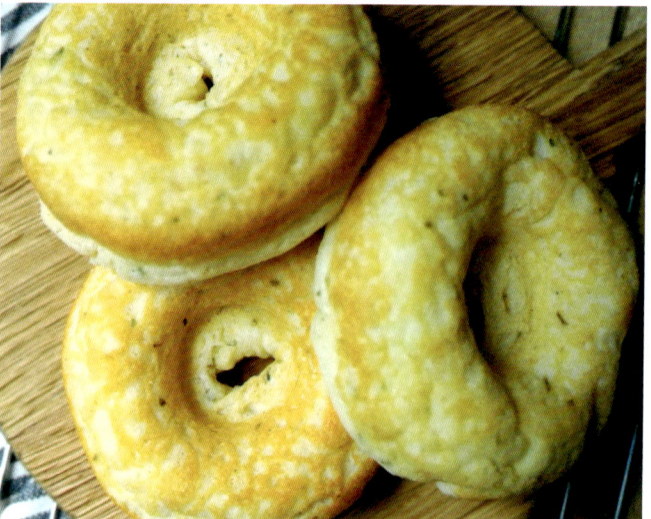

Brownie Waffles

INGREDIENTS

1 Ideal Protein chocolate caramel mug cake mix
2 T. Walden Farms chocolate syrup
2 T. water
⅛ tsp. Fudge Brownie flavor fountain extract*
   or vanilla extract
Pinch of cinnamon
Cooking spray

DIRECTIONS

1. Preheat waffle iron.
2. Add all ingredients to a mixing bowl; stir to combine. Batter will be thick.
3. Scoop batter into a sprayed waffle maker making 2 waffles. Bake according to manufacturer directions.
4. May be eaten warm or cooled. Drizzle with additional chocolate syrup, if desired.

SERVINGS

Entire recipe yield (2 brownie waffles) =
1 unrestricted

TIP: *Fudge Brownie flavor fountain extract may be purchased online at olivenation.com or amazon.com – this water-based extract adds richness, color, and flavor to the baked goods but is an optional addition.

Butter Bagels

INGREDIENTS

¼ C. shredded zucchini
1 Ideal Protein mashed potatoes mix
1 Ideal Protein crispy cereal mix
1 tsp. baking powder
1 large egg
¼ C. water
2 tsp. olive oil
1 tsp. butter extract
Cooking spray

DIRECTIONS

1. Preheat oven to 350°F degrees.
2. Blot zucchini with paper towels to absorb excess moisture; set aside.
3. Place dry ingredients in a bullet style blender or food processor; pulse to fine crumbs. Transfer to a mixing bowl.
4. Add liquid ingredients to a separate mixing bowl; whisk to mix. Stir into dry ingredients. Fold in zucchini.
5. Pour batter into a sprayed standard size 'donut' pan making 4 bagels.
6. Bake 7-9 minutes or until an inserted cake tester comes out clean. Do not overbake.
7. For best texture, remove bagels from pan and cool completely on a cooling rack before serving.

SERVINGS

4 bagels = 2 unrestricted + 1 oz. lean protein (egg) + ¼ C. veggies + 2 tsp. oil
2 bagels = 1 unrestricted + 0.5 oz. lean protein (egg) + 2 T. veggies + 1 tsp. oil

Café Au Lait Muffins

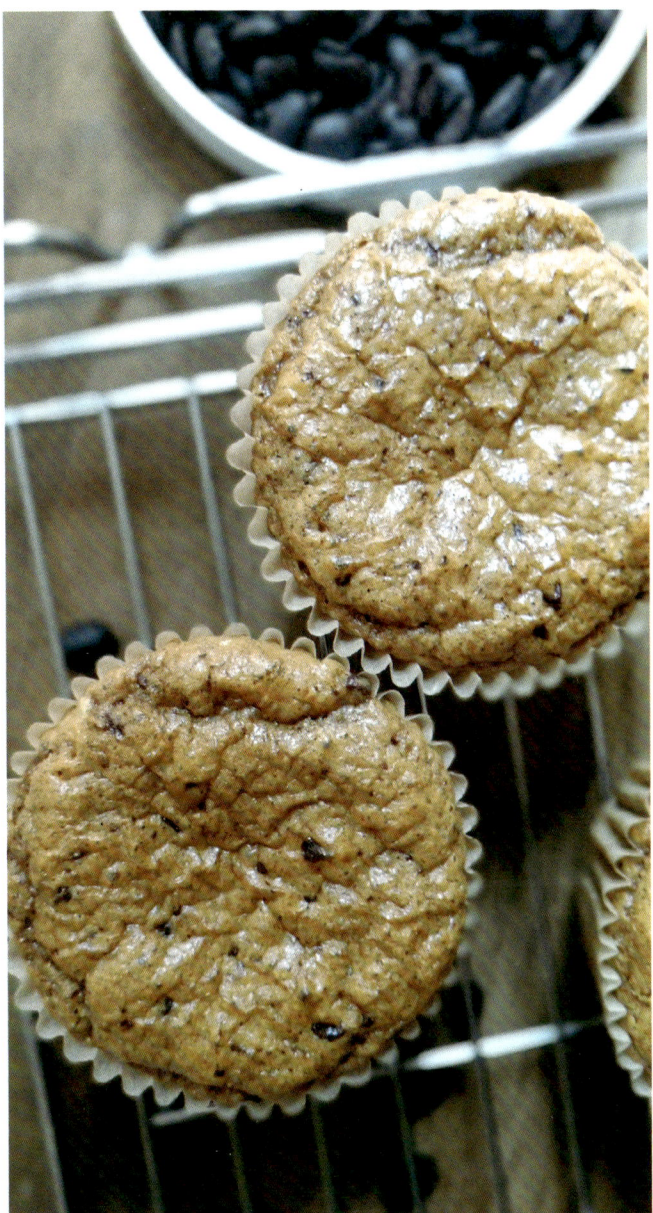

INGREDIENTS

1 Ideal Protein golden pancakes mix
1 Ideal Protein vanilla crispy bar (broken in pieces)
1 tsp. instant coffee or espresso granules
1 tsp. baking powder
1 large egg
3 T. cold coffee
1 T. half and half cream
1 tsp. vanilla
Cooking spray

DIRECTIONS

1. Preheat oven to 350°F degrees.
2. Place the dry ingredients in a bullet blender or food processor; pulse to fine crumbs. Transfer to a mixing bowl.
3. Add liquid ingredients to a separate mixing bowl; whisk to mix. Stir into dry ingredients.
4. Pour batter into a sprayed standard size muffin tin making 4 muffins.
5. Bake 8-10 minutes or until an inserted cake tester comes out clean.
6. For best texture, remove muffins from pan and cool completely on a cooling rack before serving.

SERVINGS

4 muffins = 2 unrestricted + 1 oz. lean protein (egg) + 1 T. half and half cream
2 muffins = 1 unrestricted + 0.5 oz. lean protein (egg) + 1 ½ tsp. half and half cream

Caramel Apple Muffins
Jumbo size

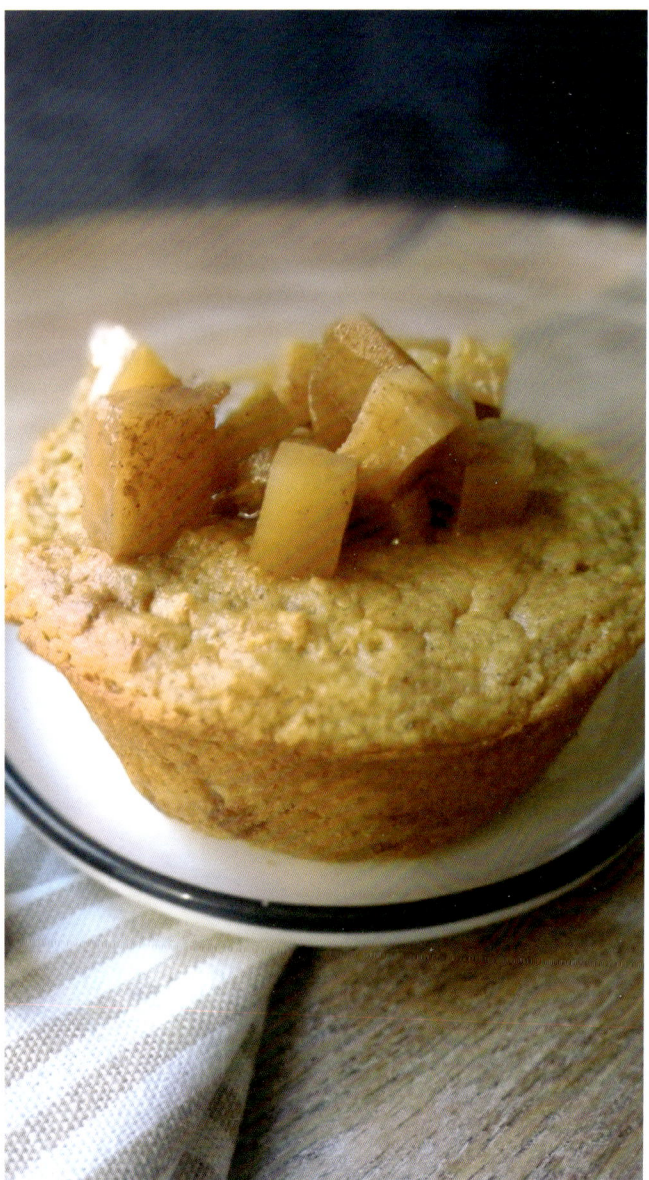

INGREDIENTS
1 pkg. Ideal Protein apple cinnamon puffs
1 Ideal Protein golden pancakes mix
1 tsp. baking powder
1 large egg
2 T. water
1 tsp. oil
¼ C. Caramel Fried Apples, finely chopped (pg. 127)
Cooking spray

DIRECTIONS
1. Preheat oven to 350°F degrees.
2. Place the dry ingredients in a bullet blender or food processor; pulse to fine crumbs. Transfer to a mixing bowl.
3. Add liquid ingredients to a separate mixing bowl (except apples); whisk to mix. Stir into dry ingredients; fold in chopped apples.
4. Pour batter into a sprayed jumbo muffin tin* making 2 muffins.
5. Bake 13-15 minutes or until an inserted cake tester comes out clean.
6. For best texture, remove muffins from pan and cool completely on a cooling rack. To serve, top with additional apples, if desired.

SERVINGS
2 jumbo muffins = 1 unrestricted + 1 restricted + 1 oz. lean protein (egg) + ¼ C. veggies + 1 tsp. oil
1 jumbo muffin = ½ unrestricted + ½ restricted + 0.5 oz. lean protein (egg) + 2 T. veggies + ½ tsp. oil

TIP: *If a jumbo muffin tin is not available, use a standard muffin tin making 4 muffins. Bake 10-12 minutes or until an inserted cake tester comes out clean.

NOTE: Because this recipe includes a restricted packet, and 1 serving (1 jumbo muffin) contains ½ restricted, I count it as 1 full restricted for the day. This ensures the carb or calorie count won't exceed protocol amounts.

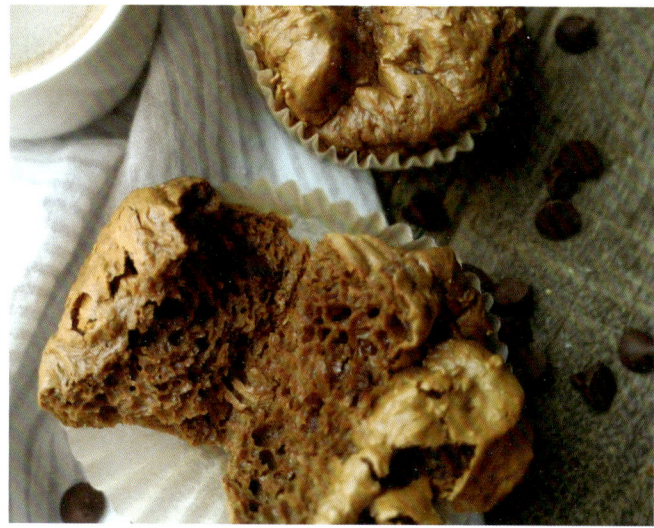

Caramel Macchiato Muffins

INGREDIENTS
1 Ideal Protein chocolate caramel mug cake mix
1 Ideal Protein vanilla smoothie mix
¼ tsp. baking soda
¼ tsp. baking powder
2 T. water
2 T. Walden Farms caramel syrup
2 T. half and half cream
1 T. instant coffee or espresso granules
1 large egg yolk
2 tsp. olive oil
1 tsp. apple cider vinegar
Cooking spray

DIRECTIONS
1. Preheat oven to 350°F degrees.
2. Add dry ingredients to a mixing bowl (except coffee granules); stir to mix.
3. Add liquid ingredients and coffee granules to a separate mixing bowl; whisk to mix. Stir into dry ingredients. Batter will be thick.
4. Scoop batter into a sprayed standard size muffin tin making 4 muffins.
5. Bake 7-9 minutes or until an inserted cake tester comes out clean.
6. Remove muffins from pan; may be served warm or cooled.

SERVINGS
4 muffins = 2 unrestricted + 0.5 oz. lean protein (egg yolk) + 2 tsp. oil + 1 oz. half and half cream
2 muffins = 1 unrestricted + 0.25 oz. lean protein (egg yolk) + 1 tsp. oil + 0.5 oz. half and half cream

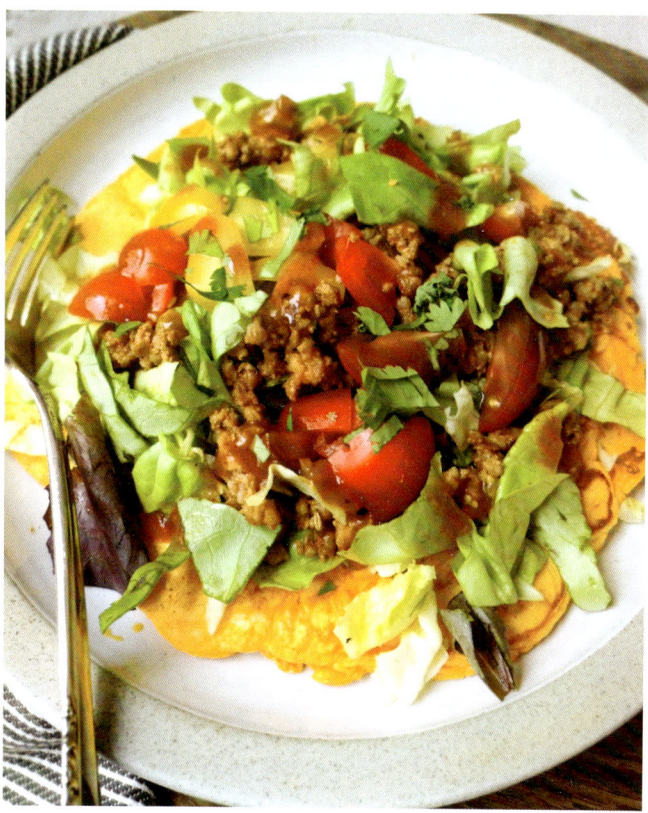

Cheesy Bread Wrap

INGREDIENTS
1 pkg. Ideal Protein cheddar cheese sauce mix
¼ tsp. baking powder
⅓ C. liquid egg whites
Cooking spray

DIRECTIONS
1. In a small bowl, combine cheese sauce mix with baking powder. Add egg whites; stir to combine.
2. Heat a skillet over medium/medium low heat. Lightly coat hot skillet with cooking spray. Add batter to skillet and spread into a 7-inch diameter 'pancake'.
3. Cook until underside is lightly browned, and edges of wrap start to look dry.
4. Flip wrap; cook until underside is lightly browned and cooked through.

SERVINGS
1 cheesy bread wrap = 1 unrestricted

NOTE: Liquid egg whites are often calculated as an 'extra' for the day. Consult your coach or clinic for egg white counts toward protocol. Fill bread wrap with desired savory fillings, and fold in half to eat.

Cheesy Breadsticks
.... Or bagels!

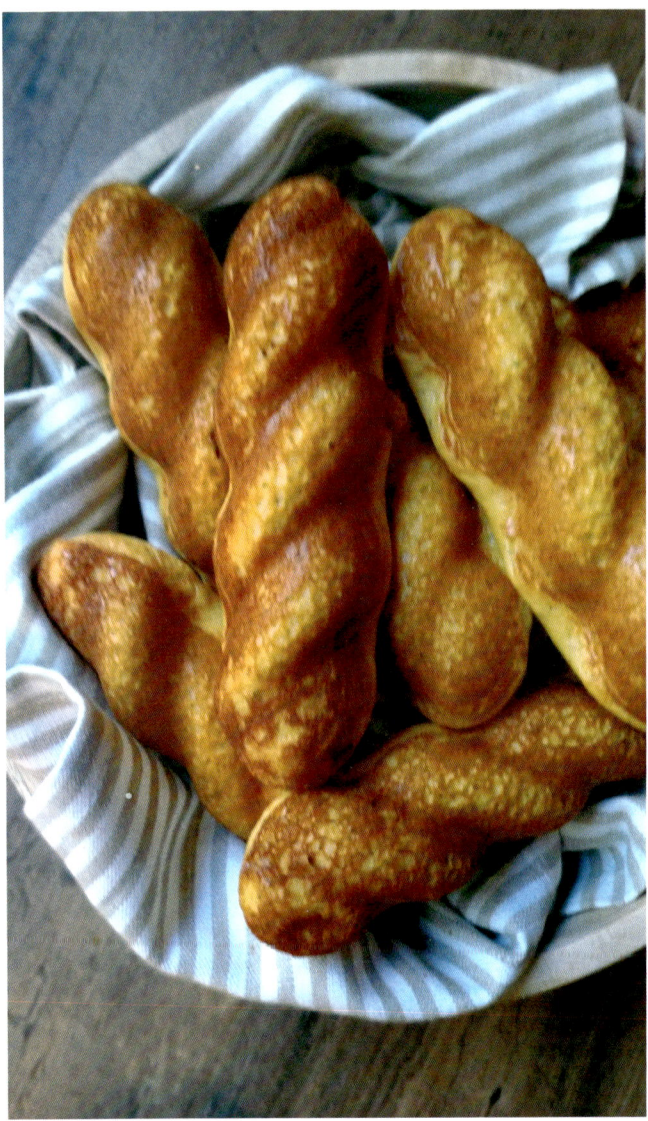

INGREDIENTS

½ C. shredded zucchini
1 Ideal Protein cheddar cheese sauce mix
1 Ideal Protein crispy cereal mix
1 Ideal Protein mashed potatoes mix
1 Ideal Protein golden pancakes mix
1 ½ tsp. baking powder
½ tsp. Italian seasoning
¼ tsp. garlic powder
¼ tsp. onion powder
1 pinch Ideal Protein salt
2 large eggs
½ C. water
2 tsp. olive oil
Cooking spray

DIRECTIONS

1. Preheat oven to 350°F degrees.
2. Blot zucchini with paper towels to absorb excess moisture; set aside.
3. Place the dry ingredients in a bullet blender or food processor; pulse to fine crumbs. Transfer to a mixing bowl.
4. Add liquid ingredients to a separate mixing bowl; whisk to mix. Stir into dry ingredients. Fold in zucchini.
5. Spoon batter into a sprayed breadstick pan (or donut twist pan) making 8 breadsticks. (Alternatively, spoon batter into a sprayed standard donut pan making 8 bagels.)
6. Bake 9-11 minutes or until an inserted cake tester comes out clean.
7. For best texture, remove bread from pan and cool completely on cooling rack before serving.

SERVING:

Entire recipe yield (8 breadsticks) = 4 unrestricted + 2 oz. lean protein (egg) + ½ C. veggies + 2 tsp. oil
¼ recipe yield (2 breadsticks) = 1 unrestricted + 0.5 oz. lean protein (egg) + 2 T. veggies + ½ tsp. oil

TIP: Excellent when sliced and lightly toasted in the toaster.

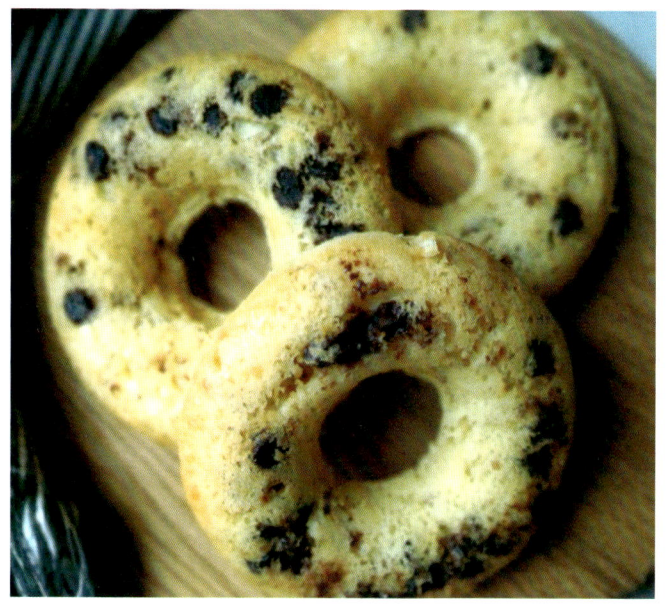

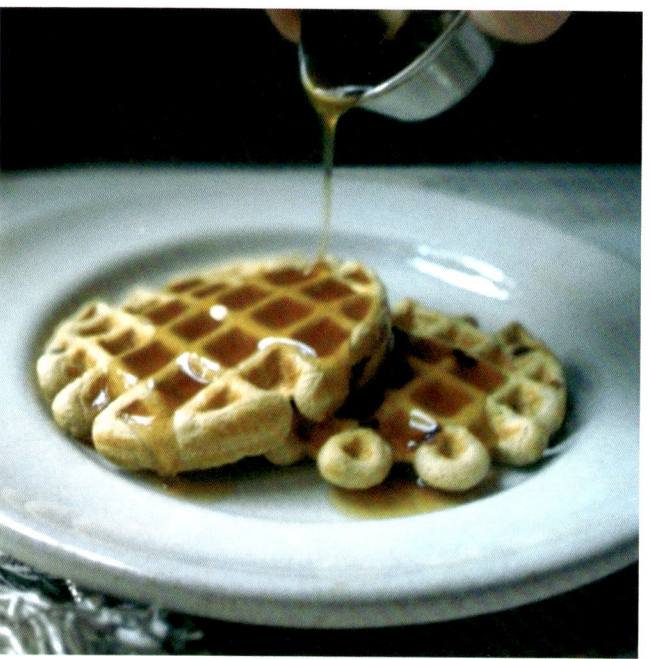

Chocolate Chip Cookie Donuts

Eggless recipe

INGREDIENTS

1 Ideal Protein chocolate caramel mug cake mix
1 Ideal Protein maple oatmeal mix
¼ tsp. baking soda
¼ tsp. baking powder
2 T. water
2 T. Ideal Protein maple syrup
2 tsp. olive oil
1 tsp. apple cider vinegar
½ tsp. vanilla extract
Cooking spray

DIRECTIONS

1. Preheat oven to 350°F degrees.
2. Add dry ingredients to a small mixing bowl; stir to mix.
3. Add liquid ingredients to a separate mixing bowl; stir to mix. Stir into dry ingredients.
4. Spoon batter into a sprayed standard size donut pan making 4 donuts.
5. Bake 5 minutes or until an inserted cake tester comes out clean.
6. Remove donuts from pan and cool completely on a cooling rack before serving.

SERVINGS

4 donuts = 2 unrestricted + 2 tsp. oil
2 donuts = 1 unrestricted + 1 tsp. oil

Chocolate Chip Zucchini Waffles

INGREDIENTS

1 Ideal Protein chocolate chip pancake mix
¼ tsp. cinnamon
2 T. water
2 T. shredded zucchini
Ideal Protein maple syrup, for topping
Cooking spray

DIRECTIONS

1. Preheat waffle iron.
2. Add all ingredients to a small bowl; stir to mix.
3. Add batter to sprayed waffle iron and bake according to manufacturer directions. Makes 2 waffles.
4. Top with maple syrup, if desired.

SERVINGS

2 waffles = 1 unrestricted + 2 T. veggies

Churro Coffee Cake
Eggless recipe

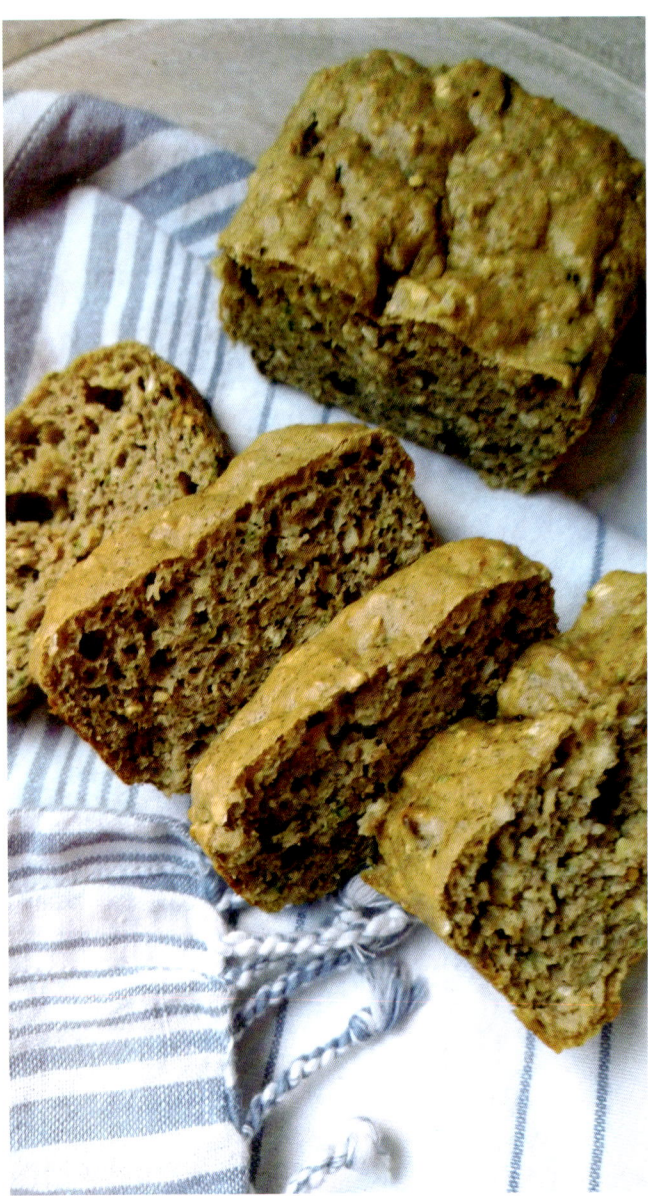

INGREDIENTS
¼ C. shredded zucchini
1 Ideal Protein golden or chocolate chip pancake mix
1 Ideal Protein maple oatmeal mix
1 tsp. dried orange peel
¼ tsp. baking soda
¼ tsp. baking powder
½ tsp. cinnamon
⅛ tsp. nutmeg
¼ C. water
2 T. Ideal Protein maple syrup
2 tsp. olive oil
1 tsp. apple cider vinegar
Cooking spray

DIRECTIONS
1. Preheat oven to 350°F degrees.
2. Blot zucchini with paper towels to absorb excess moisture; set aside.
3. Add dry ingredients to a mixing bowl; stir to mix.
4. Add liquid ingredients to a separate mixing bowl; whisk to mix. Stir into dry ingredients; fold in zucchini.
5. Pour batter into a sprayed (5 3/8 x 3 x 2 ⅛-inch) mini loaf pan; level batter.
6. Bake 16-18 minutes or until an inserted cake tester comes out clean.
7. For best texture, remove coffee cake from pan and cool completely on a cooling rack before serving.

SERVINGS
Entire coffee cake = 2 unrestricted + ¼ C. veggies + 2 tsp. oil
½ coffee cake = 1 unrestricted + 2 T. veggies + 1 tsp. oil

Cinnamon Roll Pancakes

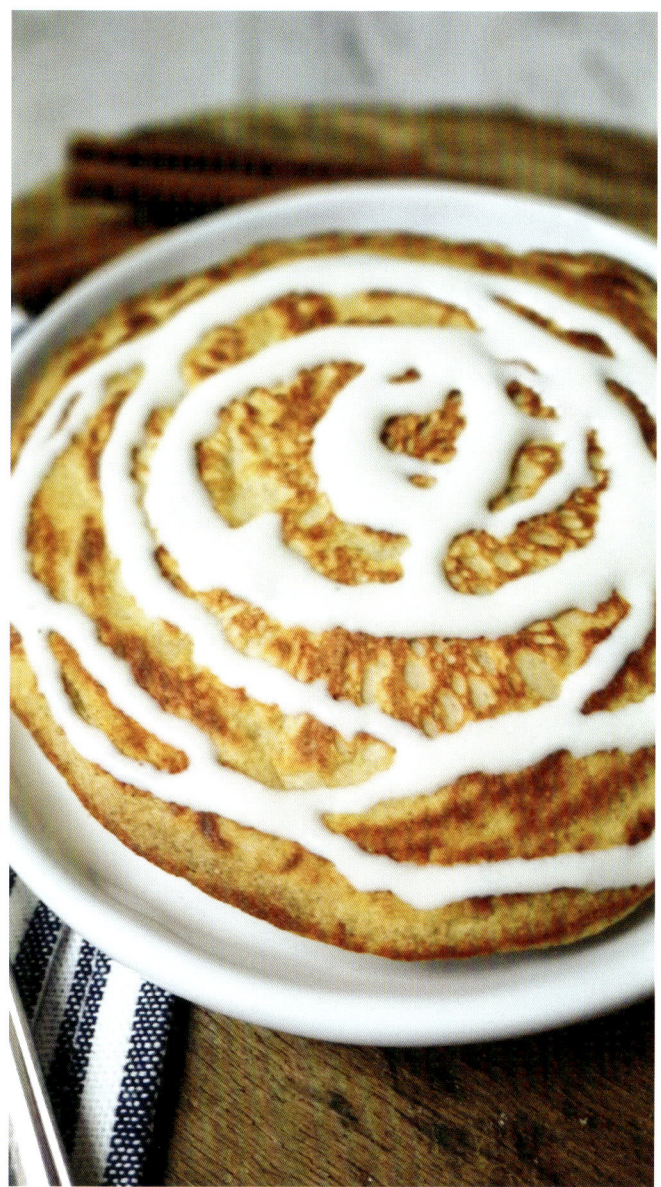

INGREDIENTS (PANCAKES)
1 Ideal Protein golden pancakes mix
¼ tsp. cinnamon
3 T. water
1 T. liquid egg whites
¼ tsp. vanilla
¼ tsp. butter extract
Cooking spray

INGREDIENTS (GLAZE)
2 tsp. Walden Farms marshmallow dip
2 tsp. Ideal Protein maple syrup

DIRECTIONS
1. Add all pancake ingredients to a mixing bowl; stir to mix.
2. Heat a skillet over medium/medium low heat. When skillet is hot, lightly coat with cooking spray and immediately pour batter into skillet making 2 pancakes.
3. Cook until undersides are lightly browned, and edges of pancakes begin to look dry. Flip and cook until undersides are lightly browned, and pancakes are cooked through.
4. In a small bowl, stir glaze ingredients until combined. Drizzle in a circular pattern over warm pancakes.

SERVINGS
Entire recipe yield (2 pancakes) = 1 unrestricted

NOTE: Liquid egg whites are often calculated as an 'extra' for the day. Consult your coach or clinic for egg white counts toward protocol.

Cinnamon Swirl Coffee Cake

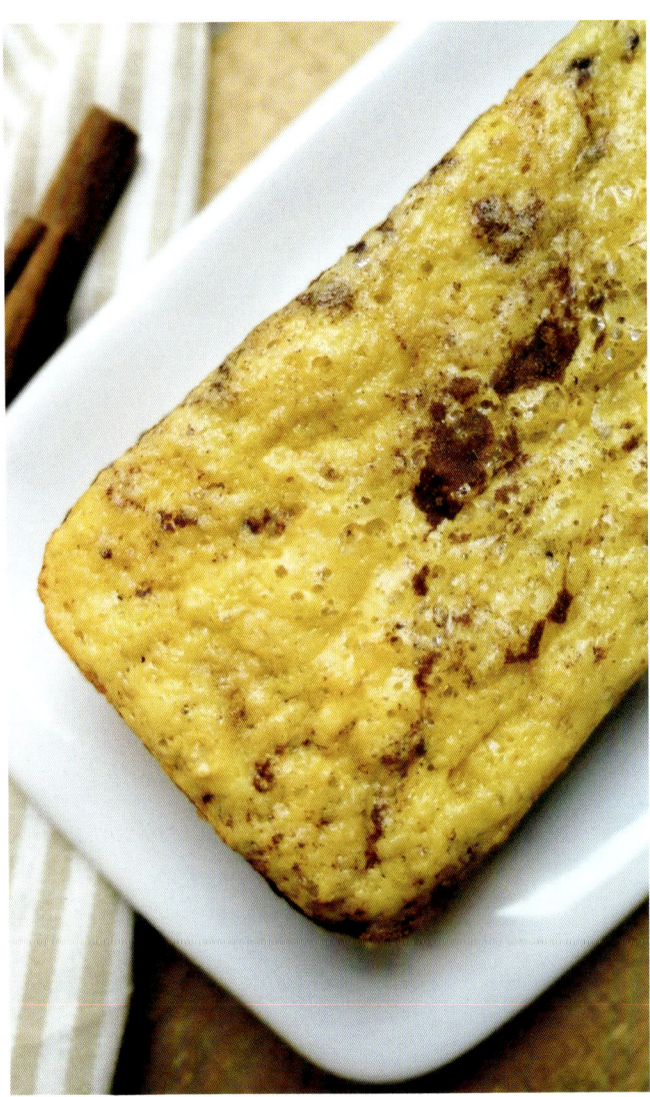

INGREDIENTS

1 Ideal Protein golden pancakes mix
1 Ideal Protein vanilla crispy square (broken in pieces)
1 tsp. baking powder
1 large egg
3 T. water
1 T. Ideal Protein maple syrup
¼ tsp. vanilla extract
Cinnamon, to taste
Cooking spray

DIRECTIONS

1. Preheat oven to 350°F degrees.
2. Place the dry ingredients (except cinnamon) in a bullet blender or food processor; pulse to fine crumbs. Transfer to a mixing bowl.
3. Add liquid ingredients to a separate mixing bowl; whisk to mix. Stir into dry ingredients.
4. Pour ½ the batter into a sprayed (5 3/8 x 3 x 2 ⅛-inch) mini loaf pan; level batter. Sprinkle a thin layer of cinnamon across the batter. Pour remaining batter into pan; level batter.
5. Starting at short end of pan, drag a table knife through batter making a zig zag pattern.
6. Bake 16-18 minutes or until an inserted cake tester comes out clean.
7. For best texture, remove coffee cake from pan and cool completely on a cooling rack before serving.

SERVINGS

Entire coffee cake = 2 unrestricted + 1 oz. lean protein (egg)
½ coffee cake = 1 unrestricted + 0.5 oz. lean protein (egg)

Cornbread Stuffing

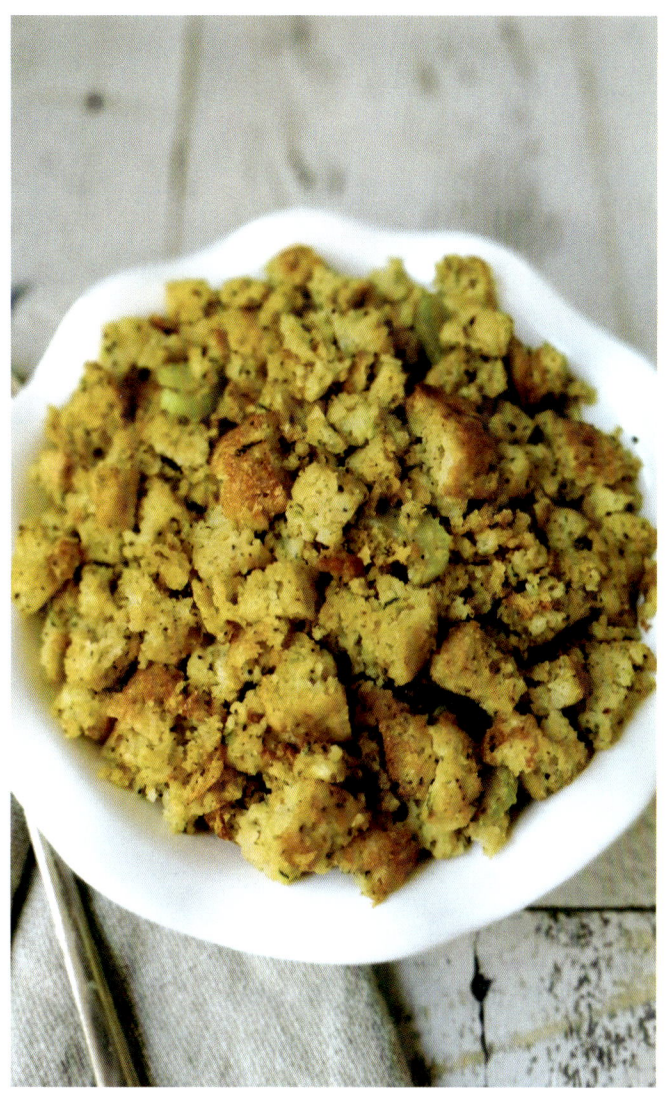

INGREDIENTS

1 pkg. Ideal Protein ranch Dorados
1 Ideal Protein mashed potatoes mix
1 tsp. baking powder
½ tsp. poultry seasoning
¼ tsp. onion powder
½ C. shredded zucchini
1 large egg
2 T. water
½ C. thinly sliced celery
1 tsp. olive oil
½ C. turkey broth or chicken broth
Ideal Protein salt and black pepper, to taste
Cooking spray

DIRECTIONS

1. Preheat oven to 350°F degrees.
2. Place Dorados, mashed potato mix, baking powder, poultry seasoning, and onion powder in a bullet blender or food processor; pulse to fine crumbs. Transfer mixture to a mixing bowl; set aside.
3. Blot zucchini with paper towels to absorb excess moisture. In a small bowl, combine zucchini, egg, and water; whisk to mix. Add to dry mixture; stir to mix. Batter will be thick.
4. Spread batter evenly into a sprayed 9 x 5-inch standard size loaf pan.
5. Bake 15-17 minutes or until inserted toothpick comes out clean.
6. Remove cornbread from pan and cool on cooling rack. Do not turn off oven.
7. Meanwhile, sauté celery in olive oil over medium heat in a small skillet; set aside.
8. Cut cornbread into small cubes and toss with cooked celery and broth; season with salt and pepper. Place stuffing mixture into the loaf pan and bake 20 minutes; gently stir stuffing once during cooking.
9. Transfer stuffing to a serving dish; scrape any bits off bottom of loaf pan and add to the top of the stuffing for extra crunch.

SERVINGS

Entire recipe yield = 2 unrestricted + 1 C. veggies + 1 oz. lean protein (egg) + 1 tsp. oil
½ recipe yield = 1 unrestricted + ½ C. veggies + 0.5 oz. lean protein (egg) + ½ tsp. oil

Cranberry Linzer Donuts

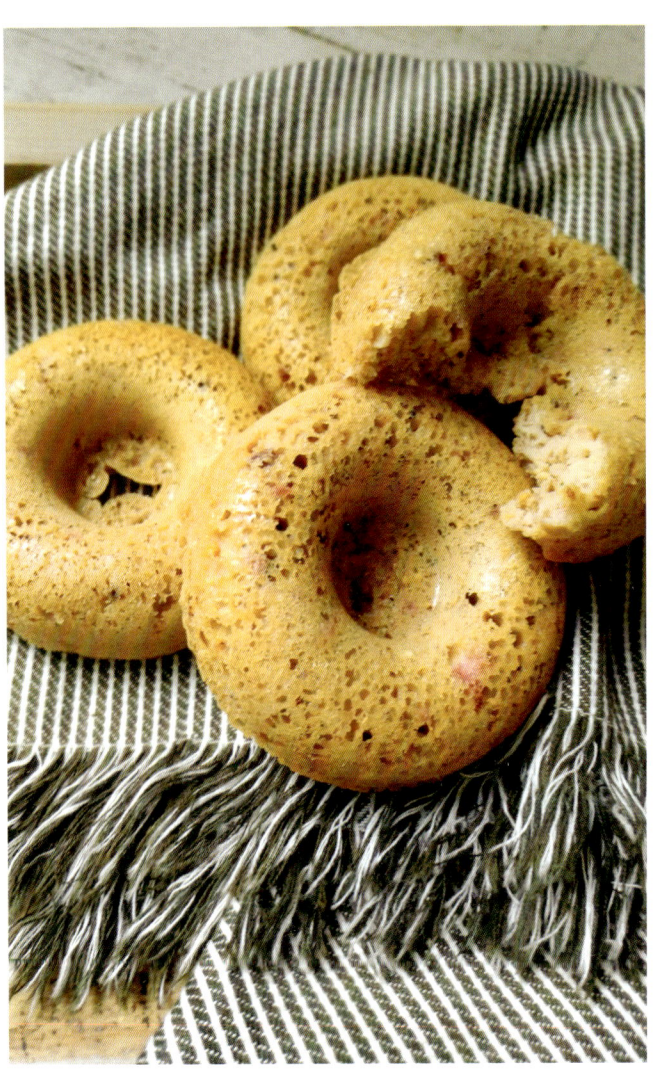

INGREDIENTS

1 Ideal Protein golden pancakes mix
1 Ideal Protein cranberry pomegranate protein bar (broken into pieces)
½ tsp. baking powder
1/8 tsp. cinnamon
2 pinches ground ginger
2 T. Walden Farms raspberry spread
1 large egg
Zest of ½ lemon
2 T. water
1 tsp. walnut oil
Cooking spray

DIRECTIONS

1. Preheat oven to 350°F degrees.
2. Place dry ingredients in a bullet blender or food processor; pulse to fine crumbs. Transfer to a mixing bowl.
3. Heat raspberry spread 15 seconds on high in microwave; stir to liquify from its jelly texture. Add egg, zest, water, and walnut oil to a separate mixing bowl; whisk to mix. While whisking, add raspberry spread and continue to whisk until combined. Stir liquid ingredients into dry ingredients.
4. Pour batter into a sprayed standard size donut pan making 4 donuts.
5. Bake 9-11 minutes or until an inserted cake tester comes out clean.
6. For best texture, remove donuts from pan and cool completely on a cooling rack.

SERVINGS

4 donuts = 1 unrestricted + 1 restricted + 1 oz. lean protein (egg) + 1 tsp. oil
2 donuts = ½ unrestricted + ½ restricted + 0.5 oz. lean protein (egg) + ½ tsp. oil

NOTE: Because this recipe includes a restricted packet, and 1 serving (2 donuts) contains ½ restricted, I count it as 1 full restricted for the day. This ensures the carb or calorie count won't exceed protocol amounts.

Double Chocolate Chip Muffins

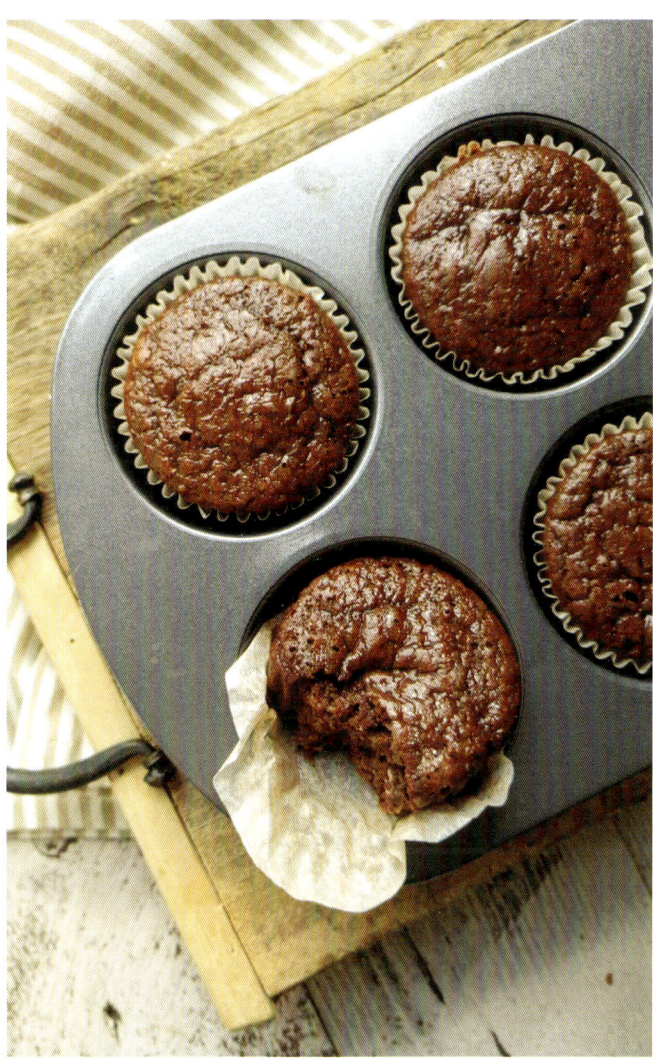

INGREDIENTS
1 Ideal Protein chocolate chip pancake mix
1 Ideal Protein chocolate crispy square (broken into pieces)
½ tsp. baking powder
1 large egg
2 T. water
2 T. Walden Farms chocolate syrup
¼ tsp. vanilla extract
¼ tsp. Fudge brownie flavor fountain extract*
Cooking spray

DIRECTIONS
1. Preheat oven to 350°F degrees.
2. Sift out chocolate chips from pancake mix; set aside.
3. Place the dry ingredients in a bullet blender or food processor; pulse to fine crumbs. Transfer to a mixing bowl.
4. Add liquid ingredients to a separate mixing bowl; whisk to mix. Stir into dry ingredients. Fold in chocolate chips.
5. Pour batter into a sprayed standard size muffin tin making 4 muffins.
6. Bake 11-13 minutes or until an inserted cake tester comes out clean.
7. For best texture, remove muffins from pan and cool completely on a cooling rack before serving.

SERVINGS
4 muffins = 2 unrestricted + 1 oz. lean protein (egg)
2 muffins = 1 unrestricted + 0.5 oz. lean protein (egg)

TIP: *Fudge brownie flavor fountain extract may be purchased online at olivenation.com or amazon.com – this water-based extract adds richness, color, and flavor to the baked goods but is an optional addition.

Farmers Market Muffins

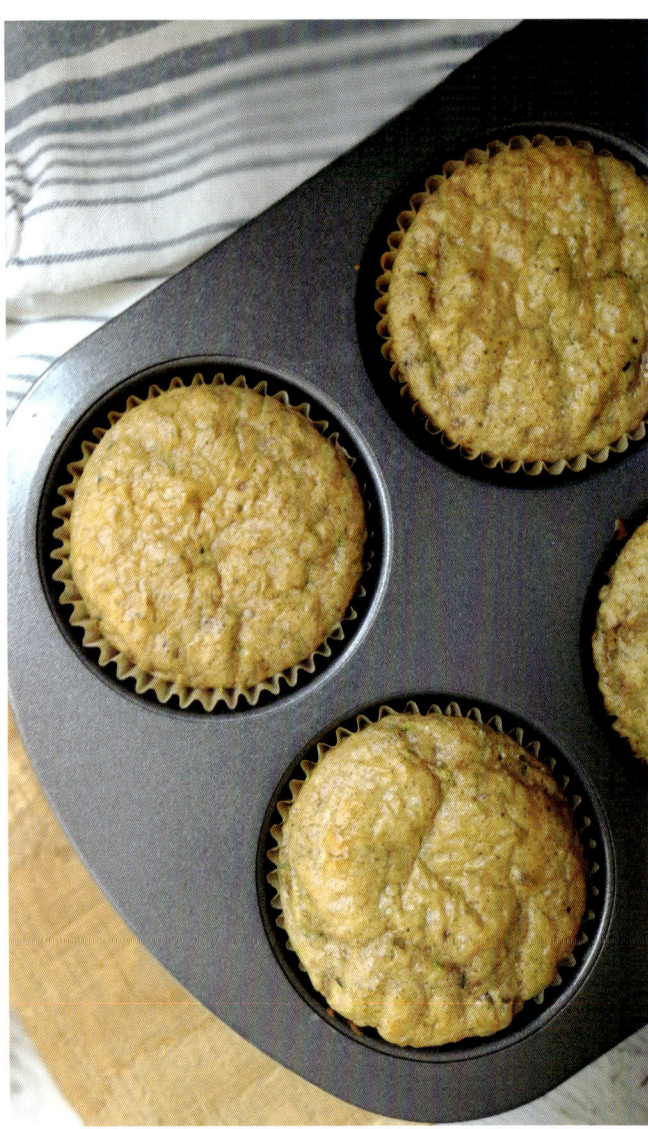

INGREDIENTS

¼ C. shredded zucchini
1 Ideal Protein golden pancakes mix
1 Ideal Protein cranberry pomegranate protein bar
   (broken in pieces)
1 tsp. baking powder
½ tsp. cinnamon or Pumpkin Pie Spice, pg. 145
1 large egg
1 T. Ideal Protein maple syrup
1 T. water
1 tsp. vanilla extract
Cooking spray

DIRECTIONS

1. Preheat oven to 350°F degrees.
2. Blot shredded zucchini with paper towels to absorb excess moisture; set aside.
3. Place the dry ingredients in a bullet blender or food processor; pulse to fine crumbs. Transfer to a mixing bowl.
4. Add liquid ingredients to a separate mixing bowl; whisk to mix. Stir into dry ingredients. Fold in zucchini.
5. Pour batter into a sprayed standard size muffin tin making 4 muffins.
6. Bake 10-12 minutes or until an inserted cake tester comes out clean.
7. For best texture, remove muffins from pan and cool completely on a cooling rack before serving.

SERVINGS

4 muffins = 1 unrestricted + 1 restricted + 1 oz. lean protein (egg) + ¼ C. veggies
2 muffins = ½ unrestricted + ½ restricted + 0.5 oz. lean protein (egg) + 2 T. veggies

NOTE: Because this recipe includes a restricted packet, and 1 serving (2 muffins) contains ½ restricted, I count it as 1 full restricted for the day. This ensures the carb or calorie count won't exceed protocol amounts.

Frost on the Pumpkin Pie Bread

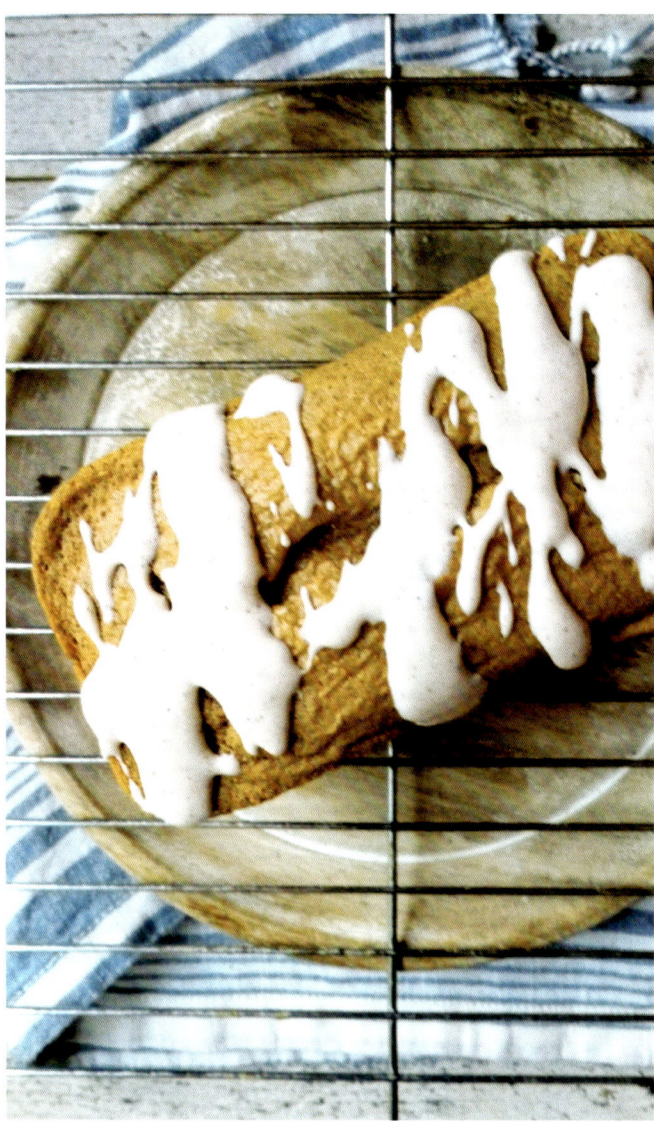

INGREDIENTS
1 pkg. Ideal Protein apple cinnamon puffs
1 Ideal Protein golden pancakes mix
1 tsp. baking powder
½ tsp. Pumpkin Pie Spice, pg. 145
1 large egg
2 T. water
1 T. Ideal Protein maple syrup
1 T. Walden Farms caramel syrup
¼ tsp. vanilla extract
Cooking spray

INGREDIENTS (GLAZE)
2 T. Walden Farms marshmallow dip
1 T. Ideal Protein maple syrup
¼ tsp. Pumpkin Pie Spice, pg. 145

DIRECTIONS
1. Preheat oven to 350°F degrees.
2. Place the dry ingredients in a bullet blender or food processor; pulse to fine crumbs. Transfer to a mixing bowl.
3. Add liquid ingredients to a separate mixing bowl; whisk to mix. Stir into dry ingredients.
4. Pour batter into a sprayed (5 3/8 x 3 x 2 ⅛-inch) mini loaf pan.
5. Bake 18-20 minutes or until an inserted cake tester comes out clean.
6. Remove bread from pan; cool completely on a cooling rack.
7. Combine glaze ingredients; drizzle over bread.

SERVINGS
Entire loaf = 1 unrestricted + 1 restricted + 1 oz. lean protein (egg)
½ loaf = ½ unrestricted + ½ restricted + 0.5 oz. lean protein (egg)

NOTE: Because this recipe includes a restricted packet, and 1 serving (½ loaf) contains ½ restricted, I count it as 1 full restricted for the day. This ensures the carb or calorie count won't exceed protocol amounts.

Garlic Zucchini Bagels

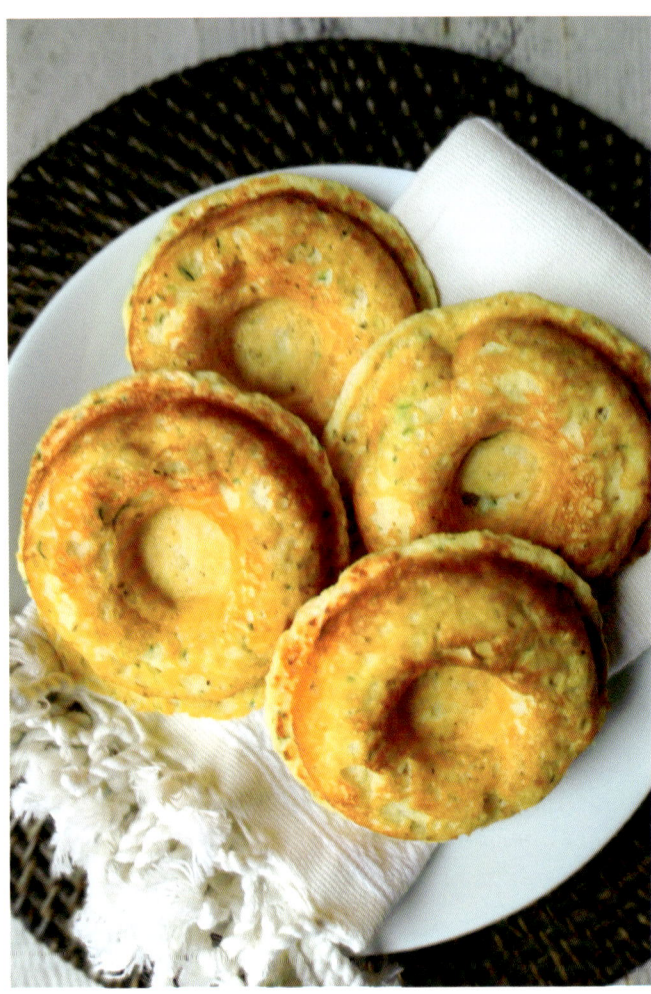

INGREDIENTS

½ C. shredded zucchini
1 Ideal Protein mashed potatoes mix
1 Ideal Protein crispy cereal mix
1 tsp. baking powder
½ tsp. garlic powder
1 large egg
1/4 C. water
2 tsp. olive oil
Cooking spray

DIRECTIONS

1. Preheat oven to 350°F degrees.
2. Blot zucchini with paper towels to absorb excess moisture; set aside.
3. Place the dry ingredients in a bullet blender or food processor; pulse to fine crumbs. Transfer to a mixing bowl.
4. Add liquid ingredients to a separate mixing bowl; whisk to mix. Stir into dry ingredients. Fold in zucchini.
5. Add batter to a sprayed standard size donut pan making 4 bagels.
6. Bake 12-14 minutes or until inserted cake tester comes out clean.
7. For best texture, remove bagels from pan and cool completely on a cooling rack before serving.

SERVINGS

4 bagels = 2 unrestricted + 1 oz. lean protein (egg) + ½ C. veggies + 2 tsp. oil
2 bagels = 1 unrestricted + 0.5 oz. lean protein (egg) + ¼ C. veggies + 1 tsp. oil

TIP: Garlic Zucchini Bagels make excellent sandwich or burger buns.

Glazed Cinnamon Rolls

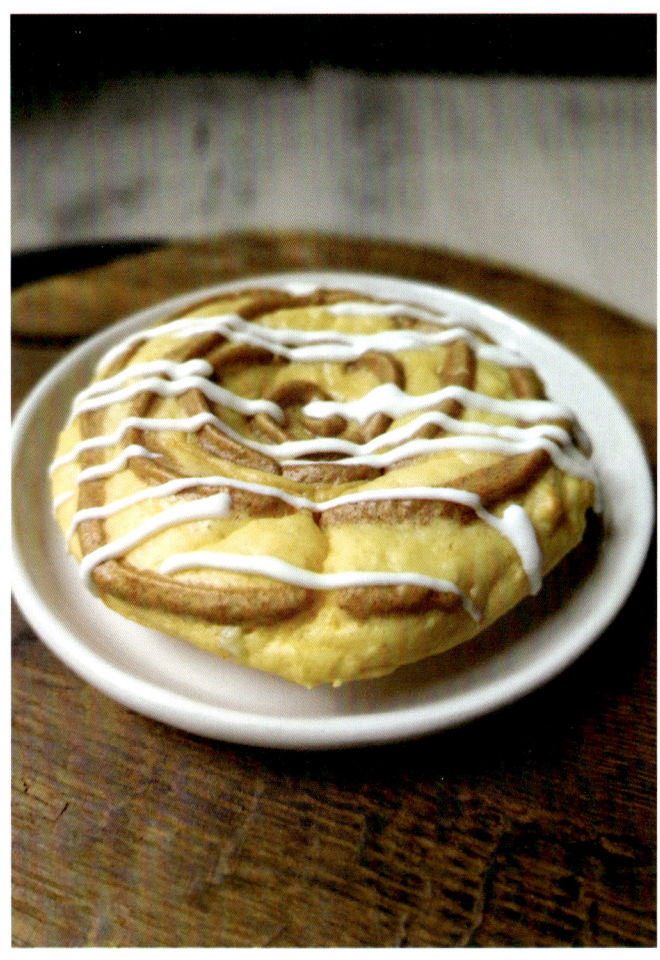

INGREDIENTS (CINNAMON ROLLS)
1 Ideal Protein vanilla smoothie mix
1 Ideal Protein golden pancakes mix
½ tsp. baking powder
1 large egg
1 large egg yolk
2 T. half and half cream
2 T. Ideal Protein maple syrup
¼ tsp. cinnamon
Cooking spray

INGREDIENTS (GLAZE)
1 T. Walden Farms marshmallow dip
1 T. Ideal Protein maple syrup
Cinnamon, to taste (optional)

DIRECTIONS
1. Preheat oven to 350° F degrees.
2. Add the cinnamon roll dry ingredients (except cinnamon) to a mixing bowl; set aside. Add cinnamon roll liquid ingredients to a separate mixing bowl; whisk to mix. Stir into dry ingredients.
3. Place approximately 1/6 of the batter into a separate bowl. Add the cinnamon and stir to mix; set aside.
4. Spoon the plain vanilla batter into a sprayed 'muffin top' pan* making 4 cinnamon rolls.
5. Place the cinnamon batter into one corner of a sandwich baggie making a piping bag. Clip ¼-inch off the plastic baggie corner and pipe the cinnamon batter onto the cinnamon rolls in a circular pattern.
6. Bake 7-8 minutes or until an inserted cake tester comes out clean. Combine glaze ingredients and drizzle over rolls.

SERVINGS
4 cinnamon rolls = 2 unrestricted + 1.5 oz. lean protein (egg + yolk) + 1 oz. half and half cream
2 cinnamon rolls = 1 unrestricted + 0.75 oz. lean protein (egg + yolk) + 0.5 oz. half and half cream

TIP: *If a muffin top pan is unavailable, make four 3-inch rounds on a parchment lined baking sheet.

Glazed Gingerbread Scones

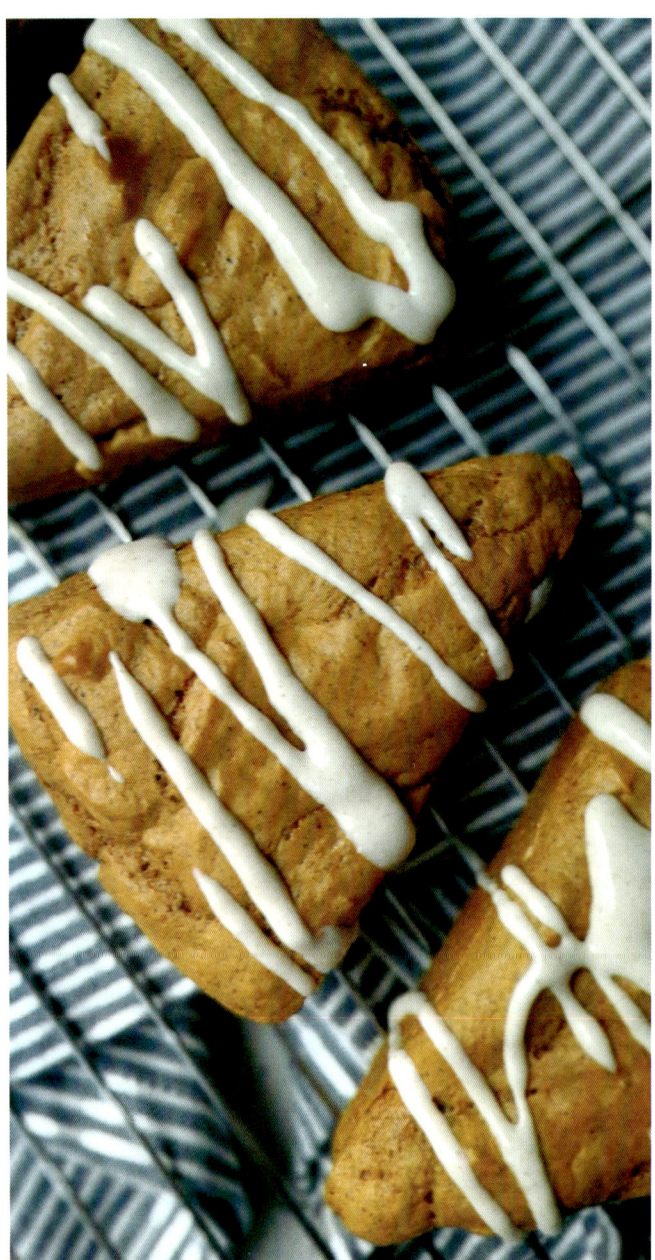

INGREDIENTS (SCONES)
1 pkg. Ideal Protein apple cinnamon puffs
1 Ideal Protein golden pancakes mix
1 tsp. baking powder
⅛ tsp. ground cloves
⅛ tsp. nutmeg
⅛ tsp. ground ginger
1 large egg
1 T. Ideal Protein maple syrup
1 T. water
Cooking spray

INGREDIENTS (GLAZE)
1 T. Walden Farms marshmallow dip
2 tsp. Ideal Protein maple syrup
Pinch of cinnamon

DIRECTIONS
1. Preheat oven to 350°F degrees.
2. Place the dry ingredients in a bullet blender or food processor; pulse to fine crumbs. Transfer to a mixing bowl.
3. Add liquid ingredients to a separate mixing bowl; whisk to mix. Stir into dry ingredients.
4. Pour batter into a sprayed scone pan making 4 scones.
5. Bake 12-14 minutes or until an inserted cake tester comes out clean.
6. Remove scones from pan and cool completely on a cooling rack.
7. Combine glaze ingredients and drizzle over scones.

SERVINGS
4 scones = 1 unrestricted + 1 restricted + 1 oz. lean protein (egg)
2 scones = ½ unrestricted + ½ restricted + 0.5 oz. lean protein (egg)

NOTE: Because this recipe includes a restricted packet, and 1 serving (2 scones) contains ½ restricted, I count it as 1 full restricted for the day. This ensures the carb or calorie count won't exceed protocol amounts.

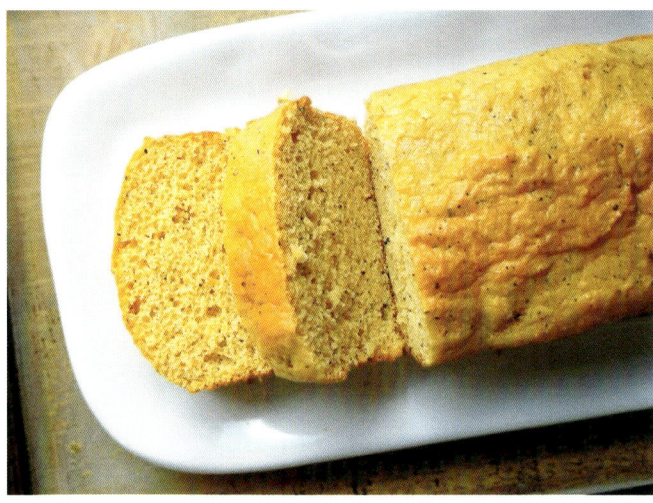

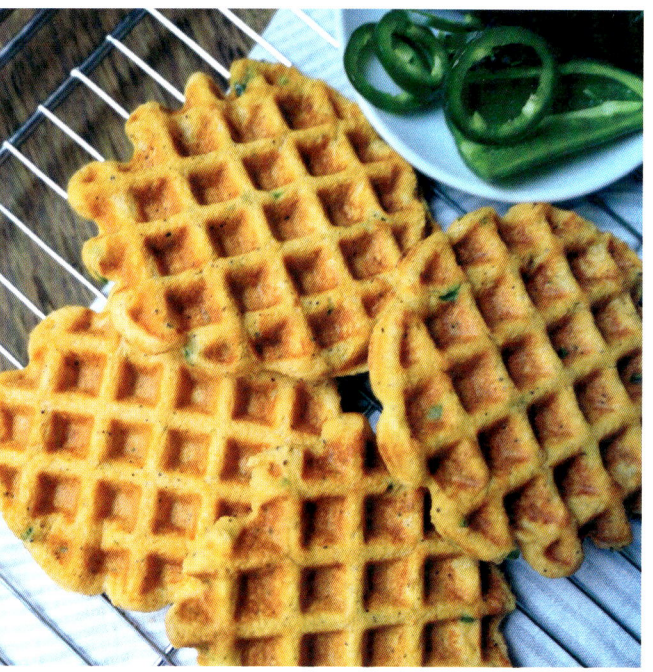

'Honey' Cornbread

INGREDIENTS

¼ C. shredded zucchini (peeled or unpeeled)
1 pkg. Ideal Protein Dorados, any flavor
1 Ideal Protein mashed potatoes mix
1 tsp. baking powder
1 large egg
1 large egg yolk
2 T. water
1 T. Ideal Protein maple syrup
⅛ tsp. cornbread extract, optional
Cooking spray

DIRECTIONS

1. Preheat oven to 350°F degrees.
2. Blot zucchini with paper towels to absorb excess moisture; set aside.
3. Place the dry ingredients in a bullet blender or food processor; pulse to fine crumbs. Transfer to a mixing bowl.
4. Add liquid ingredients to a separate mixing bowl; whisk to mix. Stir into dry ingredients. Fold in zucchini.
5. Pour batter into a sprayed (5 3/8 x 3 x 2 ⅛-inch) mini loaf pan; level batter.
6. Bake 18-20 minutes or until an inserted cake tester comes out clean.
7. For best texture, remove bread from pan and cool completely on a cooling rack before serving.

SERVINGS

Entire loaf = 2 unrestricted + 1.5 oz. lean protein (egg and yolk) + ¼ C. veggies
½ loaf = 1 unrestricted + 0.75 oz. lean protein (egg and yolk) + 2 T. veggies

Jalapeño Cornbread Waffles

INGREDIENTS

1 pkg. Ideal Protein Dorados, any flavor
1 Ideal Protein mashed potatoes mix
1 tsp. baking powder
1 large egg
¼ C. water
2 tsp. minced jalapeño pepper
Cooking spray

DIRECTIONS

1. Heat waffle iron.
2. Place the dry ingredients in a bullet blender or food processor; pulse to fine crumbs. Transfer to a mixing bowl.
3. Add liquid ingredients to a separate mixing bowl; whisk to mix. Stir into dry ingredients.
4. Spray waffle iron with cooking spray; add cornbread batter making 4 waffles. (This may have to be done in batches.)
5. Bake waffles according to manufacturer directions.

SERVINGS

4 waffles = 2 unrestricted + 1 oz. lean protein (egg) + 2 tsp. veggies
2 waffles = 1 unrestricted + 0.5 oz. lean protein (egg) + 1 tsp. veggies

TIP: Delicious as savory sandwich buns.

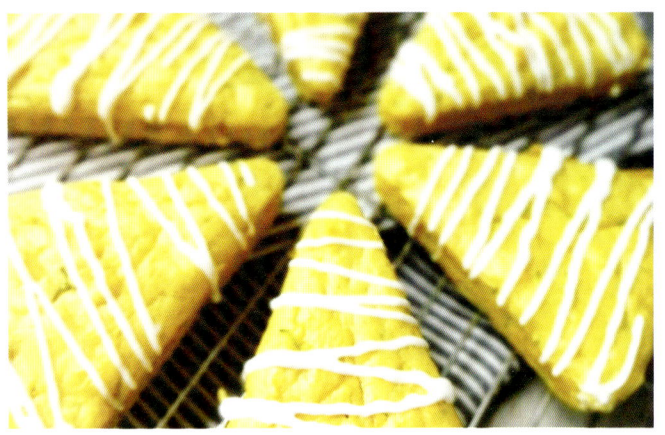

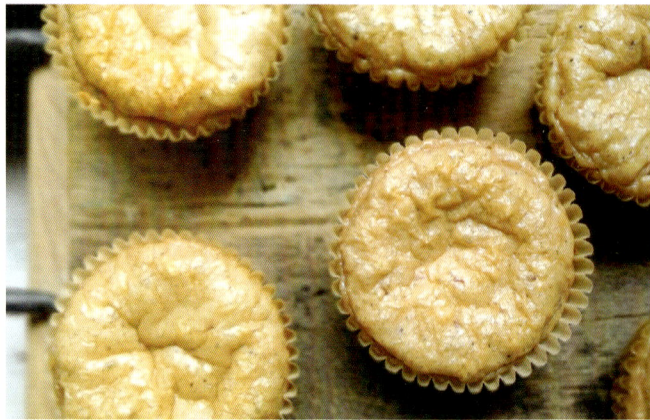

Lemon Zucchini Scones

INGREDIENTS (SCONES)

¼ C. shredded zucchini
1 pkg. (2 squares) Ideal Protein lemon wafers, crushed
1 Ideal Protein chocolate caramel mug cake mix
½ tsp. baking powder
1 large egg
¼ C. water
Zest of ½ lemon (I use a Meyer lemon)
Cooking spray

INGREDIENTS (GLAZE)

1 T. Walden Farms marshmallow dip
2 tsp. Ideal Protein maple syrup

DIRECTIONS

1. Preheat oven to 350°F degrees.
2. Blot zucchini with paper towels to absorb excess moisture; set aside.
3. Add dry ingredients to a mixing bowl; stir to mix.
4. Add liquid ingredients to a separate mixing bowl; whisk to mix. Stir into dry ingredients. Fold in zucchini.
5. Add batter to a sprayed scone pan making 4 scones.
6. Bake 12-14 minutes or until an inserted cake tester comes out clean.
7. Remove scones from pan and cool completely on a cooling rack.
8. Combine glaze ingredients and drizzle over scones.

SERVINGS

4 scones = 2 unrestricted + 1 oz. lean protein (egg) + ¼ C. veggies
2 scones = 1 unrestricted + 0.5 oz. lean protein (egg) + 2 T. veggies

Mixed Berry Muffins
Eggless recipe

INGREDIENTS

1 Ideal Protein cranberry pomegranate bar (broken into pieces)
2 Ideal Protein golden pancakes mix
1 Ideal Protein berry smoothie mix
½ tsp. baking powder
¼ tsp. baking soda
½ C. water
2 T. Walden Farms blueberry syrup
2 T. Walden Farms strawberry syrup
1 T. + 1 tsp. olive oil
1 tsp. apple cider vinegar
Cooking spray

DIRECTIONS

1. Preheat oven to 350°F degrees.
2. Place the dry ingredients in a bullet blender or food processor; pulse to fine crumbs. Transfer to a mixing bowl.
3. Add liquid ingredients to a separate mixing bowl; whisk to mix. Stir into dry ingredients.
4. Pour batter into a sprayed standard size muffin tin making 8 muffins.
5. Bake 9-11 minutes or until an inserted cake tester comes out clean.
6. For best texture, remove muffins from pan and cool completely on a cooling rack before serving.

SERVINGS

8 muffins = 3 unrestricted + 1 restricted + 4 tsp. oil
2 muffins = ¾ unrestricted + ¼ restricted + 1 tsp. oil

NOTE: Because this recipe includes a restricted packet, and 1 serving (2 muffins) contains ¼ restricted, I count it as 1 full restricted for the day. This ensures the carb or calorie count won't exceed protocol amounts.

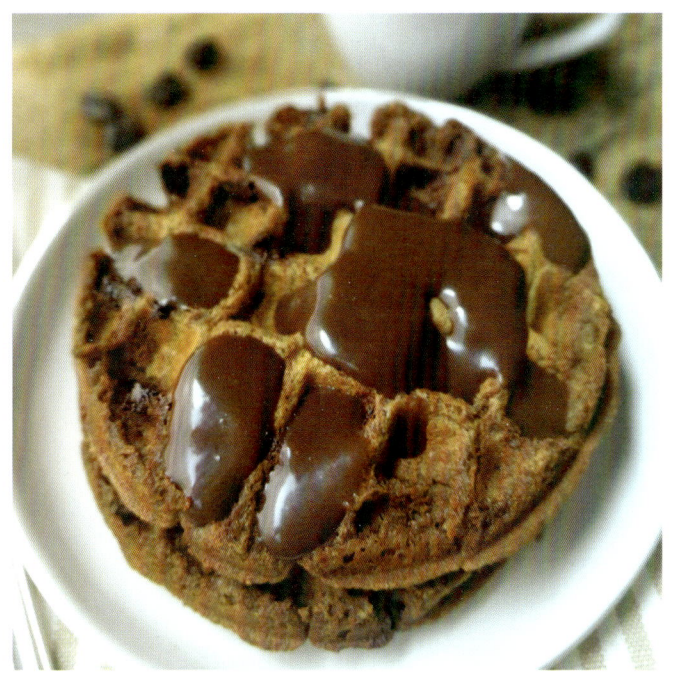

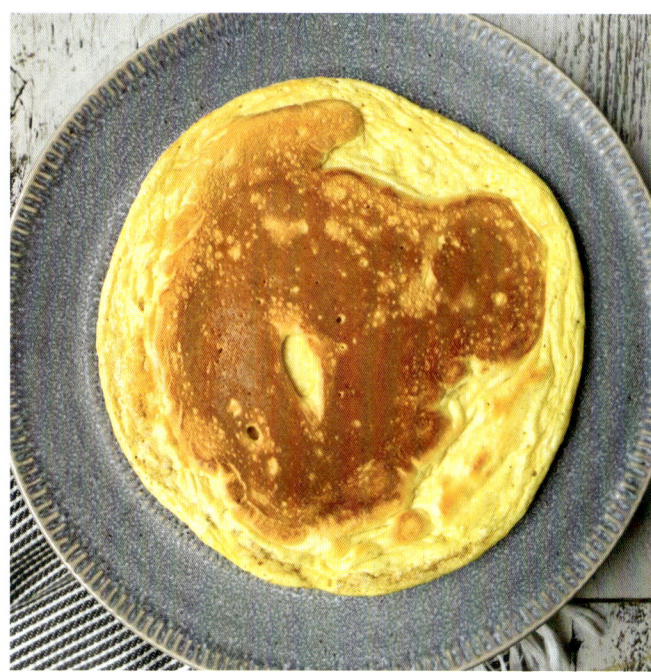

Mocha Waffles

INGREDIENTS
1 Ideal Protein chocolate caramel mug cake mix
3 T. cold coffee or espresso
1 T. Walden Farms chocolate syrup
Cooking spray

DIRECTIONS
1. Preheat waffle iron.
2. Add all ingredients to a small bowl; stir to mix.
3. Add batter to sprayed waffle iron and bake according to manufacturer directions. Makes 2 waffles.
4. Top with additional chocolate syrup, if desired.

SERVINGS
Entire recipe yield (2 waffles) = 1 unrestricted

Naan Bread

INGREDIENTS
1 Ideal Protein mashed potatoes mix
¼ tsp. baking powder
½ tsp. yellow curry spice
⅓ C. liquid egg whites
1 tsp. olive oil
Cooking spray

DIRECTIONS
1. In a small bowl, mix the dry ingredients. Add liquid ingredients; stir to mix.
2. Heat a skillet over medium heat. Lightly coat with cooking spray; add batter and spread into the size of a large pancake.
3. Cook until underside is lightly browned. Flip bread; cook until underside is lightly browned and bread is cooked through.
4. Let cool slightly on cooling rack. Add veggies, dressing and/or lean protein down center of bread; fold to eat.

SERVINGS
Entire recipe yield = 1 unrestricted + 1 tsp. oil

NOTE: Liquid egg whites are often calculated as an 'extra' for the day. Consult your coach or clinic for egg white counts toward protocol.

Peanut Butter Banana Bread

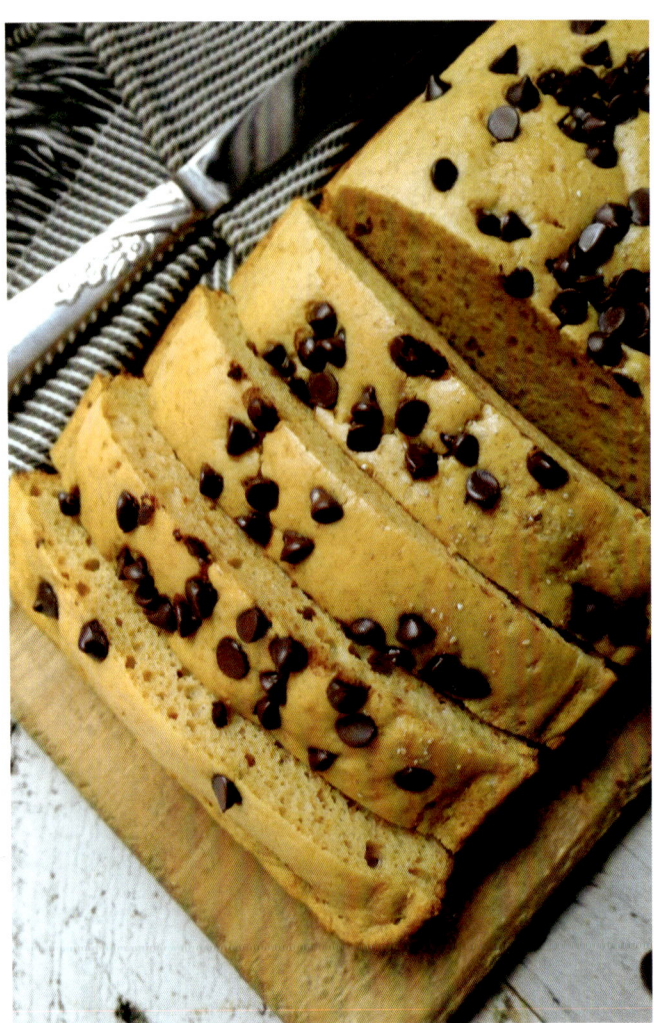

INGREDIENTS

2 Ideal Protein chocolate caramel mug cake mix
2 Ideal Protein peanut butter protein bars (broken into pieces)
1 tsp. baking powder
2 large eggs
¼ C. water
2 T. Ideal Protein maple syrup
2 T. half and half cream
¾ tsp. banana extract
Cooking spray

DIRECTIONS

1. Preheat oven to 350°F degrees.
2. Sift chocolate chips out of mug cake mixes; set chips aside.
3. Place the dry ingredients in a bullet blender or food processor; pulse to fine crumbs. Transfer to a mixing bowl.
4. Add liquid ingredients to a separate mixing bowl; stir to mix. Stir into dry ingredients.
5. Pour batter into a sprayed 9 x 5-inch metal loaf pan. Sprinkle chocolate chips over batter.
6. Bake 18-19 minutes or until an inserted cake tester comes out clean.
7. For best texture and flavor, remove bread from pan and cool completely on a cooling rack before serving.

SERVINGS

Entire loaf = 2 unrestricted + 2 restricted + 2 oz. lean protein (eggs) + 1 oz. half and half cream
¼ loaf = ½ unrestricted + ½ restricted + 0.5 oz. lean protein (eggs) + 0.25 oz. half and half cream

NOTE: Because this recipe includes both restricted and unrestricted packets, and 1 serving (¼ loaf) contains ½ restricted, I count it as 1 full restricted for the day. This ensures the carb or calorie count won't exceed protocol amounts.

Peanut Butter Cup Donuts

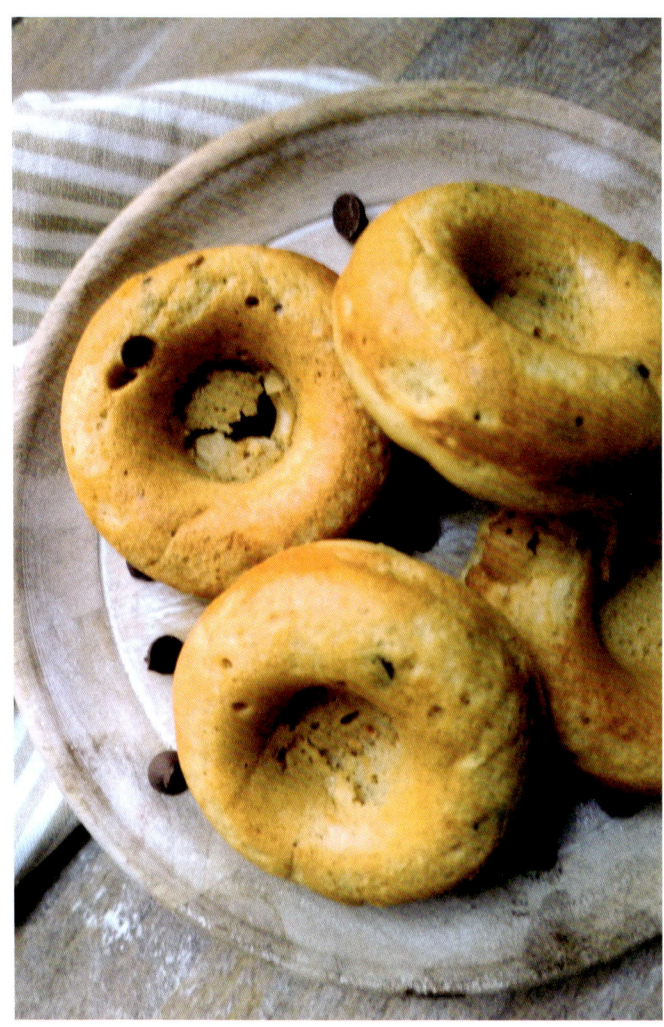

INGREDIENTS

1 Ideal Protein chocolate caramel mug cake mix
1 Ideal Protein peanut butter protein bar (broken into pieces)
½ tsp. baking powder
1 large egg
¼ C. water
¼ tsp. vanilla extract
Cooking spray

DIRECTIONS

1. Preheat oven to 350°F degrees.
2. Sift chocolate chips out of mug cake mix; set chips aside.
3. Place the dry ingredients in a bullet blender or food processor; pulse to fine crumbs. Transfer to a mixing bowl.
4. Add liquid ingredients to a separate mixing bowl; whisk to mix. Stir into dry ingredients; fold in chocolate chips.
5. Pour batter into a sprayed standard size donut pan making 4 donuts.
6. Bake 9-10 minutes or until an inserted cake tester comes out clean.
7. Remove donuts from molds and serve warm or cooled.

SERVINGS

4 donuts = 1 unrestricted + 1 restricted + 1 oz. lean protein (egg)
2 donuts = ½ unrestricted + ½ restricted + 0.5 oz. lean protein (egg)

NOTE: Because this recipe includes a restricted packet, and 1 serving (2 donuts) contains ½ restricted, I count it as 1 full restricted for the day. This ensures the carb or calorie count won't exceed protocol amounts.

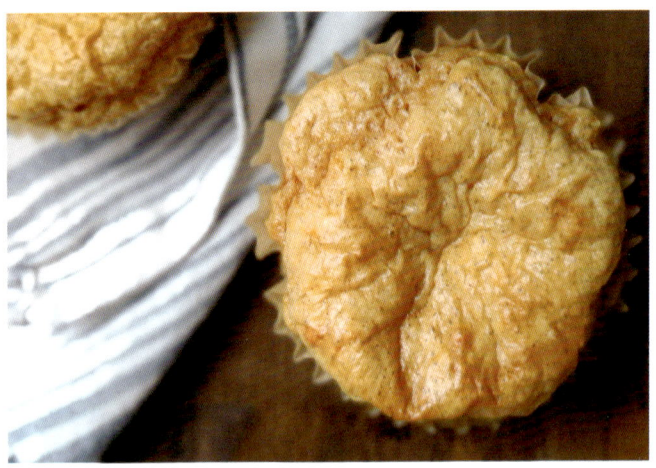
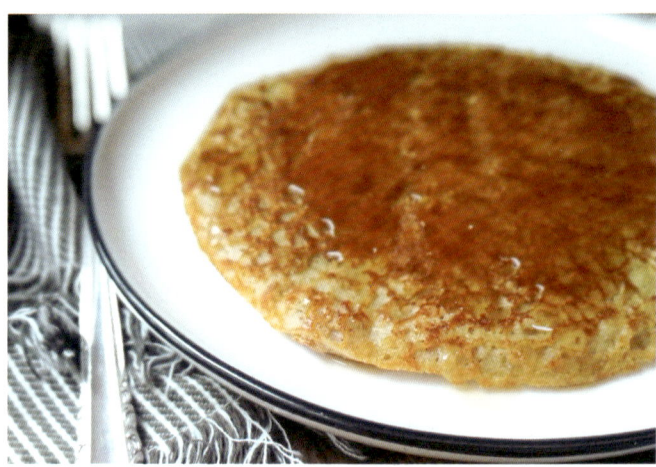

Peanut Butter Muffins

INGREDIENTS
1 Ideal Protein golden pancakes mix
1 Ideal Protein peanut butter protein bar (broken into pieces)
1 tsp. baking powder
1 large egg
2 T. Ideal Protein maple syrup
2 T. water
Cooking spray

DIRECTIONS
1. Preheat oven to 350°F degrees.
2. Place the dry ingredients in a bullet blender or food processor; pulse to fine crumbs. Transfer to a mixing bowl.
3. Add liquid ingredients to a separate mixing bowl; whisk to mix. Stir into dry ingredients.
4. Pour batter into a sprayed standard size muffin tin making 4 muffins.
5. Bake 7-8 minutes or until an inserted cake tester comes out clean.
6. Remove muffins from pan – may be eaten warm or cooled.

SERVINGS
4 muffins = 1 unrestricted + 1 restricted + 1 oz. lean protein (egg)
2 muffins = ½ unrestricted + ½ restricted + 0.5 oz. lean protein (egg)

NOTE: Because this recipe includes a restricted packet, and 1 serving (2 muffins) contains ½ restricted, I count it as 1 full restricted for the day. This ensures the carb or calorie count won't exceed protocol amounts.

Peanut Butter Pancakes

INGREDIENTS
1 Ideal Protein peanut butter protein bar (broken into pieces)
1 Ideal Protein golden or chocolate chip pancake mix
¼ tsp. baking soda
¼ C. + 1 T. water
½ tsp. apple cider vinegar
Cooking spray

DIRECTIONS
1. Place dry ingredients in a bullet blender or food processor; pulse to fine crumbs. Transfer to a small mixing bowl.
2. Add liquid ingredients to bowl; stir to mix.
3. Heat a skillet over medium/medium low heat. Lightly coat with cooking spray; pour batter into skillet making two pancakes.
4. Cook until underside is lightly browned and edges of pancakes look 'dry'. Flip pancakes and cook until underside is lightly browned and pancake is cooked through.

SERVINGS
Entire recipe yield (2 pancakes) = 1 restricted + 1 unrestricted
½ recipe yield (1 pancake) = ½ restricted + ½ unrestricted

NOTE: Because this recipe includes a restricted packet, and 1 serving (1 pancake) contains ½ restricted, I count it as 1 full restricted for the day. This ensures the carb or calorie count won't exceed protocol amounts.

Pumpkin Chocolate Chip Zucchini Bread

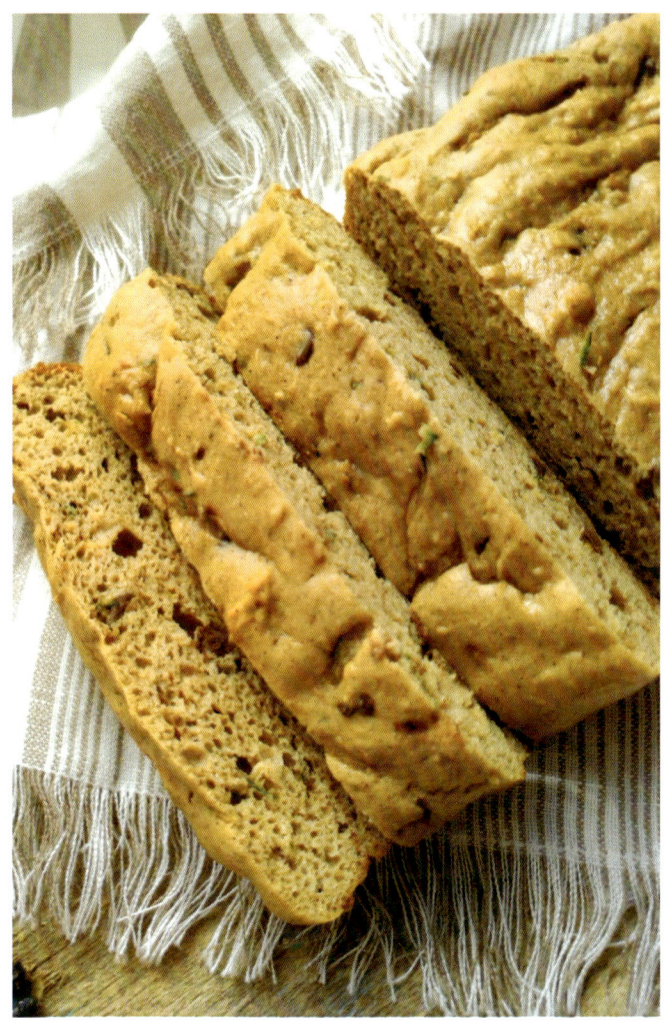

INGREDIENTS
½ C. shredded zucchini
2 Ideal Protein chocolate caramel mug cake mix
2 pkgs. Ideal Protein apple cinnamon puffs
1 tsp. baking powder
1 tsp. Pumpkin Pie Spice, pg. 145
2 large eggs
¼ C. water
2 T. Ideal Protein maple syrup
2 T. half and half cream
Cooking spray

DIRECTIONS
1. Preheat oven to 350°F degrees.
2. Blot or squeeze zucchini with paper towels to remove excess moisture; set aside. Sift chocolate chips out of mug cake mixes; set chips aside.
3. Place the dry ingredients in a bullet blender or food processor; pulse to fine crumbs. Transfer to a mixing bowl.
4. Add liquid ingredients to a separate mixing bowl (including zucchini); whisk to mix. Stir into dry ingredients. Fold in chocolate chips.
5. Pour batter into a sprayed metal (9 x 5-inch) loaf pan; level batter.
6. Bake 19-21 minutes or until an inserted cake tester comes out clean.
7. For best texture, remove bread from pan and cool completely on a cooling rack before serving.

SERVINGS
Entire loaf = 2 unrestricted + 2 restricted + 2 oz. lean protein (egg) + ½ C. veggies + 1 oz. half and half cream
¼ loaf = ½ unrestricted + ½ restricted + 0.5 oz. lean protein (egg) + 2 T. veggies + 0.25 oz. half and half cream

NOTE: Because this recipe includes both restricted and unrestricted packets, and 1 serving (¼ loaf) contains ½ restricted, I count it as 1 full restricted for the day. This ensures the carb or calorie count won't exceed protocol amounts.

Pumpkin Pie Pancakes

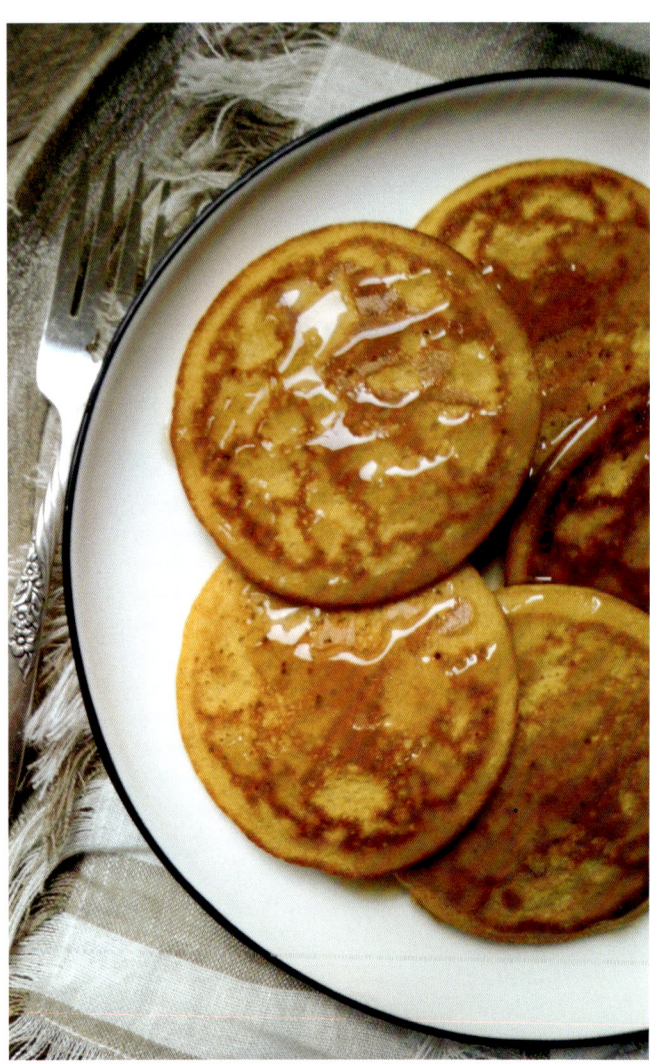

INGREDIENTS

1 Ideal Protein golden pancakes mix
⅛ tsp. Pumpkin Pie flavor fountain* or ¼ tsp. Pumpkin Pie Spice, pg. 145
⅛ tsp. butter extract
3 T. water
1 large egg yolk
Cooking spray
Ideal Protein maple syrup (for topping)

DIRECTIONS

1. Mix all ingredients in a small bowl.
2. Heat a large skillet over medium/medium low heat.
3. Lightly coat skillet with cooking spray; pour batter into skillet making 5 mini pancakes (or 2 larger pancakes).
4. Cook pancakes until edges start to look dry and underside is lightly browned. Flip and cook until underside is lightly browned and pancake is cooked through.
5. Serve topped with maple syrup, if desired.

SERVINGS

Entire recipe yield = 1 unrestricted + 0.5 oz. lean protein (egg yolk)

TIP: *Pumpkin Pie flavor fountain extract may be purchased online at olivenation.com or amazon.com – this water-based extract adds richness, color, and flavor to the baked goods but is an optional addition.

Rhuberry Bread

Eggless recipe

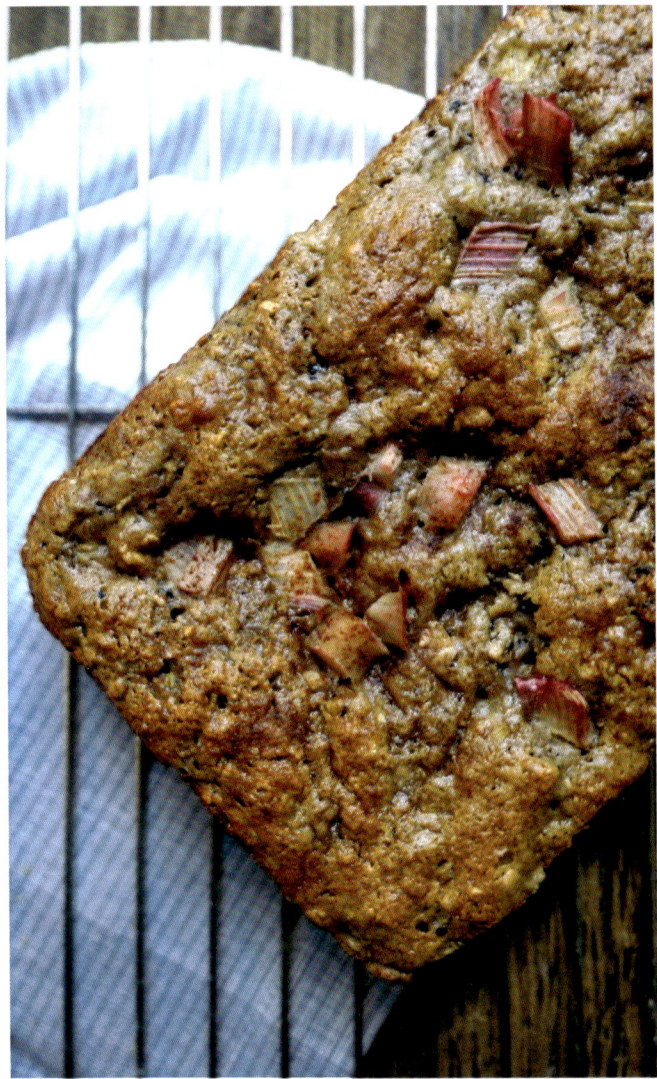

INGREDIENTS

1 Ideal Protein apple cinnamon oatmeal mix
2 Ideal Protein golden pancakes mix
1 Ideal Protein blueberry muffin mix
½ tsp. baking soda
1 tsp. cinnamon
½ C. finely chopped rhubarb
¼ C. water
¼ C. Walden Farms strawberry syrup
1 T. + 1 tsp. olive oil
2 tsp. apple cider vinegar
Cooking spray

INGREDIENTS (TOPPING)

½ C. coarsely chopped rhubarb
Cinnamon (to taste)
Sugar free sweetener, granular (to taste)

DIRECTIONS

1. Preheat oven to 350°F degrees.
2. Add dry ingredients to a mixing bowl; stir to mix. Set aside.
3. Blot finely chopped rhubarb with paper towels to absorb excess moisture, and place in a separate mixing bowl; add remaining (liquid) ingredients. Stir to mix.
4. Combine liquid and dry ingredients; stir to mix.
5. Pour batter into a sprayed 9 x 5-inch loaf pan; level batter.
6. Evenly top batter with chopped rhubarb; lightly sprinkle with cinnamon and sugar free sweetener.
7. Bake 18-20 minutes or until an inserted cake tester comes out clean. (Do not overbake.)
8. For best texture, remove bread from pan and cool completely on a cooling rack before serving.

SERVINGS

Entire loaf = 4 unrestricted + ½ C. veggies + 4 tsp. oil
1/4 loaf = 1 unrestricted + 2 T. veggies + 1 tsp. oil

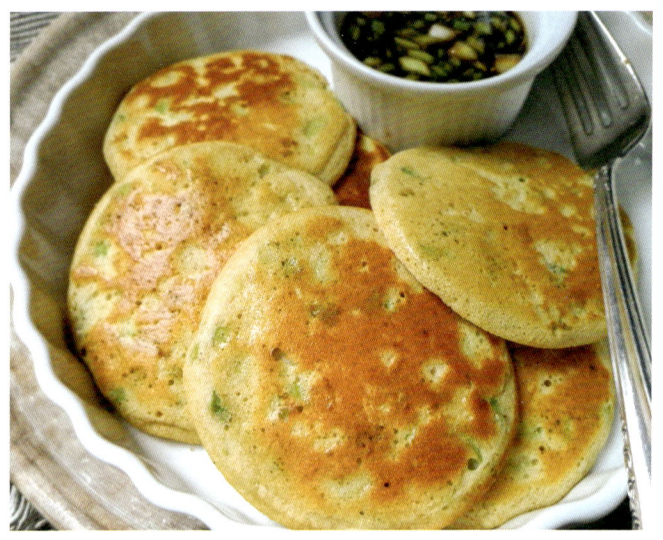

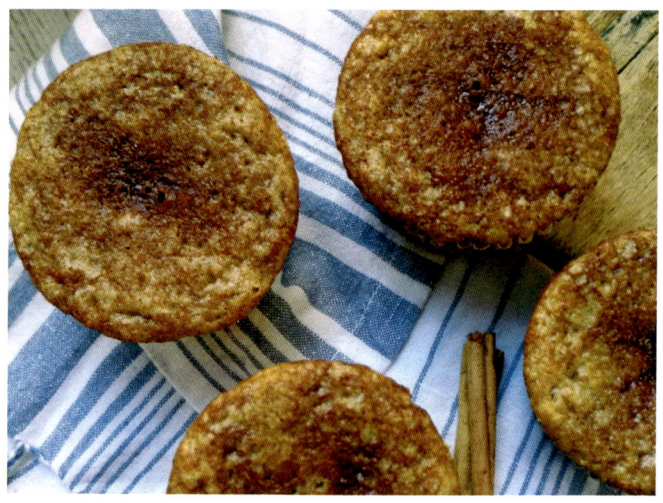

Scallion Pancakes

INGREDIENTS (DIPPING SAUCE)
1 T. white vinegar
1 T. sugar free sweetener, granular
1 T. low sodium soy sauce
¼ tsp. minced fresh ginger
1 T. chopped green onion

INGREDIENTS (PANCAKES)
1 Ideal Protein golden pancakes mix
1 large egg
2 T. water
3 T. chopped green onion
1 tsp. toasted sesame oil

DIRECTIONS
1. Add dipping sauce ingredients to a small bowl; stir to mix. Set aside.
2. Add pancake mix, egg, and water to a mixing bowl; stir to mix. Fold in chopped green onion.
3. Brush a large skillet with sesame oil; heat over medium/medium low. Pour batter into skillet making 6 mini pancakes or 2 larger pancakes.
4. Cook until edges of pancakes begin to look dry, and underside is lightly browned; flip and cook until underside is lightly browned.
5. Serve with dipping sauce.

SERVINGS
Entire recipe yield (6 mini pancakes) = 1 unrestricted + 1 oz. lean protein (egg) + 1 tsp. oil + ¼ C. veggies

TIP: Place cooked chicken and/or veggies in the center of pancakes; fold and dip in sauce – amazing!

Snickerdoodle Muffins

INGREDIENTS (CINNAMON & SUGAR TOPPING)
1 tsp. sugar free sweetener, granular
⅛ tsp. cinnamon

INGREDIENTS (MUFFINS)
1 Ideal Protein golden pancakes mix
1 Ideal Protein vanilla crispy square (broken into pieces)
1 tsp. cinnamon
½ tsp. baking powder
1 large egg
2 T. water
2 T. Ideal Protein maple syrup
1 tsp. vanilla extract
Cooking spray

DIRECTIONS
1. Preheat oven to 350° F degrees.
2. Prepare topping by mixing sweetener and cinnamon in a small bowl; set aside.
3. To prepare muffins, add dry muffin ingredients to a mixing bowl; stir to mix.
4. Add liquid ingredients to a separate mixing bowl; whisk to mix. Stir into dry ingredients.
5. Spoon batter into a sprayed standard size muffin tin making 4 muffins; sprinkle muffins with cinnamon and sugar topping.
6. Bake 11-13 minutes or until an inserted cake tester comes out clean.
7. For best texture, remove muffins from pan and cool completely on a cooling rack before serving.

SERVINGS
4 muffins = 2 unrestricted + 1 oz. lean protein (egg)
2 muffins = 1 unrestricted + 0.5 oz. lean protein (egg)

Soup Bagels

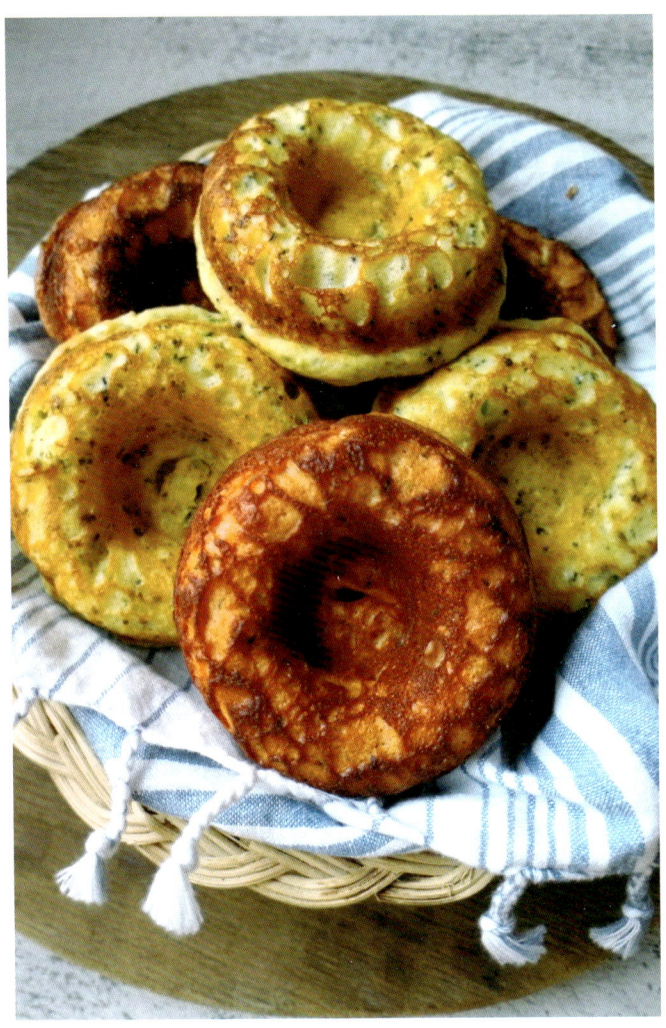

INGREDIENTS
¼ C. shredded zucchini
1 Ideal Protein mashed potatoes mix
1 Ideal Protein soup mix, any flavor
1 tsp. baking powder
¼ tsp. garlic powder
1 large egg
3 T. water*
2 T. Ideal Protein honey Dijon dressing
2 tsp. olive oil
Cooking spray

DIRECTIONS
1. Preheat oven to 350°F degrees.
2. Blot zucchini with paper towels to absorb excess moisture; set aside.
3. Place the dry ingredients in a bullet blender or food processor; pulse to fine crumbs. Transfer to a mixing bowl.
4. Add liquid ingredients to a separate mixing bowl; whisk to mix. Stir into dry ingredients. Fold in zucchini.
5. Add batter to a sprayed standard size donut pan making 4 bagels.
6. Bake 8-12 minutes or until inserted cake tester comes out clean. (Bake time varies based on soup flavor used in recipe.)
7. Remove bagels from pan – may be served warm or cooled.

SERVINGS
4 bagels = 2 unrestricted + 1 oz. lean protein (egg) + ¼ C. veggies + 2 tsp. oil
2 bagels = 1 unrestricted + 0.5 oz. lean protein (egg) + 2 T. veggies + 1 tsp. oil

TIP: *Batter should be thick but not stiff – some soups will create a stiff batter; add more water to thin the batter as necessary (batter should not be so thin that it pours out of mixing bowl).

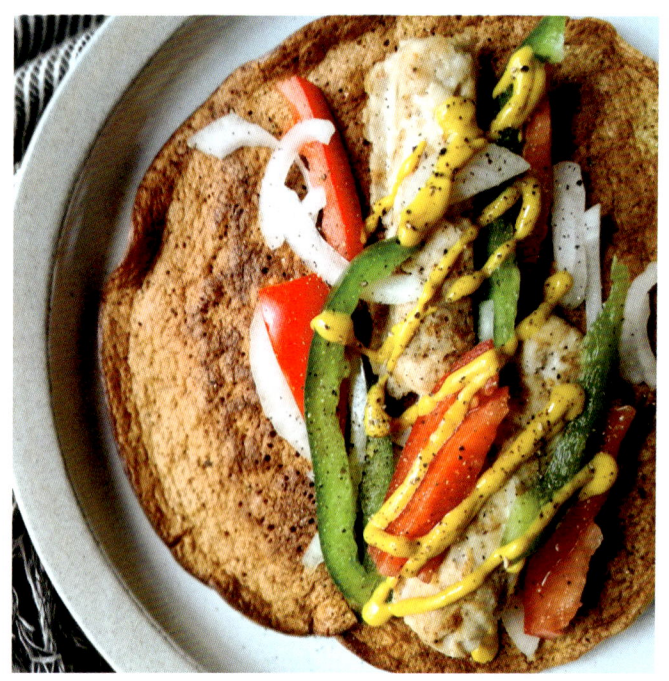

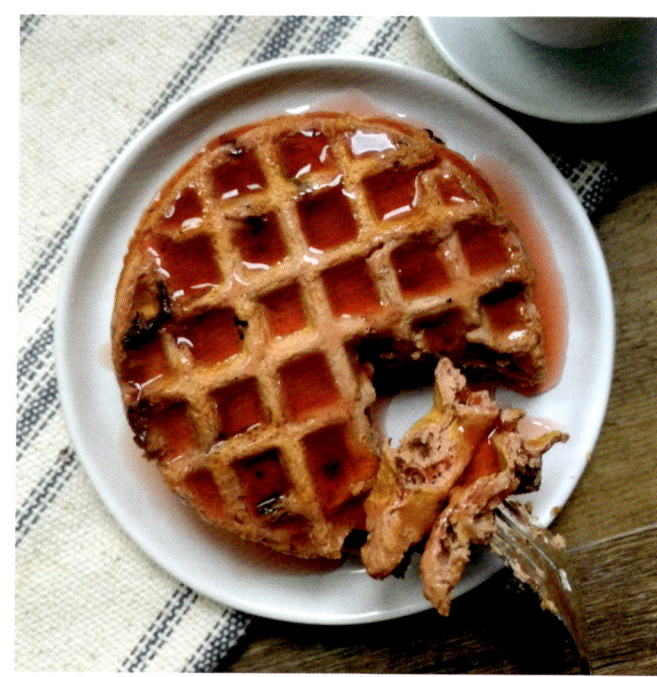

Soup Pitas

INGREDIENTS
1 Ideal Protein soup mix, any flavor
¼ tsp. baking powder
2 egg whites, lightly beaten
1 tsp. olive oil
Cooking spray

DIRECTIONS
1. Add soup mix and baking powder to a mixing bowl; stir to mix.
2. Add remaining ingredients; stir to mix.
3. Heat a skillet over medium heat. Lightly coat skillet with cooking spray and pour batter into pan making a 7-inch (diameter) 'pancake'.
4. Cook until underside is lightly browned and edges begin to look dry; flip and cook until underside is lightly browned and cooked through.
5. Let cool slightly on cooling rack. Stuff with veggies, dressing and/or lean protein; fold to eat.

SERVINGS
1 pita wrap = 1 unrestricted + 1 tsp. oil

NOTE: Liquid egg whites are often calculated as an 'extra' for the day. Consult your coach or clinic for egg white counts toward protocol.

Strawberry Chocolate Chip Waffles

INGREDIENTS
1 Ideal Protein chocolate caramel mug cake mix
2 T. Walden Farms strawberry syrup
2 T. water
⅛ tsp. strawberry extract
3 drops red food coloring, optional
Cooking spray

DIRECTIONS
1. Preheat waffle iron.
2. In a small mixing bowl, mix all ingredients to combine. Batter will be thick.
3. Scoop batter into a sprayed waffle maker making 2 waffles. Bake according to manufacturer directions.
4. Drizzle with additional strawberry syrup, if desired.

SERVINGS
Entire recipe yield (2 waffles) = 1 unrestricted

Texas Turtle Muffins
Jumbo size

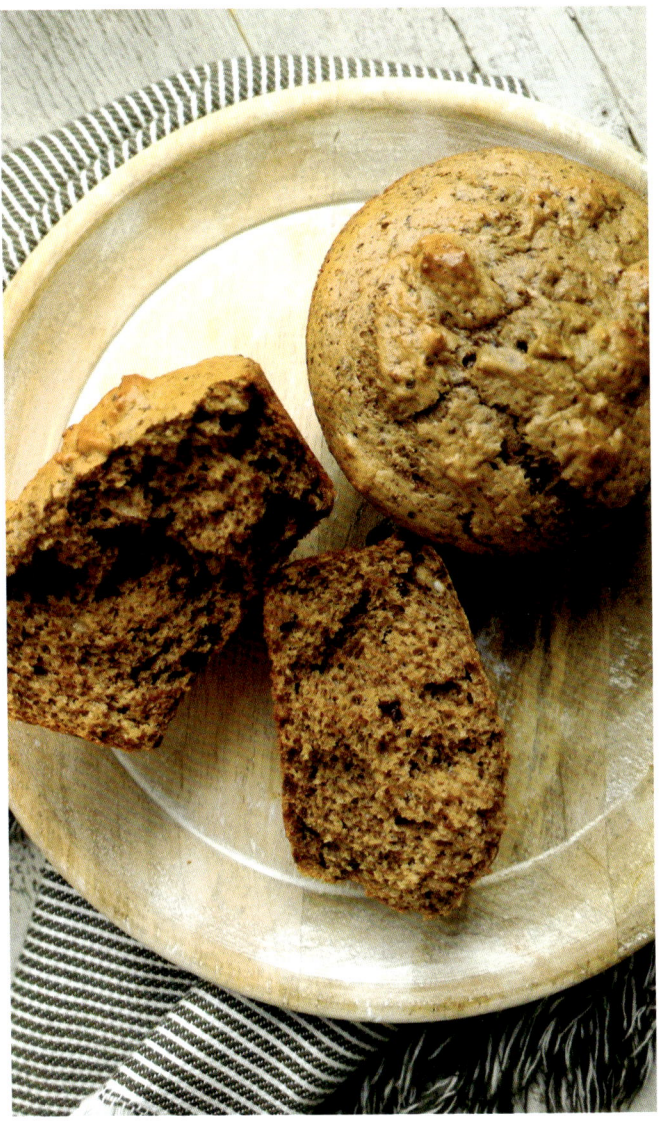

INGREDIENTS
1 Ideal Protein chocolate caramel mug cake mix
1 Ideal Protein chocolate crispy square (broken in pieces)
1 tsp. baking powder
1 large egg
3 T. water
1 T. Walden Farms caramel syrup
1 T. Walden Farms chocolate syrup
½ tsp. vanilla extract
Cooking spray

DIRECTIONS
1. Preheat oven to 350°F degrees.
2. Place the dry ingredients in a bullet blender or food processor; pulse to fine crumbs. Transfer to a mixing bowl.
3. Add liquid ingredients to a separate mixing bowl; whisk to mix. Stir into dry ingredients.
4. Pour batter into a sprayed jumbo size muffin tin* making 2 muffins.
5. Bake 14-16 minutes or until an inserted cake tester comes out clean.
6. For best texture, remove muffins from pan and cool completely on a cooling rack before serving.

SERVINGS
2 jumbo muffins = 2 unrestricted + 1 oz. lean protein (egg)
1 jumbo muffin = 1 unrestricted + 0.5 oz. lean protein (egg)

TIP: *If a jumbo muffin tin is not available, use a standard muffin tin making 4 muffins; bake approximately 9-11 minutes or until an inserted cake tester comes out clean.

Vanilla Chocolate Chip Muffins

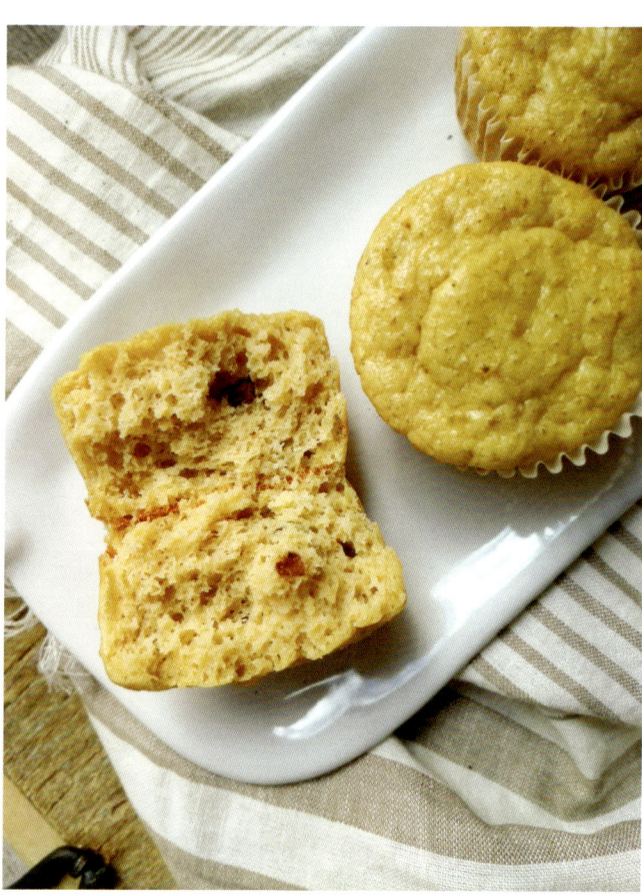

INGREDIENTS

1 Ideal Protein chocolate chip pancake mix
1 Ideal Protein vanilla crispy square (broken into pieces)
½ tsp. baking powder
1 large egg
2 T. water
1 T. Ideal Protein maple syrup
1 T. half and half cream
½ tsp. vanilla extract
Cooking spray

DIRECTIONS

1. Preheat oven to 350°F degrees.
2. Sift out chocolate chips from pancake mix; set chips aside.
3. Place the dry ingredients in a bullet blender or food processor; pulse to fine crumbs. Transfer to a mixing bowl.
4. Add liquid ingredients to a separate mixing bowl; whisk to mix. Stir into dry ingredients. Fold in chocolate chips.
5. Pour batter into a sprayed standard size muffin tin making 4 muffins.
6. Bake 11-13 minutes or until an inserted cake tester comes out clean.
7. For best texture, remove muffins from pan and cool completely on a cooling rack before serving.

SERVINGS

4 muffins = 2 unrestricted + 1 oz. lean protein (egg) + 0.5 oz. half and half cream
2 muffins = 1 unrestricted + 0.5 oz. lean protein (egg) + 0.25 oz. half and half cream

Zesty Italian Bagels

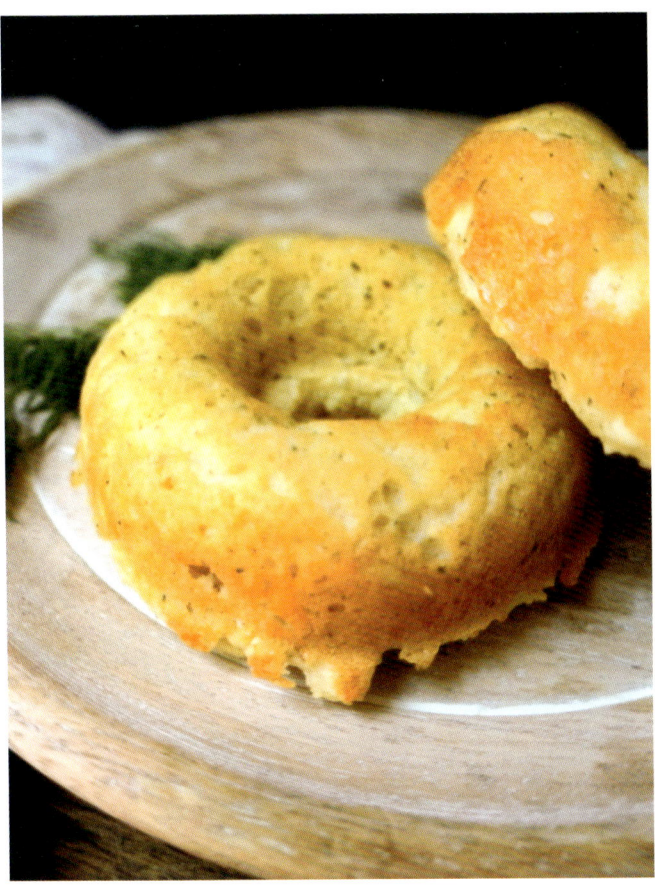

INGREDIENTS

½ C. shredded zucchini
1 Ideal Protein mashed potatoes mix
1 Ideal Protein crispy cereal mix
1 tsp. baking powder
½ tsp. Italian seasoning
¼ tsp. crushed red pepper
1 large egg
2 T. water
2 T. Ideal Protein Italian dressing
2 tsp. olive oil
Cooking spray

DIRECTIONS

1. Preheat oven to 350°F degrees.
2. Blot zucchini with paper towels to absorb excess moisture; set aside.
3. Place the dry ingredients in a bullet blender or food processor; pulse to fine crumbs. Transfer to a mixing bowl.
4. Add liquid ingredients to a separate mixing bowl; whisk to mix. Stir into dry ingredients. Fold in zucchini.
5. Add batter to a sprayed standard size donut pan making 4 bagels.
6. Bake 12-14 minutes or until inserted cake tester comes out clean.
7. For best texture, remove bagels from pan and cool completely on a cooling rack before serving.

SERVINGS

4 bagels = 2 unrestricted + 1 oz. lean protein (egg) + ½ C. veggies + 2 tsp. oil
2 bagels = 1 unrestricted + 0.5 oz. lean protein (egg) + ¼ C. veggies + 1 tsp. oil

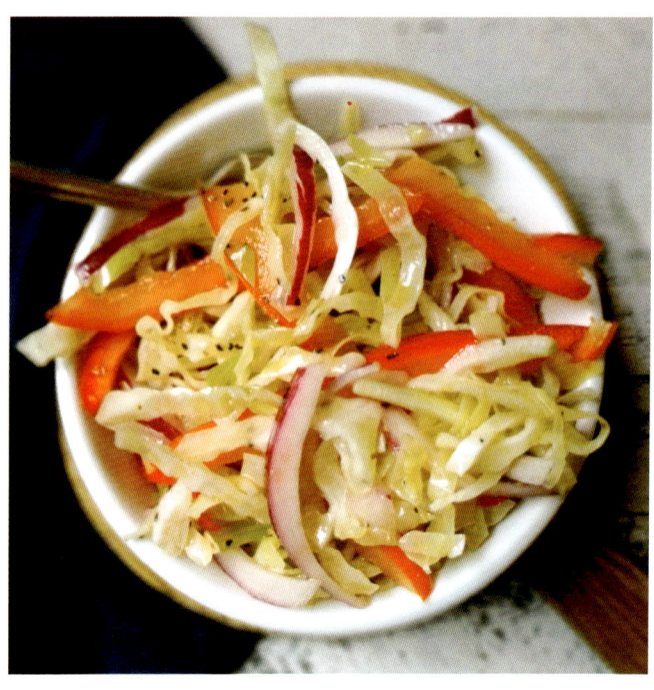

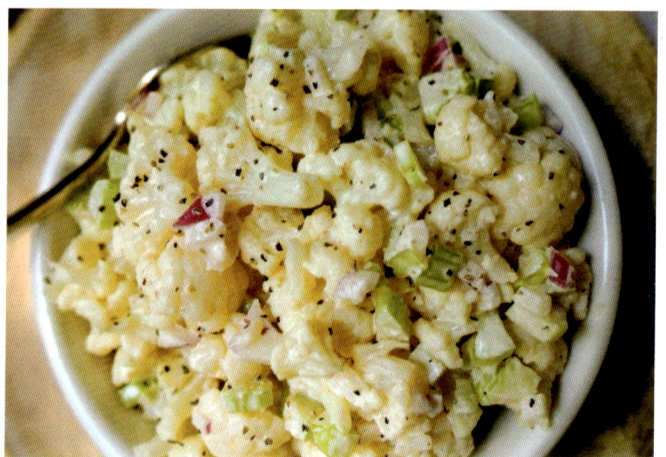

Carolina Cabbage Slaw

INGREDIENTS (SLAW)
4 ½ C. finely sliced green cabbage
1 C. (5.3 oz.) thinly sliced red bell pepper
½ C. thinly sliced red onion

INGREDIENTS (DRESSING)
2 T. extra virgin olive oil
1 T. + 2 tsp. apple cider vinegar
¼ tsp. kosher salt
Black pepper, to taste

DIRECTIONS
1. Place slaw ingredients in a large bowl.
2. Add dressing ingredients to slaw; toss to coat.
3. Marinate in fridge at least 15 minutes. Toss before serving.

SERVINGS
Entire recipe yield = 6 C. veggies + 2 T. oil
⅓ recipe yield = 2 C. veggies + 2 tsp. oil

TIP: A perfect side dish for serving with slow cooker meats.

Cauliflower Fauxtato Salad

INGREDIENTS (DRESSING)
2 T. Janeva's mayonnaise, pg. 141
1 tsp. apple cider vinegar
1 tsp. lemon juice
½ tsp. sugar free sweetener, granular
⅛ tsp. ground mustard
Pinch of smoked paprika

INGREDIENTS (SALAD)
4 C. cauliflower florets (cut in 1-inch pieces)
½ C. chopped celery
2 T. minced red onion
Salt & pepper, to taste

DIRECTIONS
1. In a small mixing bowl, whisk all dressing ingredients to combine. Store in fridge until ready to use.
2. Place cauliflower florets in a microwave proof bowl and add 1" inch of water. Cover and microwave on high 8 minutes or until fork tender. Drain and cool in fridge.
3. Combine cooled florets and remaining salad ingredients in a medium mixing bowl; gently fold to mix.
4. Pour dressing over salad mixture and fold to coat.

SERVINGS
Entire recipe yield = 4 C. and 2 T. veggies + 4 tsp. olive oil (mayonnaise); raw celery not counted
½ recipe yield = 2 C. and 1 T. veggies + 2 tsp. olive oil (mayonnaise); raw celery not counted

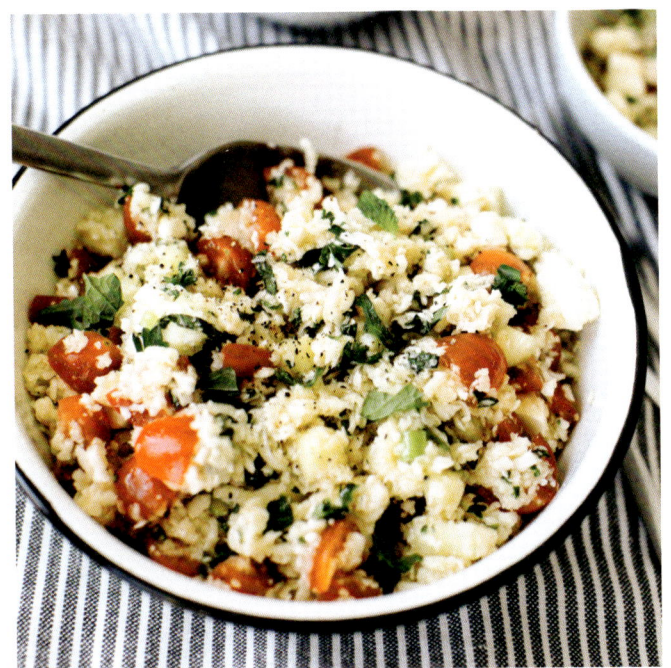
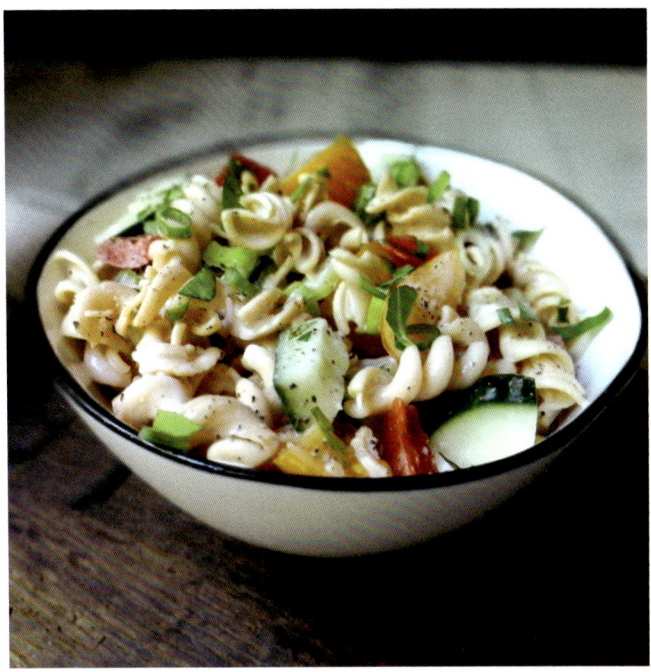

Cauliflower Tabouli Salad

INGREDIENTS (SALAD)
3 C. (10.5 oz.) cauliflower florets, riced
1 C. grape tomatoes, quartered
¾ C. cucumber (peeled and chopped)
¼ C. chopped green onion
¼ C. chopped fresh parsley
2 T. chopped fresh mint
Salt and pepper, to taste

INGREDIENTS (DRESSING)
⅓ C. lemon juice
3 T. + 1 tsp. olive oil
1 T. soy sauce

DIRECTIONS
1. In a large bowl, gently toss salad ingredients. Set aside.
2. In a medium bowl, whisk together the dressing ingredients. Store salad and dressing separately in fridge until ready to serve.
3. Just before serving, pour dressing over cauliflower mixture and fold to coat salad.
4. Cover and refrigerate any leftovers.

SERVINGS
Entire recipe yield = 5 C. veggies + 3 T. and 1 tsp. oil
⅕ recipe yield = 1 C. veggies + 2 tsp. oil

Garden Rotini Salad

INGREDIENTS
1 pkg. Ideal Protein rotini pasta
1 T. Janeva's Mayonnaise, pg. 141
1 T. Ideal Protein Italian Herb or Honey Dijon dressing
½ C. diced English cucumber (unpeeled)
½ C. diced Roma tomatoes
3 T. diced bell pepper (assorted colors)
1 T. chopped green onion
Salt & pepper, to taste

DIRECTIONS
1. Prepare rotini pasta according to package directions; drain and set aside.
2. In a small bowl, whisk together the mayonnaise and dressing.
3. Add pasta, veggies, and dressing mixture to a large bowl; gently fold to coat. Season with salt and pepper.

SERVINGS
Entire recipe yield = 1 unrestricted + 1 ¼ C. veggies + 2 tsp. oil (mayonnaise)

Green Bean & Tomato Salad

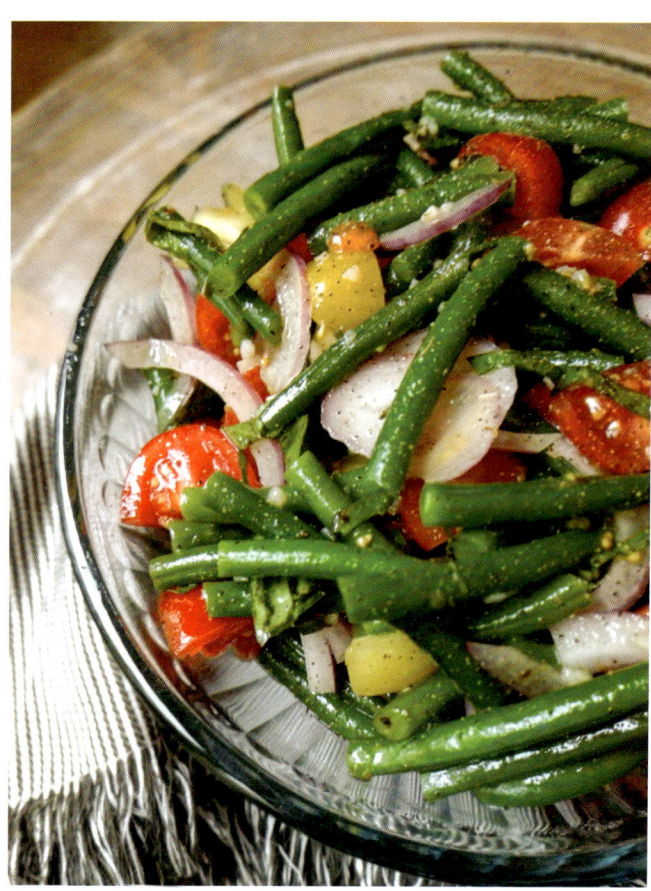

INGREDIENTS (DRESSING)
3 T. extra virgin olive oil
2 T. lemon juice
2 tsp. minced garlic
½ tsp. sea salt
½ tsp. dried oregano

INGREDIENTS (SALAD)
4 C. French-style fresh green beans (cut in 2-inch pieces; ends removed)
1 large bowl ice water
1 C. thinly sliced red onion
2 C. quartered baby heirloom or cherry tomatoes
⅓ C. chopped fresh basil
Salt and pepper, to taste

DIRECTIONS
1. Place all dressing ingredients in a small bowl and whisk to mix; set aside.
2. Place a steamer basket in a large saucepan or Dutch oven. Add 1-inch water and heat to a low boil. Add green beans to basket, cover, and steam green beans over medium high heat 5 minutes or until tender crisp (the beans should be par-cooked, do not cook until tender).
3. Immediately transfer beans into ice water. Cool beans 2 minutes, drain, and transfer to a large bowl.
4. Add remaining salad ingredients to bowl. Pour dressing over salad and gently fold to coat. Season with additional salt and pepper, if desired.
5. Serve chilled or room temperature. Store covered in fridge.

SERVINGS
Entire recipe yield = 7 C. veggies + 3 T. oil
½ recipe yield = 1 C. veggies + 1 ¼ tsp. oil

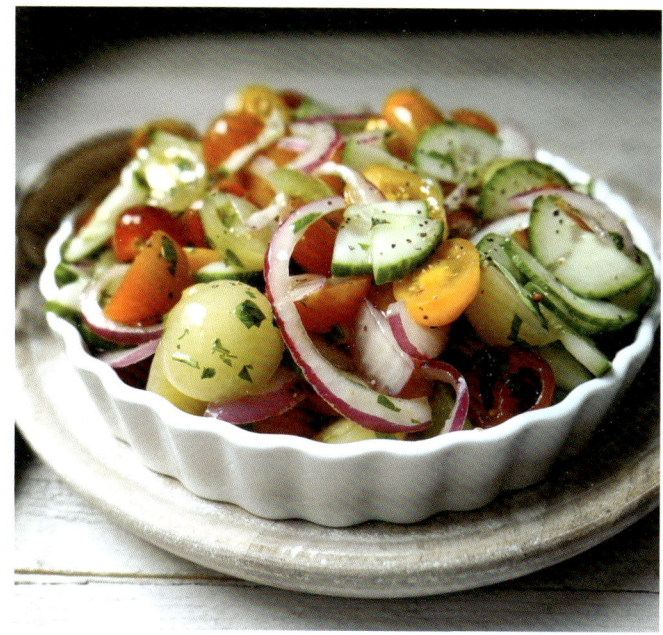

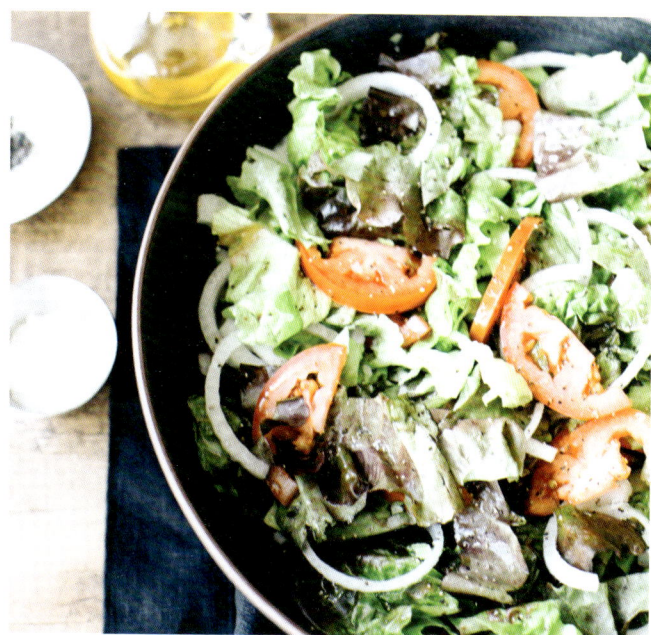

Heirloom Tomato Cucumber Salad

INGREDIENTS

4 C. baby heirloom tomatoes, halved
2 ½ C. half-moon slices English cucumber (unpeeled)
½ C. thinly sliced red onion
2 T. chopped fresh cilantro
¼ C. Ideal Protein honey Dijon dressing
Black pepper, to taste

DIRECTIONS

1. Add all ingredients to a large bowl; fold to coat veggies with dressing.
2. Store covered in fridge.

SERVINGS

Measure amount being used and count that amount toward the daily veggie protocol. For example, 1 C. salad = 1 C. veggies.

Janeva's Simple Salad

INGREDIENTS

8 C. chopped red leaf lettuce
2 ½ C. thinly sliced Roma tomatoes
1 ½ C. thinly sliced yellow onion
2 T + 2 tsp. olive oil
2 T. apple cider vinegar
¼ tsp. sea salt
⅛ tsp. coarsely ground black pepper

DIRECTIONS

1. Add lettuce to a large salad bowl; set aside.
2. Cut round tomato and onion slices in half. Add to lettuce; gently toss.
3. Just before serving, drizzle olive oil and vinegar over salad. Sprinkle with salt and pepper. Gently toss.

SERVINGS

Entire recipe yield = 12 C. veggies + 2 T. oil
¼ recipe yield (3 C. salad) = 1 C. veggies + 1 ½ tsp. oil + 2 C. lettuce, unlimited (see NOTE below)

NOTE: Lettuce is unlimited and does not need to be counted; the only veggies that are necessary to count in this salad are the tomatoes and onion.

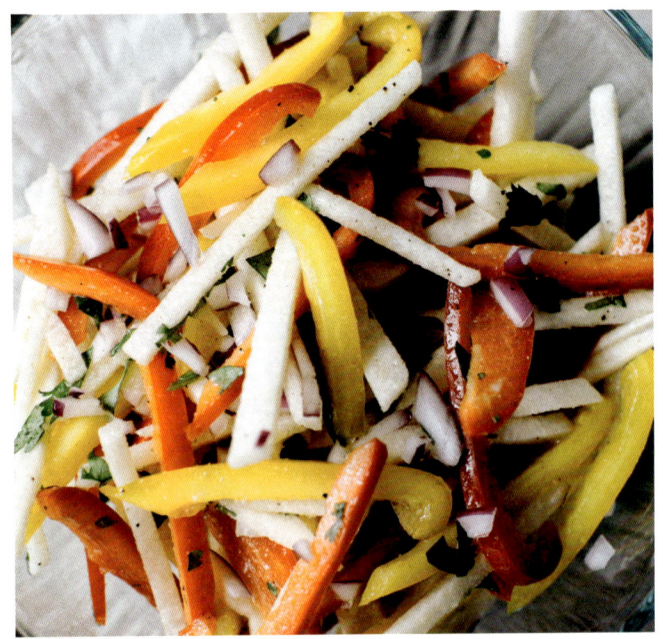

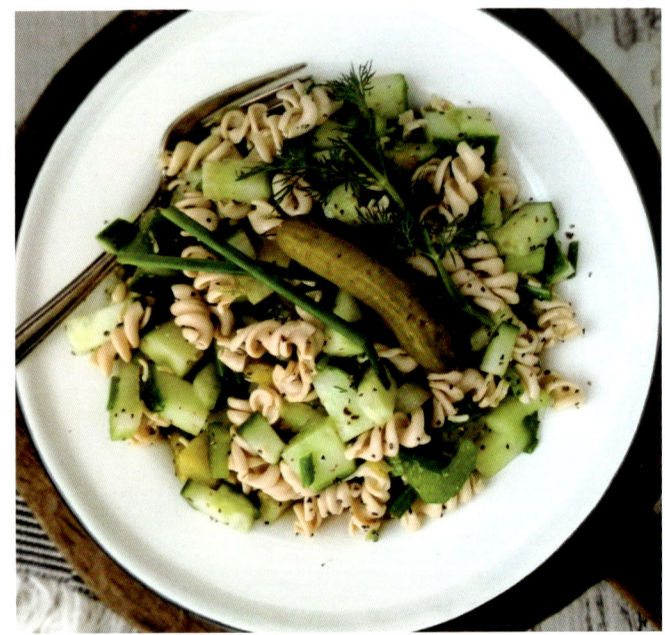

Jicama Sweet Pepper Slaw

INGREDIENTS

2 C. julienned jicama (cut the size of matchsticks)
1 C. julienned bell pepper (red and yellow)
2 T. olive oil
1 T. apple cider vinegar
1 T. Ideal Protein maple syrup
1 T. minced red onion
½ tsp. garlic powder
¼ tsp. ground cumin
2 T. finely chopped fresh cilantro
Salt & pepper, to taste

DIRECTIONS

1. Place the jicama and bell pepper in a large bowl; set aside.
2. In a small bowl, whisk the remaining ingredients until mixed.
3. Pour the dressing over the jicama and bell pepper; fold to coat.
4. Keep refrigerated until use. Toss before serving.

SERVINGS

Entire recipe yield = 3 C. and 1 T. veggies + 2 T. olive oil
⅓ recipe yield = 1 C. veggies and 1 tsp. veggies + 2 tsp. olive oil

Pickle Pasta Salad

INGREDIENTS

2 pkg. Ideal Protein rotini pasta
2 T. Dill Pickle Vinaigrette, pg. 139
2 C. chopped English cucumber (unpeeled)
1 C. chopped baby dill pickles
1 C. thinly sliced celery
¼ C. chopped fresh chives
¼ tsp. red pepper flakes, optional
Salt & black pepper, to taste

DIRECTIONS

1. Prepare pasta according to package directions; drain. Place pasta in medium mixing bowl; cover and store in fridge until cooled.
2. Meanwhile, prepare vinaigrette. Add vinaigrette and remaining salad ingredients to cooled pasta; gently toss to coat.
3. Season with salt and pepper; store refrigerated. Serve chilled.

SERVINGS

Entire recipe yield = 2 unrestricted + 4 C. veggies + 4 tsp. oil (portion in vinaigrette)
½ recipe yield = 1 unrestricted + 2 C. veggies + 2 tsp. oil (portion in vinaigrette)

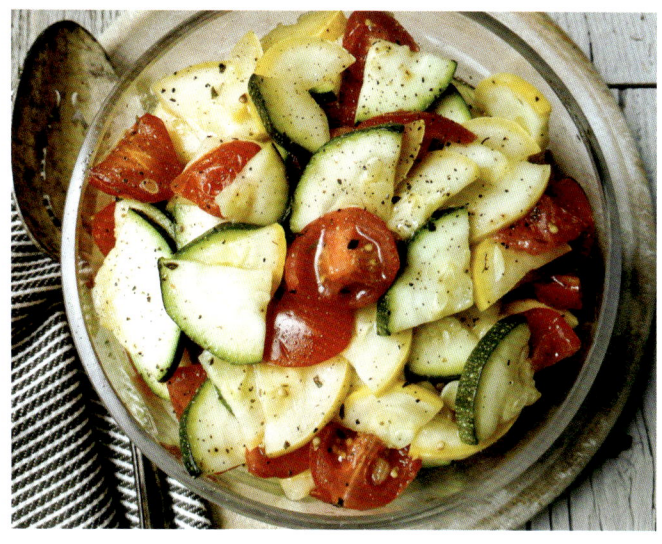

Summer Squash Salad

INGREDIENTS (DRESSING)
¼ C. apple cider vinegar
3 T. olive oil
2 T. sugar free sweetener, granular
½ tsp. dried basil
¼ tsp. dried thyme leaves
¼ tsp. garlic powder
Pinch of sea salt & black pepper

INGREDIENTS (SALAD)
2 C. sliced and quartered zucchini squash
2 C. sliced and quartered yellow summer squash
1 large bowl ice water
1 C. quartered cherry or grape tomatoes

DIRECTIONS
1. In a small bowl, whisk together dressing ingredients; set aside.
2. Place a steamer basket in a large saucepan or Dutch oven. Add 1 inch water and heat to a low boil. Add squash to basket, cover, and steam squash over medium high heat 1-2 minutes or until tender crisp (the squash should be par-cooked, do not cook until tender.)
3. Immediately transfer squash into ice water. Cool squash 2 minutes; drain.
4. Place squash and tomatoes in a large clean bowl; pour dressing over the top and fold to coat.
5. Cover and refrigerate; serve chilled.

SERVINGS
Entire recipe yield = 5 C. veggies + 3 T. oil
⅕ recipe yield = 1 C. veggies + 1 ¾ tsp. oil

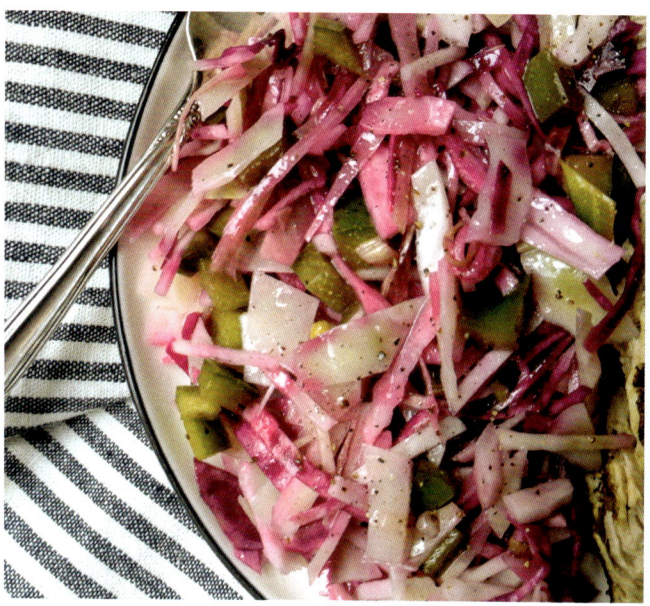

Sweet & Sour Chop Slaw

INGREDIENTS (SLAW)
3 C. chopped green cabbage
1 ¾ C. chopped red cabbage
1 C. chopped green pepper
¼ C. chopped green onion

INGREDIENTS (SWEET & SOUR DRESSING)
½ C. sugar free sweetener, granular
½ C. apple cider vinegar
¼ C. olive oil
1 tsp. ground mustard
½ tsp. celery seed
Salt and pepper, to taste

DIRECTIONS
1. Toss slaw ingredients in a large mixing bowl.
2. Add all dressing ingredients to a medium mixing bowl; whisk to mix.
3. Pour dressing over slaw and toss to coat. Allow flavors to meld together by refrigerating 3 hours before serving; toss occasionally to coat during marinating.
4. Cover and store refrigerated; serve chilled.

SERVINGS
Entire recipe yield = 6 C. slaw + 4 T. oil
⅙ recipe yield = 1 C. veggies + 2 tsp. oil

TIP: This slaw is excellent served as a side and perfectly complements any pork recipes.

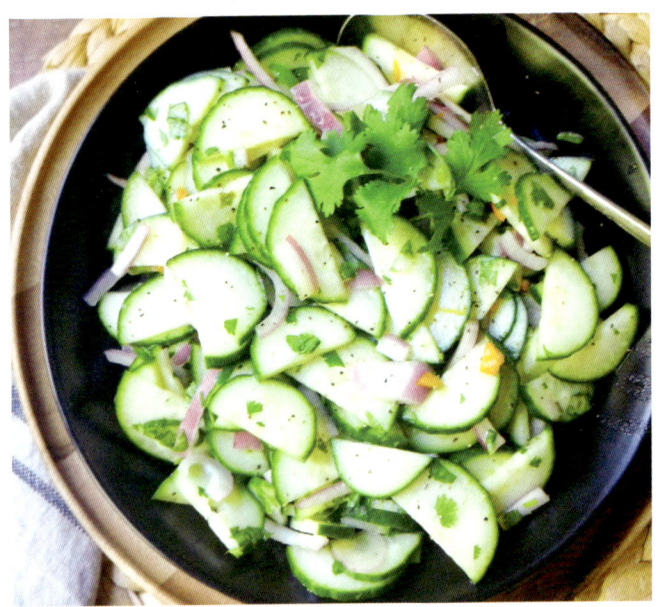

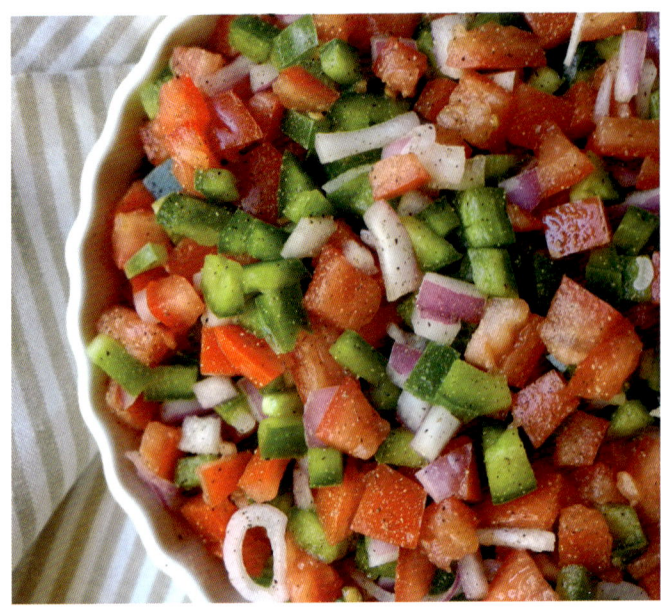

Thai Cucumber Salad

INGREDIENTS (DRESSING)
½ C. + 1 tsp. white vinegar
½ C. sugar free sweetener, granular
½ tsp. salt
2 T. Walden Farms peanut butter

INGREDIENTS (SALAD)
2 English cucumbers (unpeeled)
2 serrano peppers (seeded, finely chopped)
½ medium red onion, thinly sliced
¼ C. chopped fresh cilantro

DIRECTIONS
1. In a medium mixing bowl, whisk dressing ingredients. Add dressing to a small saucepan and heat on medium just until mixture starts to steam, stirring frequently. Remove from heat and transfer to a bowl. Refrigerate until cool.
2. Meanwhile, cut ends off cucumbers and slice lengthwise, then thinly slice crosswise into half-moons.
3. Place all salad ingredients in a bowl. Pour chilled dressing over salad; gently toss. Store refrigerated.

SERVINGS
Entire recipe yield = 5 C. veggies (approximately) – measure amount desired; for example: 1 C. salad = 1 C. veggies

Tomato Bell Pepper Salad

INGREDIENTS (DRESSING)
2 T. apple cider vinegar
1 T. sugar free sweetener, granular
½ tsp. fine sea salt
⅛ tsp. black pepper

INGREDIENTS (SALAD)
2 C. chopped Roma tomatoes (pulp and seeds removed)
1 C. chopped green bell pepper
½ C. chopped red onion
½ C. thinly sliced celery

DIRECTIONS
1. Add all dressing ingredients to a small bowl; whisk to blend.
2. Place all salad ingredients in a large mixing bowl.
3. Pour dressing over salad; fold to coat.
4. Store in refrigerator; fold to coat before serving. Serve with a slotted spoon.

SERVINGS
Entire recipe yield = 4 C. veggies
½ recipe yield = 2 C. veggies

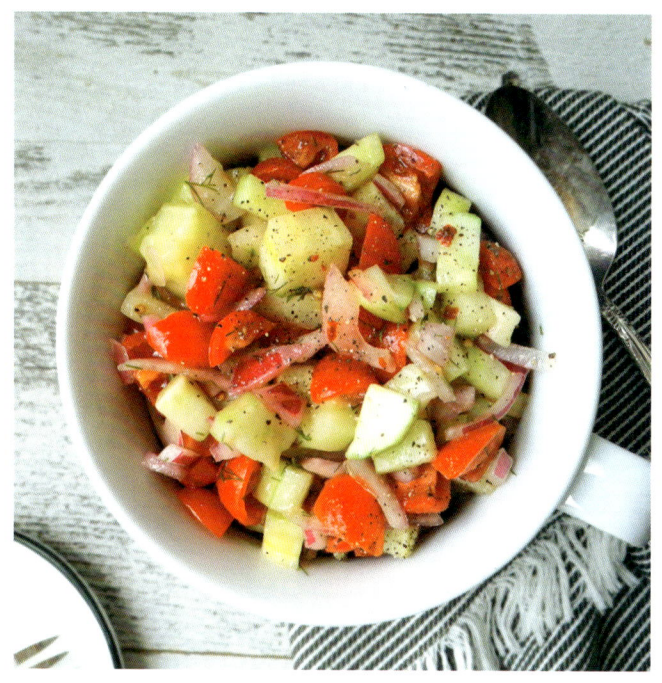
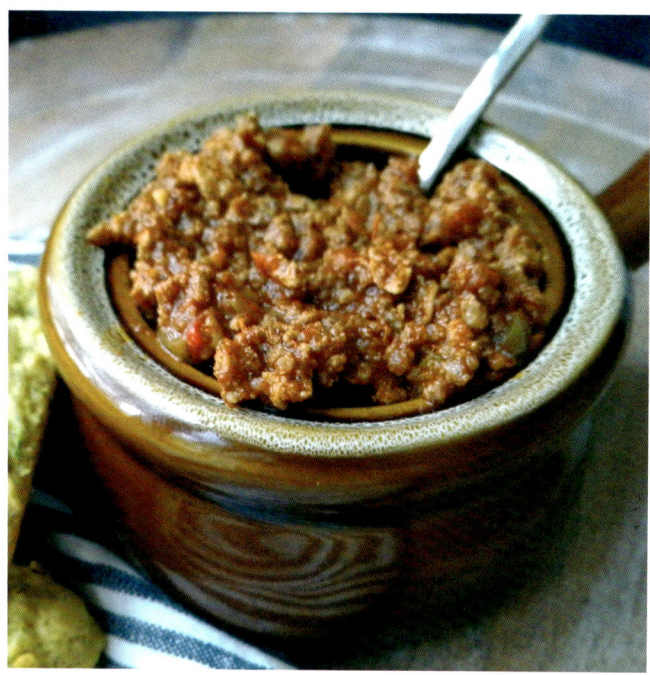

Zesty Cucumber Salad

INGREDIENTS

3 T. apple cider vinegar
2 T. olive oil
1 tsp. sugar free sweetener, granular
2 English cucumbers, peeled and diced
10 oz. grape tomatoes, quartered
½ medium chopped yellow or red onion
1 T. chopped fresh dill or cilantro
½ tsp. crushed red pepper flakes
Salt & pepper, to taste

DIRECTIONS

1. In a large bowl, whisk vinegar, oil, and sweetener until mixed.
2. Add remaining ingredients. Fold to coat; marinate 20 minutes before serving.
3. Cover and store in fridge.

SERVINGS

Entire recipe yield = 7 C. veggies + 2 T. oil
½ recipe yield = 1 C. veggies + ¾ tsp. oil

Chili Con Carne

INGREDIENTS

2 T. olive oil
1 C. sliced fresh mushrooms
1 C. diced green bell pepper
3 tsp. minced garlic
36 oz. lean ground beef, turkey, or chicken
28 oz. can crushed tomatoes
7 oz. can mild green chiles
3 T. ground cumin
1 ½ T. chili powder
1 tsp. salt
¼ tsp. black pepper

DIRECTIONS

1. Heat oil in a Dutch oven or soup pot on medium heat; add mushrooms, green pepper, and garlic. Stir fry until lightly browned. Transfer mixture to a bowl; set aside.
2. Add ground beef to hot pot; brown over medium heat.
3. Transfer mushroom mixture back into pot along with remaining ingredients; stir to mix.
4. Reduce heat; cover and simmer 15 minutes. Remove lid and simmer to desired thickness of sauce.

SERVINGS

Entire recipe yield = 36 oz. lean protein + 9 C. veggies + 2 T. oil
⅙ recipe yield = 6 oz. lean protein + 1 ½ C. veggies + 1 tsp. oil

Chinese Chicken Cabbage Soup

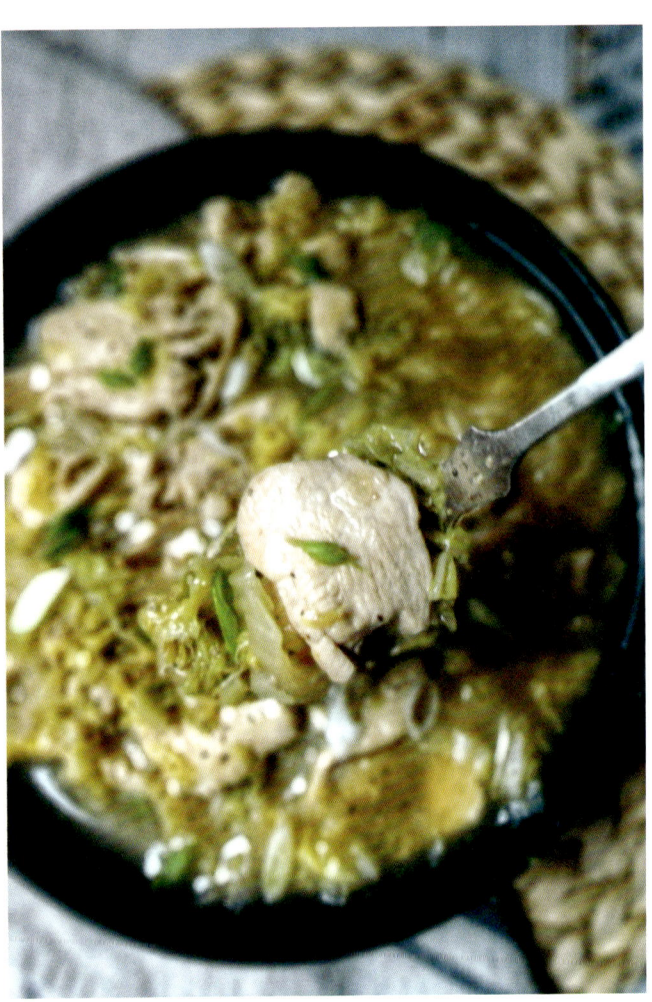

INGREDIENTS

24 oz. chicken breasts or thighs, boneless & skinless
Salt and pepper, to taste
1 T. + 1 tsp. olive oil
2 T. soy sauce
1 tsp. minced garlic
1 tsp. minced fresh ginger
¼ tsp. red pepper flakes
4 C. chicken broth
8 C. thinly sliced Chinese (napa) cabbage
Chopped green onions, optional (for topping)

DIRECTIONS

1. Slice chicken into thin, bite size strips; season with salt and pepper.
2. In a Dutch oven or soup pot, heat oil over medium/medium high heat. When oil is hot, add chicken. Cook 7-9 minutes or until lightly browned, stirring occasionally.
3. Add soy sauce, garlic, ginger, and red pepper flakes. Stir fry one minute to coat chicken.
4. Add chicken broth and cabbage to pot; stir. Bring to a low boil; reduce heat and simmer 10 minutes. Taste and adjust seasonings, if necessary.
5. Serve topped with green onions, if desired.

SERVINGS

Entire recipe yield = 24 oz. lean protein + 8 C. veggies + 4 tsp. oil
¼ recipe yield = 6 oz. lean protein + 2 C. veggies + 1 tsp. oil

Creamy Cauliflower & Red Pepper Soup

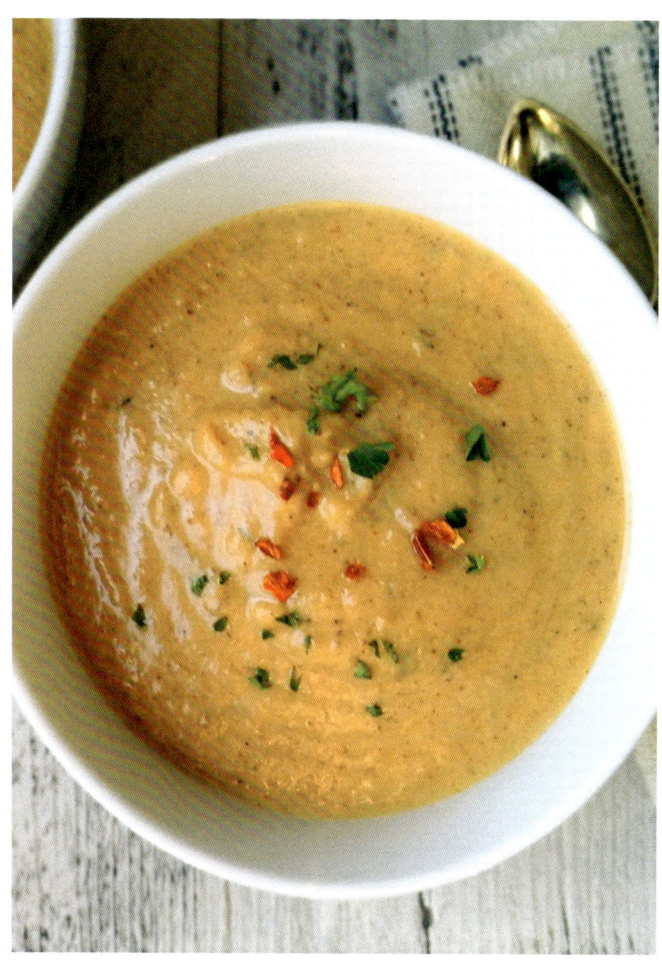

INGREDIENTS

6 C. cauliflower florets (cut in bite size pieces)
2 C. red bell pepper (cut in bite size pieces)
2 T. olive oil
1 tsp. garlic powder
1 tsp. salt
½ tsp. pepper
3 ½ C. chicken broth
1 T. dried minced onion
1 tsp. smoked paprika
½ tsp. dried thyme
½ C. half and half cream

DIRECTIONS

1. Preheat oven to 425°F degrees.
2. Place cauliflower florets, red pepper and oil in a large resealable plastic bag. Seal bag and shake gently to coat veggies with oil.
3. Spread veggies evenly on a rimmed baking sheet. Sprinkle with garlic powder, salt and pepper.
4. Place baking sheet on lower shelf of oven and roast 20-25 minutes. Turn veggies over and roast an additional 15 minutes.
5. Place roasted veggies in a large saucepan; add chicken broth, dried minced onion, paprika and thyme. Stir.
6. Bring to a low boil and reduce heat to medium low; simmer 10 minutes.
7. Using an immersion blender, blend until smooth. Stir in half and half cream and heat through. Adjust seasonings to taste, if necessary.

SERVINGS

Entire recipe yield = 8 C. veggies + 2 T. oil + ½ C. (4 oz.) half and half cream
¼ recipe yield = 2 C. veggies + 1 ½ tsp. oil + 2 T. (1 oz.) half and half cream

TIP: If you do not have an immersion blender, you may use a standard blender or food processor. Cool soup before blending as the heat can blow the top off small appliances.

Greek Chicken Soup

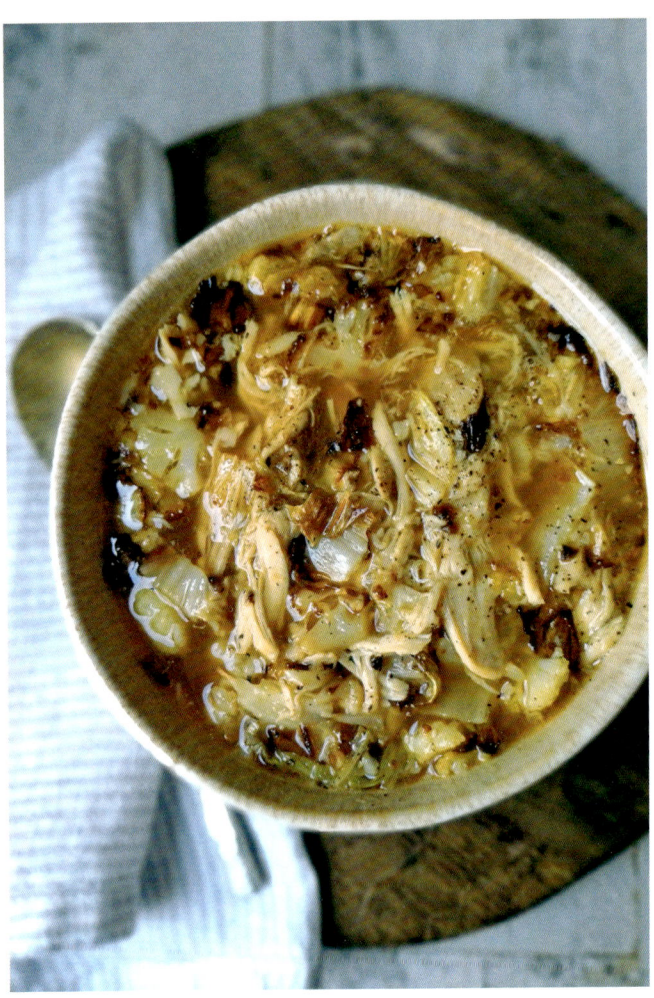

INGREDIENTS

2 C. cauliflower florets, cut in bite size pieces
2 C. thinly sliced cabbage
2 tsp. olive oil
Salt and pepper, to taste
2 – 6 oz. chicken breasts, skinless & boneless
2 C. chicken broth
1 T. Greek seasoning, pg. 141

DIRECTIONS

1. Preheat oven to 425˚ F degrees.
2. Toss cauliflower and cabbage with olive oil, salt, and pepper. Place on a rimmed baking sheet; spread evenly. Roast approximately 20 minutes or until lightly browned, turning once during roasting.
3. Meanwhile, add chicken breasts, chicken broth, and Greek seasoning to a Dutch oven or soup pot. Bring to a low boil; reduce heat and simmer 15 minutes or until chicken is cooked through.
4. Remove chicken and shred using two forks; add back to pot. Add roasted veggies to pot; simmer 5 minutes. Add more chicken broth if necessary.

SERVINGS

Entire recipe yield = 12 oz. lean protein + 4 C. veggies
½ recipe yield = 6 oz. lean protein + 2 C. veggies

Hamburger Soup

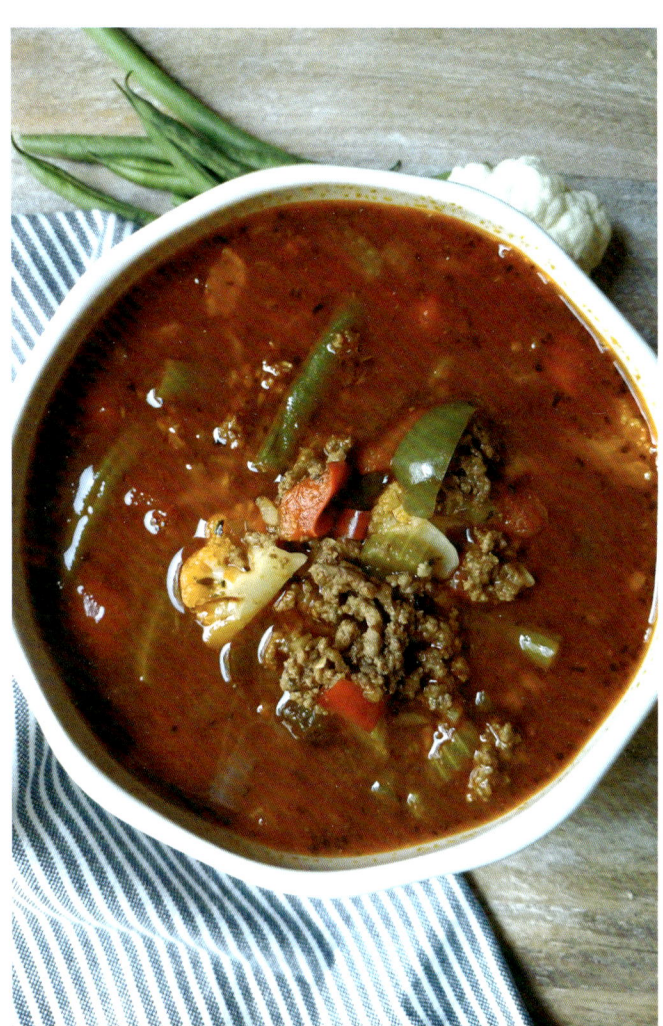

INGREDIENTS

1 T. + 2 tsp. olive oil
1 C. diced celery
½ C. diced red bell pepper
½ C. diced green bell pepper
1 lb. 14 oz. lean ground beef
1 ½ tsp. minced garlic
1 T. Italian seasoning
2 tsp. sea salt
½ tsp. black pepper
8 C. beef broth
1 tsp. garlic powder
1 tsp. smoked paprika
2 C. cauliflower florets (cut in bite size pieces)
2 C. green beans (cut in 1 ½ inch pieces)
14.5 oz. can petite diced tomatoes (undrained)
¼ C. tomato paste

DIRECTIONS

1. Heat olive oil over medium heat in a large Dutch oven or soup pot. Add celery and bell peppers. Sauté until fork tender (about 13-15 minutes), stirring often. Remove from heat and transfer veggies to a plate.

2. To the same stock pot, add ground beef, minced garlic, Italian seasoning, salt, and pepper. Brown ground beef over medium/medium high heat; stir to break up meat.

3. Add all remaining ingredients to the pot (including celery and peppers); stir. Bring to a low boil, reduce heat and simmer 35-40 minutes, uncovered.

SERVINGS

Entire recipe yield = 30 oz. lean protein + 10 C. veggies + 5 tsp. oil
⅕ recipe yield = 6 oz. lean protein + 2 C. veggies + 1 tsp. oil

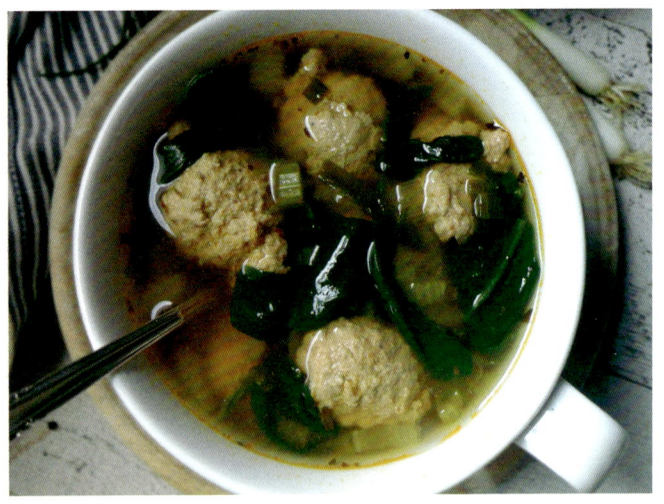
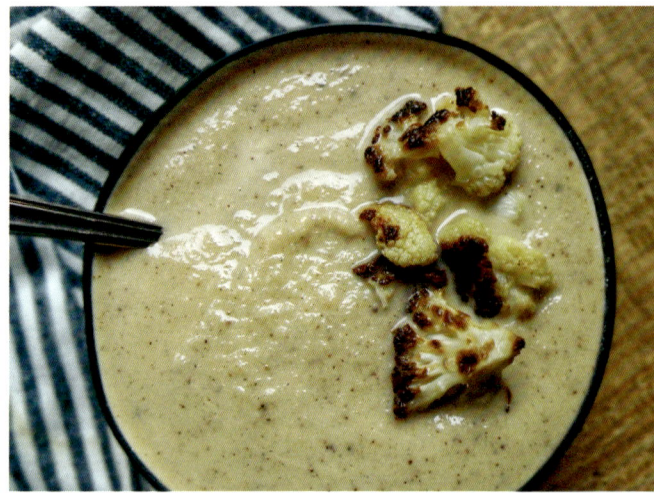

Italian Wedding Soup

INGREDIENTS (MEATBALLS)
18 oz. lean ground chicken or turkey
⅓ C. liquid egg whites
1 T. Sausage Seasoning, pg. 147

INGREDIENTS (SOUP)
8 C. chicken broth
1 tsp. dried basil leaves
2 tsp. garlic powder
1 tsp. kosher salt
¼ tsp. black pepper
1 ½ C. chopped celery
½ C. chopped green onion
4 C. fresh spinach leaves, destemmed

DIRECTIONS
1. In a large bowl, mix meatball ingredients until combined. Refrigerate 1 hour.
2. Form chilled mixture into 1 ½ inch meatballs using a small cookie dough scoop (or roll with hands to that size). Set aside.
3. In a Dutch oven or soup pot, combine broth and seasonings. Bring to a boil over high heat. Drop meatballs into boiling soup; add celery and onions.
4. Reduce heat and simmer 25 minutes, uncovered. Stir occasionally.
5. Add fresh spinach and continue to cook 3-5 minutes or until wilted. Taste and season with additional salt and pepper, if necessary.

SERVINGS
Entire recipe yield = 18 oz. lean protein + 6 C. veggies
⅓ recipe yield = 6 oz. lean protein + 2 C. veggies

Roasted Cauliflower Soup

INGREDIENTS
21 oz. (6 C.) cauliflower florets (cut in bite size pieces)
2 T. olive oil
¾ tsp. garlic powder
1 tsp. ground cumin
3 C. chicken broth
3 oz. (6 T.) half and half cream
Salt and pepper, to taste

DIRECTIONS
1. Preheat oven to 400°F degrees.
2. Add cauliflower and olive oil to a large resealable bag; toss to coat.
3. Spread cauliflower out on a large, rimmed baking sheet; season with garlic powder and cumin.
4. Place baking sheet on bottom rack of oven and roast 20 minutes flipping cauliflower halfway through roasting time.
5. Add cauliflower and chicken broth to a medium saucepan. Heat to boiling; reduce heat and simmer 10 minutes.
6. Remove pan from heat and add half and half cream. Using a stick blender, blend mixture until creamy.
7. Season well with salt and pepper; stir, taste, and adjust if necessary.

SERVINGS
Entire recipe yield = 6 C. veggies + 2 T. oil + 3 oz. half and half cream
⅓ recipe yield = 2 C. veggies + 2 tsp. oil + 1 oz. half and half cream

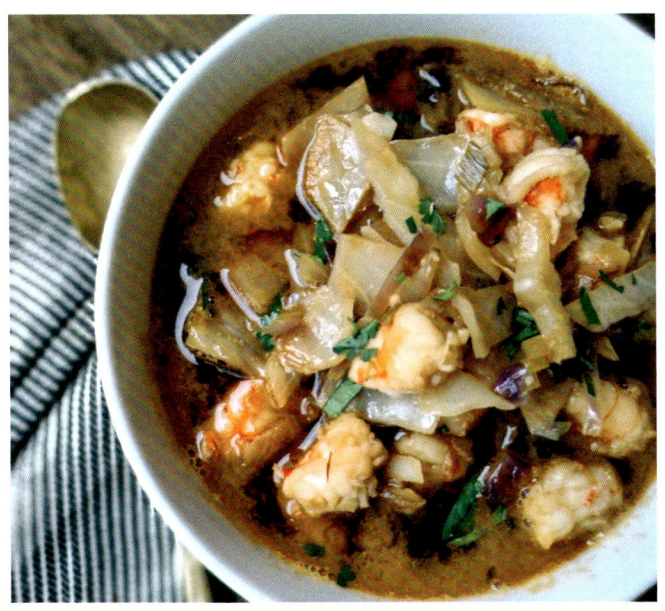

Shrimp Egg Roll Soup

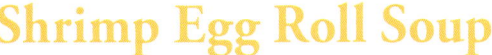

INGREDIENTS

12 oz. large cooked shrimp, deveined and tail off
¼ c. soy sauce
2 tsp. chili garlic sauce
2 tsp. white vinegar
½ tsp. ground ginger
1 tsp. sugar free sweetener, granular
1 T. + 1 tsp. toasted sesame oil
3 ½ C. shredded green or red cabbage
½ C. chopped green onion
Salt and pepper, to taste
3 C. chicken broth

DIRECTIONS

1. Cut shrimp in bite size pieces; set aside.
2. In a small bowl, combine soy sauce, chili garlic sauce, vinegar, ground ginger, and sweetener. Stir to mix; set aside.
3. Heat oil in a Dutch oven or soup pot over medium/medium high heat. Add cabbage and green onion; season with salt and pepper. Stir fry until cabbage is slightly wilted and tender.
4. Add soy sauce mixture to pot and give it a quick stir to coat the cabbage.
5. Stir in chicken broth and bring to a low boil; reduce heat and simmer 5 minutes. Add shrimp and heat through.

SERVINGS

Entire recipe yield = 12 oz. lean protein + 4 C. veggies
½ recipe yield = 6 oz. lean protein + 2 C. veggies

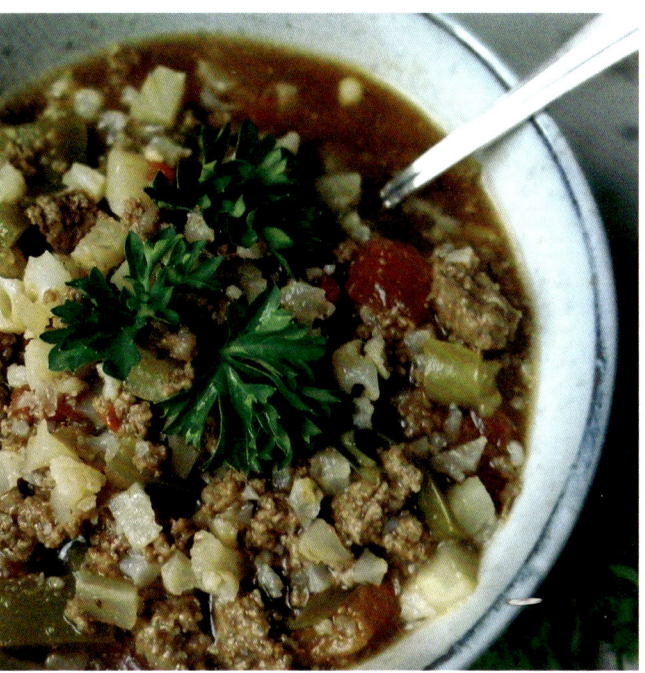

Stuffed Pepper Soup

INGREDIENTS

18 oz. lean ground beef
½ tsp. salt
¼ tsp. black pepper
1 T. dried minced onion
1 tsp. minced garlic
2 C. chopped green pepper
10 oz. can Rotel® tomatoes and green chiles
32 oz. beef broth
2 tsp. soy sauce
1 tsp. apple cider vinegar
¼ tsp. red pepper flakes
3 C. cauliflower florets, coarsely chopped

DIRECTIONS

1. To a Dutch oven or soup pot, add ground beef, salt, pepper, dried minced onion and garlic. Brown beef over medium heat; stir to break up meat.
2. Add remaining ingredients (except cauliflower.) Bring to a boil, reduce heat and simmer 25 minutes. Stir occasionally.
3. Add cauliflower; simmer an additional 5-7 minutes or until cauliflower is tender. Season with additional salt and pepper, if desired.

SERVINGS

Entire recipe yield = 18 oz. lean protein + 6 C. veggies
⅓ recipe yield = 6 oz. lean protein + 2 C. veggies

Tortilla Soup

This recipe submitted by Sarah Hansel

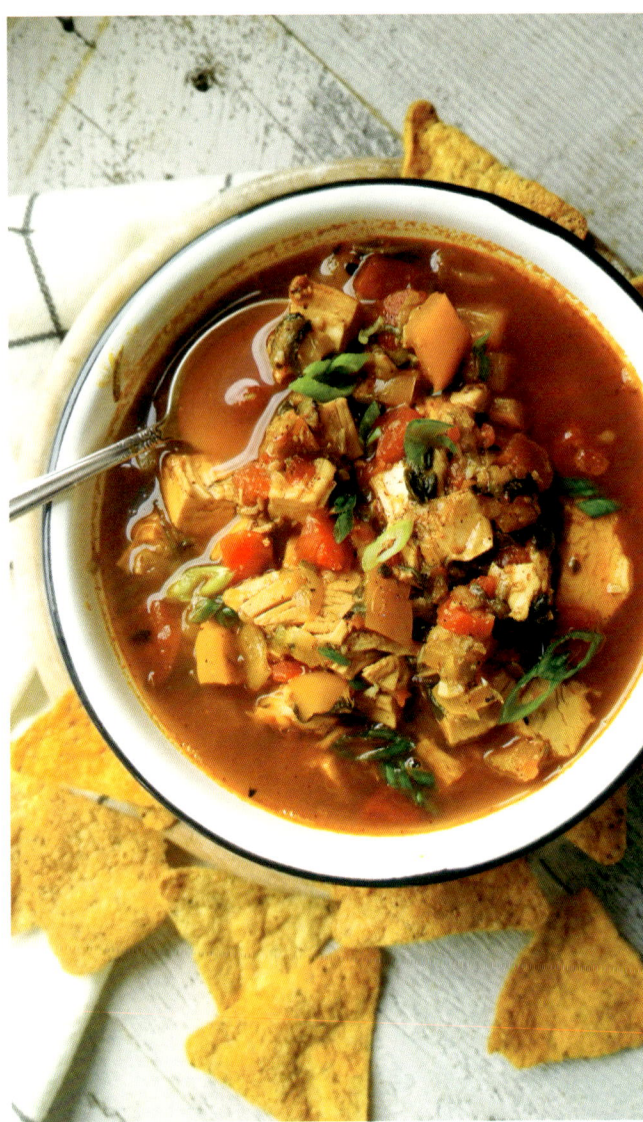

INGREDIENTS

1 T. olive oil
1 C. diced bell pepper (yellow, orange, or red)
1 C. shredded zucchini
1 C. kale or spinach leaves, destemmed and chopped
½ C. finely chopped green onion
1 T. diced jalapeno pepper, seeded (optional)
1 ½ tsp. minced garlic
1 - 10 oz. can Rotel® tomatoes and green chilies
4 C. chicken broth
13.5 oz. cooked and diced chicken breast
2 T. soy sauce
1 T. chili powder
2 tsp. cumin
Salt and pepper, to taste

DIRECTIONS

1. In a Dutch oven or soup pot, heat oil over medium heat. When oil is hot, add bell pepper, zucchini, kale, onion, jalapeno, and garlic. Stir fry until peppers soften.
2. Add remaining ingredients.
3. Reduce heat and simmer 20 minutes.

SERVINGS

Entire recipe yield = 18 oz. lean protein + 6 C. veggies + 1 T. oil
⅓ recipe yield = 6 oz. lean protein + 2 C. veggies + 1 tsp. oil

TIPS: In the serving size, 18 oz. lean protein (raw) = 13.5 oz. lean protein (cooked). If you are unable to find the Rotel® tomatoes and chilies in the same can, use 1 ¼ C. chopped tomatoes + ¼ C. green chiles.

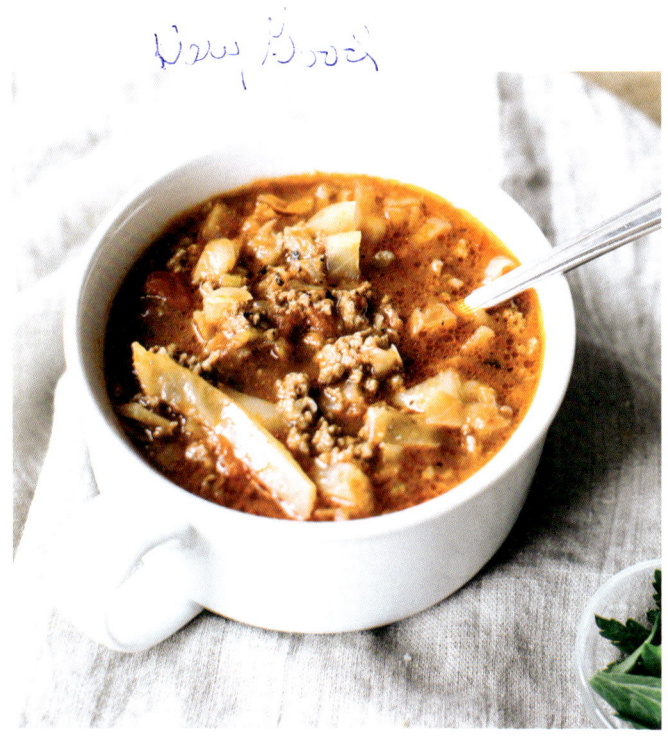

Navy Broth

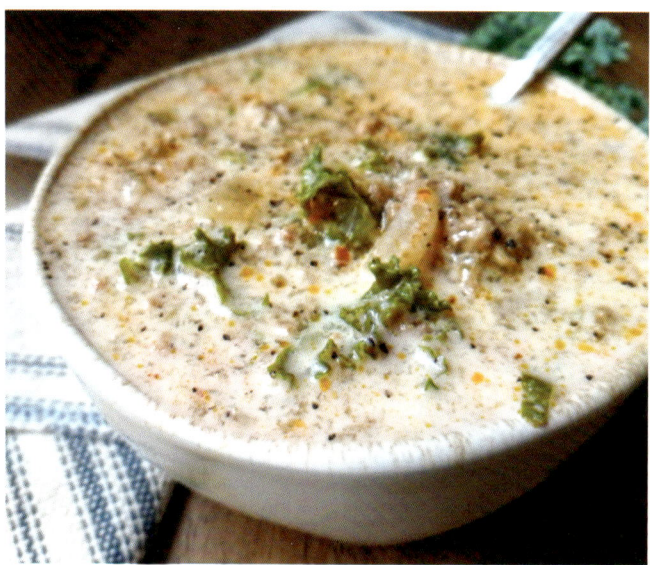

Zuppa Toscana

INGREDIENTS

1 1/2 lbs. lean ground pork or turkey
2 T. Sausage Seasoning, pg. 147
⅓ C. dried minced onions
6 ½ C. chicken broth, divided
1 C. cauliflower florets (cut in bite size pieces)
3 C. kale (destemmed and cut in bite size pieces)
2 C. diced radishes
3 oz. half and half cream
Salt and pepper, to taste

DIRECTIONS

1. Add pork, sausage seasoning and minced onion to a large skillet; brown over medium heat. Set aside.
2. Meanwhile, add 2 C. chicken broth to a medium saucepan; bring to a low boil. Add cauliflower florets; reduce heat and simmer until cauliflower is fork tender (approximately 15 minutes). Set aside to cool slightly.
3. Place remaining 4 ½ C. chicken broth, ground pork mixture, kale, and radishes into a Dutch oven or soup pot. Bring to a low boil; cover and reduce heat. Simmer 20 minutes.
4. Place the cauliflower (with broth) in a blender; puree. Add puree and half and half cream to the soup; stir and heat through. Season with salt and pepper.

SERVINGS

Entire recipe yield = 24 oz. lean protein + 6 C. veggies + 3 oz. half and half cream
¼ recipe yield = 6 oz. lean protein + 1 ½ C. veggies + 0.75 oz. half and half cream

Unstuffed Beef Cabbage Roll Soup

INGREDIENTS

1 ½ lbs. lean ground beef
2 T. dried minced onions
2 tsp. onion powder
4 ½ C. thinly sliced cabbage
2 (14.5 oz.) cans fire roasted diced tomatoes
1 tsp. minced garlic
2 tsp. Ideal Protein salt
1 tsp. black pepper
3 C. beef broth

DIRECTIONS

1. Heat a Dutch oven or soup pot over medium high heat. Add ground beef; brown. Halfway through browning, add minced onions and onion powder.
2. Add remaining ingredients and stir to mix.
3. Bring soup to a low boil. Cover and reduce heat; simmer 30 minutes. Additional beef broth may be added, if necessary.

SERVINGS

Entire recipe yield = 24 oz. lean protein + 8 C. veggies
¼ recipe yield = 6 oz. lean protein + 2 C. veggies

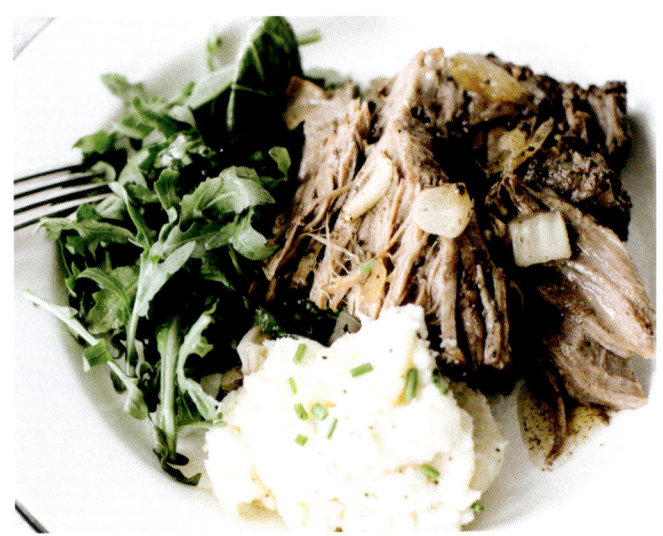 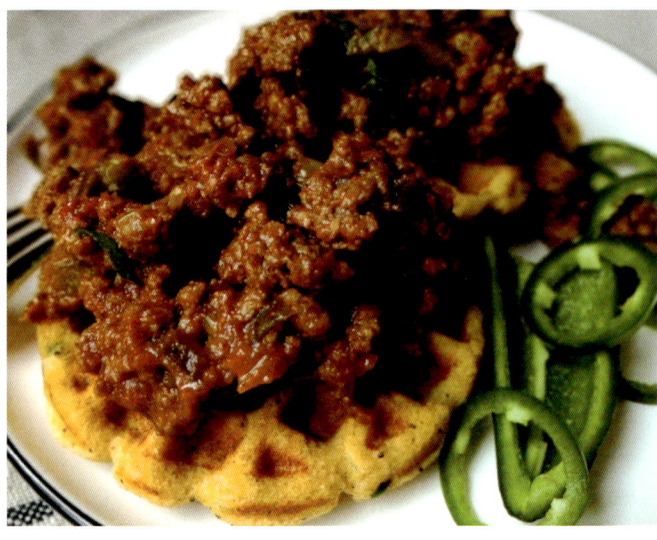

Balsamic Beef Roast

Slow cooker recipe

INGREDIENTS
3 lb. boneless chuck roast
1 T. kosher salt
1 tsp. black pepper
1 tsp. garlic powder
1 T. + 1 tsp. olive oil
½ C. Ideal Protein balsamic dressing
2 C. beef broth
2 T. dried minced onion
Chopped fresh yellow onion, optional (for topping)

DIRECTIONS
1. Season entire roast with salt, pepper, and garlic powder.
2. Heat oil in a large skillet over medium/medium high heat. Add roast and brown 3-4 minutes each side.
3. Place roast in slow cooker; add remaining ingredients around roast.
4. Cover and cook on low 8 hours, or on high 6 hours. Serve drizzled with juices.

SERVINGS
Entire recipe yield = 48 oz. lean protein + ½ C. veggies (dried minced onion) + 4 tsp. oil
⅛ recipe yield = 6 oz. lean protein + 1 T. veggies (dried minced onion) + ½ tsp. oil

BBQ Sloppy Joes

INGREDIENTS
18 oz. ground beef, chicken, or turkey
2 tsp. onion powder
1 tsp. salt
½ C. chopped green onion
½ C. chopped green bell pepper
1 C. canned diced tomatoes, undrained
½ C. Sassy BBQ Sauce, pg. 147
1 tsp. lemon juice
1 tsp. white vinegar
1 tsp. yellow mustard

DIRECTIONS
1. To a large skillet, add ground beef, onion powder and salt. Brown over medium heat; halfway through browning add green onion and bell pepper.
2. Meanwhile, add remaining ingredients to a blender; blend until smooth.
3. Add blender sauce mixture to the browned meat mixture. Heat till bubbling; reduce heat and simmer uncovered 20-25 minutes or until thickened. Stir occasionally while simmering.

SERVINGS
Entire recipe yield = 18 oz. lean protein + 3 C. veggies (includes tomato count in BBQ sauce)
⅓ recipe yield = 6 oz. lean protein + 1 C. veggies (includes tomato count in BBQ sauce)

Beef & Broccoli

Better than takeout

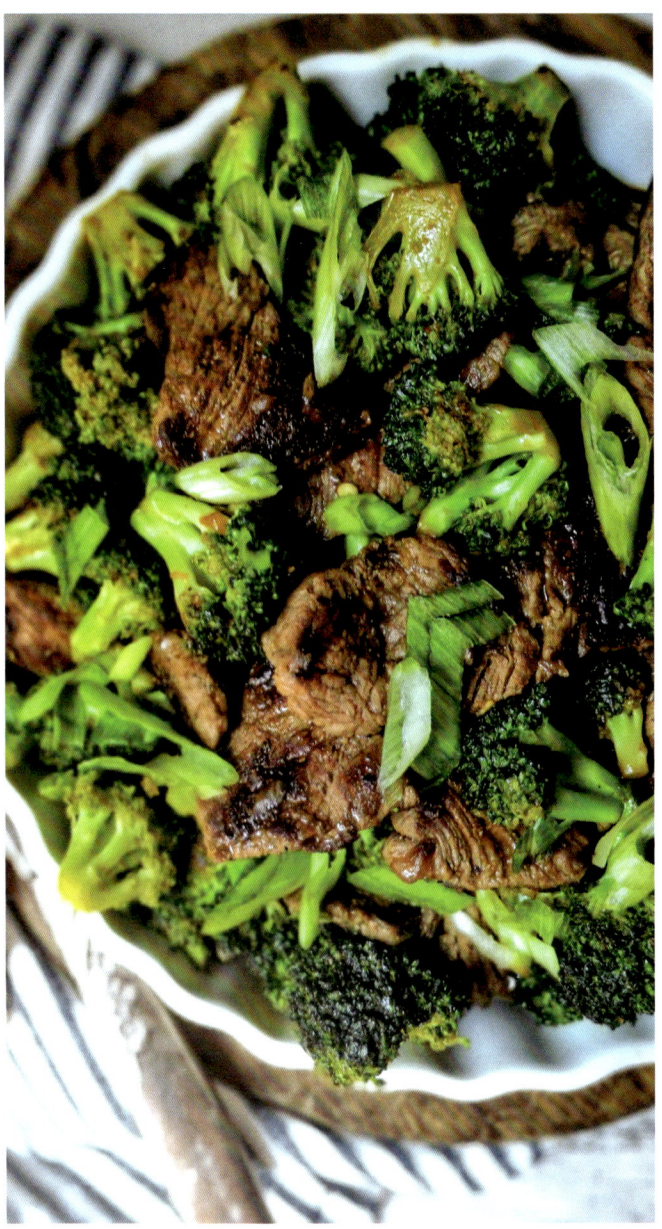

INGREDIENTS (SAUCE)

¼ C. soy sauce
1 T. Ideal Protein maple syrup
1 T. Ideal Protein honey Dijon dressing
1 tsp. minced ginger
½ tsp. garlic powder
¼ tsp. red pepper flakes

INGREDIENTS (BEEF & BROCCOLI)

4 tsp. olive oil, divided
12 oz. sliced flank, top sirloin, or chuck steak
    (¼" x 3" slices cut across grain)
¼ tsp. black pepper
4 C. fresh broccoli florets
¼ C. water
Sliced green onion, for topping (optional)

DIRECTIONS

1. Add sauce ingredients to a small bowl; stir to combine. Set aside.
2. Brush the bottom of a large skillet with 2 tsp. oil; heat over medium/medium high heat.
3. When oil is hot, add beef strips and season with black pepper. Stir fry until beef is lightly browned and cooked medium well.
4. Transfer beef to a plate; cover to keep warm. Using a paper towel, wipe frying pan clean (doesn't need to be perfect).
5. Brush the bottom of the skillet with the remaining 2 tsp. oil; heat over medium/medium high heat. When oil is hot, add broccoli and stir to coat with oil. Add water and stir fry 3 minutes or until broccoli is tender crisp.
6. Return beef to pan; drizzle with sauce. Stir to heat through.
7. Serve topped with green onion, if desired.

SERVINGS

Entire recipe yield = 12 oz. lean protein + 4 C. veggies + 4 tsp. oil
½ recipe yield = 6 oz. lean protein + 2 C. veggies + 2 tsp. oil

Beefy Mushroom Salisbury Steak

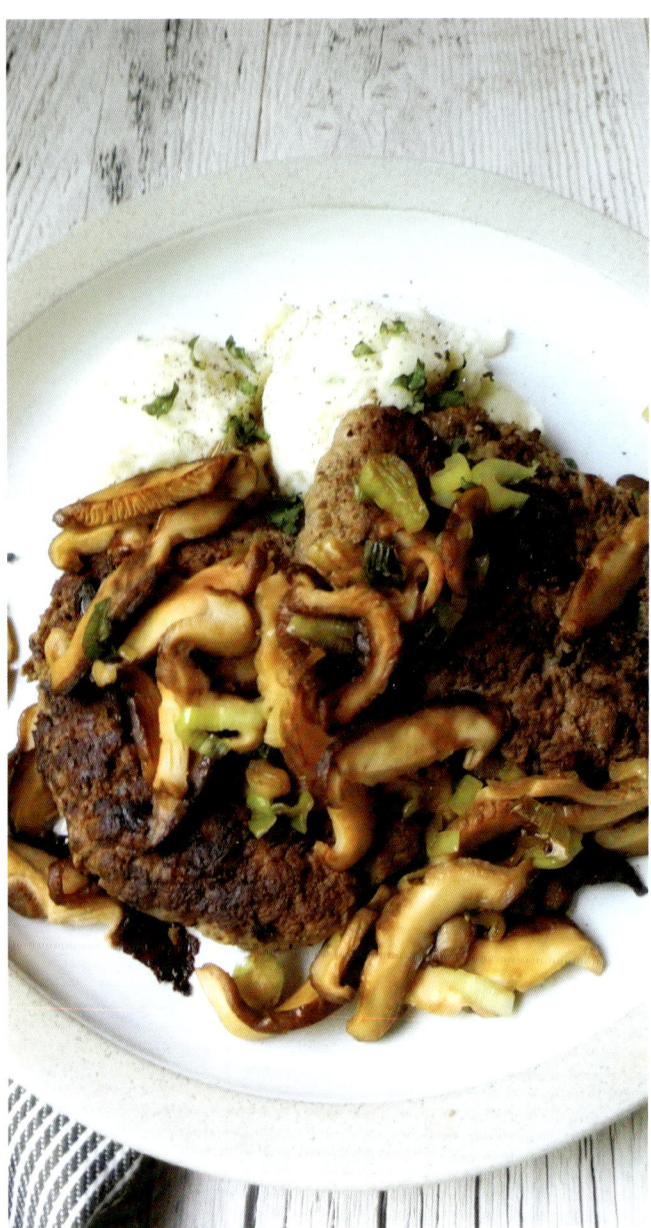

INGREDIENTS (SALISBURY STEAK)
18 oz. lean ground beef
3 T. liquid egg whites
½ tsp. soy sauce
1 T. Dijon mustard
2 T. Heinz No Sugar Added Ketchup

INGREDIENTS (MUSHROOMS)
1 T. olive oil
2 ¼ C. sliced fresh mushrooms (any variety)
½ C. sliced green onion
2 T. soy sauce
1 T. water

DIRECTIONS
1. To a large bowl, add all ingredients for the Salisbury steak; mix with hands. Form 4 equal patties; set aside.
2. Heat oil in a large skillet over medium heat. When oil is hot, add remaining mushroom ingredients. Stir fry until mushrooms are lightly browned and green onions are slightly limp. Transfer to a plate; cover to keep warm.
3. In same skillet over medium heat, cook Salisbury steaks about 3-4 minutes each side or until done.
4. Plate Salisbury steaks; top with mushroom mixture.

SERVINGS
Entire recipe yield = 18 oz. lean protein + 3 C. veggies (includes ketchup) + 1 T. oil
⅓ recipe yield = 6 oz. lean protein + 1 C. veggies (includes ketchup) + 1 tsp. oil

TIP: Delicious served over Cauliflower Mash, pg. 112.

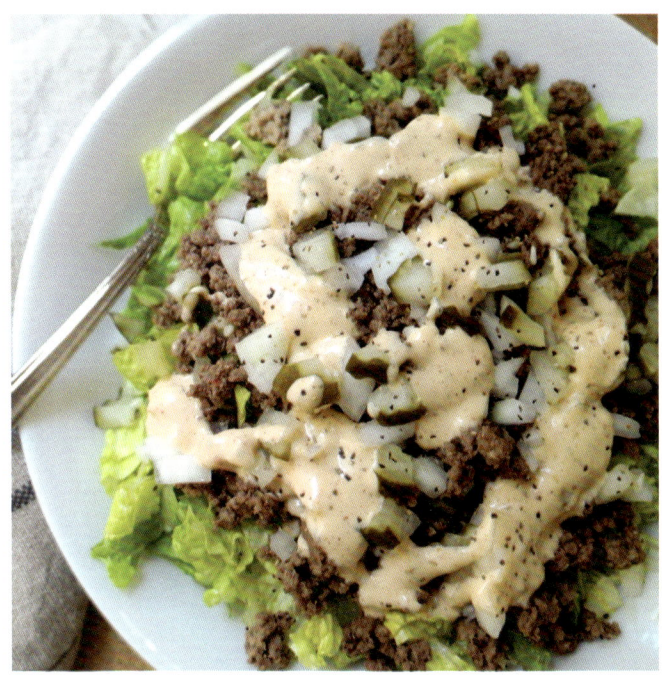

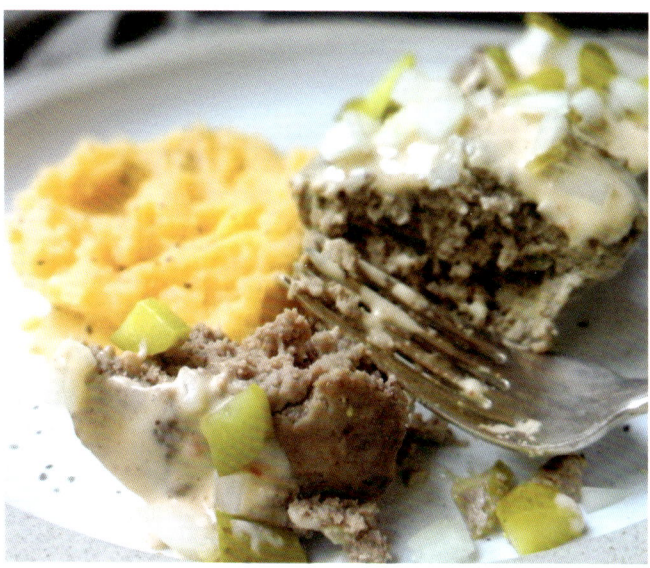

Big Mack in a Bowl

INGREDIENTS
6 oz. lean ground beef
Salt and pepper, to taste
Shredded lettuce, unlimited
¼ C. chopped yellow onion
¼ C. chopped dill pickles
2 T. Walden Farms Thousand Island dressing

DIRECTIONS
1. In a medium skillet, season the ground beef with salt and pepper, and brown over medium heat; stir to break up the meat.
2. Place desired amount of lettuce in a large salad bowl. Add ground beef, onion, and pickles.
3. Serve topped with dressing.

SERVINGS
Entire recipe yield = 6 oz. lean protein + ½ C. veggies (Lettuce is unlimited and is not in calculation.)

Big Mack Meatloaf Muffins

INGREDIENTS (MEATLOAF)
17 oz. lean ground beef
1 egg, lightly beaten
⅓ C. finely chopped pickles
1 T. Heinz No Sugar Added Ketchup
1 T. Dijon mustard
1 tsp. onion powder
½ tsp. Ideal Protein salt
¼ tsp. black pepper
Cooking spray

INGREDIENTS (TOPPINGS)
Walden Farms Thousand Island dressing, to taste
⅔ C. chopped yellow onions
Chopped pickles, optional

DIRECTIONS
1. Preheat oven to 425° F degrees.
2. Add all meatloaf ingredients to a large mixing bowl; mix with hands until combined. (Avoid over working the mixture.)
3. Press meat mixture into a sprayed muffin tin making 6 meatloaf muffins. Bake 18-20 minutes or until beef is cooked through.
4. Serve topped with Thousand Island dressing, onions, and additional chopped pickles, if desired.

SERVINGS
Entire recipe yield (6 meatloaf muffins) = 18 oz. lean protein + 1 C. veggies
⅓ recipe yield (2 meatloaf muffins) = 6 oz. lean protein + ⅓ C. veggies

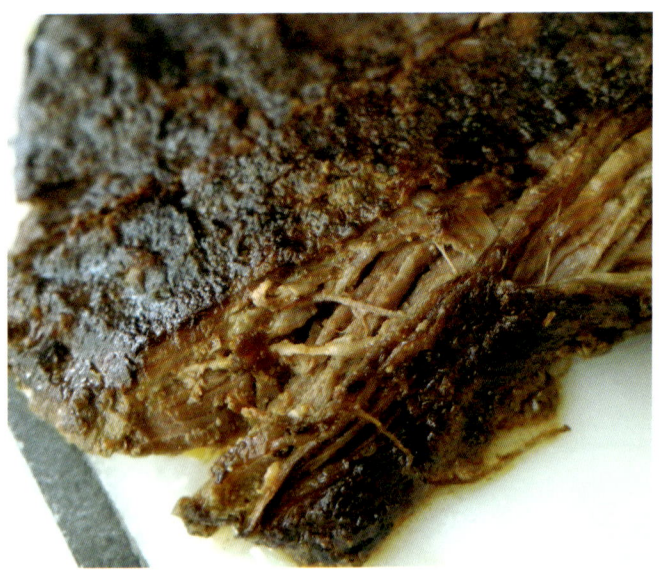

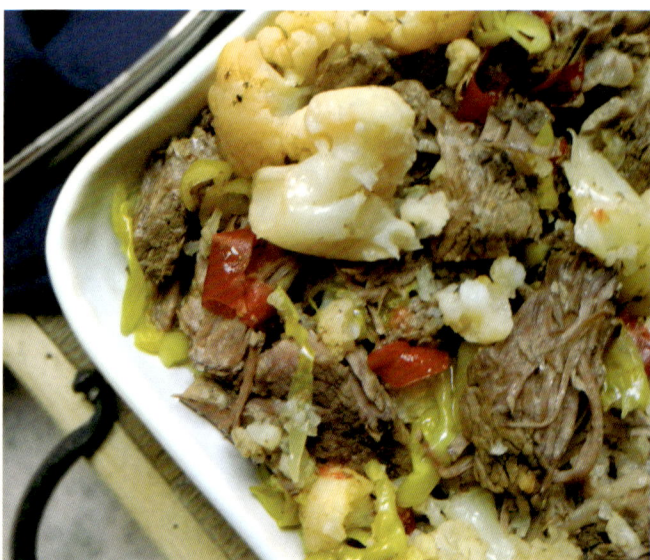

Carne Asada Skirt Steak
Slow cooker recipe

INGREDIENTS
1 ½ lbs. skirt or flank steak
1 T. + 1 tsp. soy sauce
2 tsp. apple cider vinegar
2 T. olive oil
1 T. oregano
1 T. garlic powder
1 ½ tsp. ground cumin
1 ½ tsp. paprika
½ tsp. salt
¼ tsp. black pepper

DIRECTIONS
1. Add all ingredients to slow cooker except skirt steak. Using a rubber spatula, stir to mix.
2. Place skirt steak into slow cooker; using the spatula, spread mix on both sides of steak.
3. Cover and cook on low 8 hours. Cut steak across the grain to serve.

SERVINGS
Entire recipe yield = 24 oz. lean protein + 2 T. oil
¼ recipe yield = 6 oz. lean protein + 1 ½ tsp. oil

TIP: Try serving chopped Carne Asada in butter lettuce wraps topped with Pico de Gallo (pg. 145), Mock-amole (pg. 143), and fresh chopped cilantro; fold and eat like a taco. The Carne Asada is also delicious served over Cilantro Lime Cauliflower Rice (pg. 115).

Chicago-Style Italian Beef
Slow cooker recipe

INGREDIENTS
14 oz. beef broth
3 lb. boneless chuck roast
1 envelope zesty Italian salad dressing mix* (I use Good Seasons®)
1 – 16 oz. jar Dilled Cauliflower Flowerettes, drained (I use Mezzetta®)
1 C. jarred Pepperoncini Pepper Slices, drained (Mezzetta®)

DIRECTIONS
1. Place beef broth in a slow cooker.
2. Cut chuck roast into 8 large chunks and add to the slow cooker.
3. Sprinkle dressing mix over chuck roast.
4. Add cauliflower and pepperoncini slices to slow cooker.
5. Cook on high 5-6 hours or low 8-9 hours.
6. Shred with a fork and serve drizzled with juices.

SERVINGS
Entire recipe yield = 48 oz. lean protein + 3 C. veggies
⅛ recipe yield = 6 oz. lean protein + ¼ C. + 2 T. veggies

NOTE: *The dressing mix has a minute amount of sugar and has been carefully considered in this recipe. The seasoning adds a great amount of flavor; for each 6 oz. serving, seasoning adds less than <1 carb.

Coffee Crusted Beef Roast

Slow cooker and Instant Pot method included below

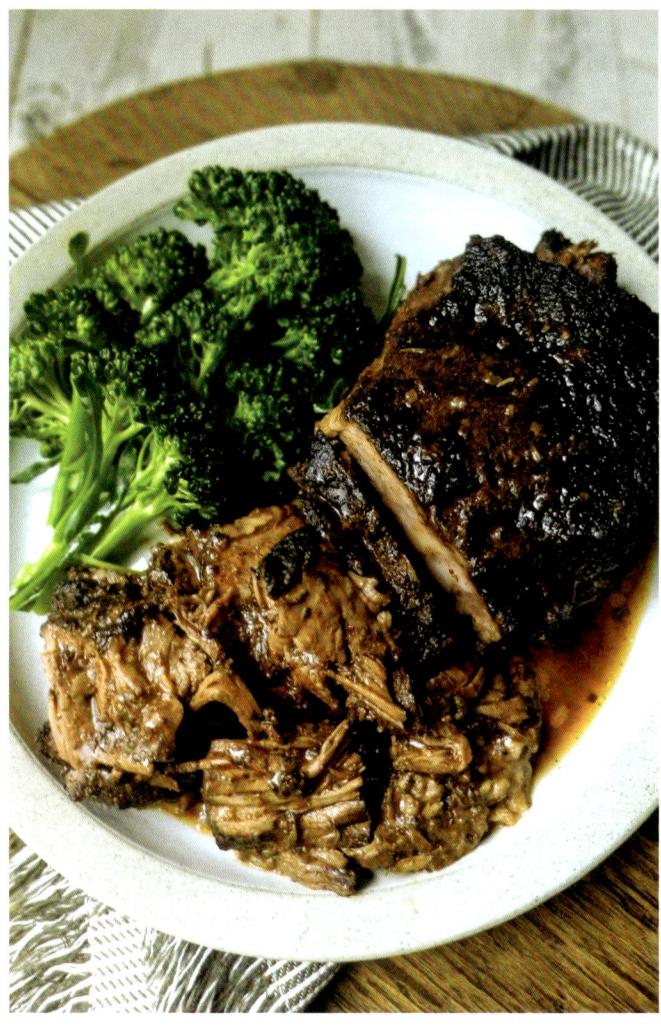

INGREDIENTS (SAUCE)
½ C. brewed decaf espresso or coffee
3 T. tomato paste
1 T. white vinegar
1 tsp. sugar substitute, granular
1 tsp. minced garlic
¼ tsp. black pepper

INGREDIENTS (ROAST)
3 lbs. chuck roast
Coffee Spice Rub, pg. 139 (use entire recipe)
2 T. olive oil

DIRECTIONS (INSTANT POT METHOD)
1. Prepare sauce by adding all ingredients to a bowl; lightly whisk until blended. Set aside.
2. Using both hands, massage (rub) the entire roast with the Coffee Spice Rub.
3. Place oil in instant pot and turn to sauté mode. When oil is hot, add roast and sear 18-20 minutes flipping roast once while searing. (This will form a crust on both sides of roast.)
4. Pour sauce over roast; cover and seal instant pot. Cook on high pressure 45 minutes; natural release for 20 minutes. Quick release and serve.

DIRECTIONS (SLOW COOKER)
1. Follow directions 1-2 above.
2. Add oil to a large skillet and heat over medium/ medium high heat. When oil is hot, add roast and sear 8-10 minutes flipping roast once while searing. (This will form a crust on both sides of roast.)
3. Place roast in slow cooker, pour sauce over roast. Cook on low 8 hours.

SERVINGS
Entire recipe yield = 48 oz. lean protein + 2 T. oil + 1 C. veggies (tomato paste)
⅛ recipe yield = 6 oz. lean protein + ¾ tsp. oil + 2 T. veggies (tomato paste)

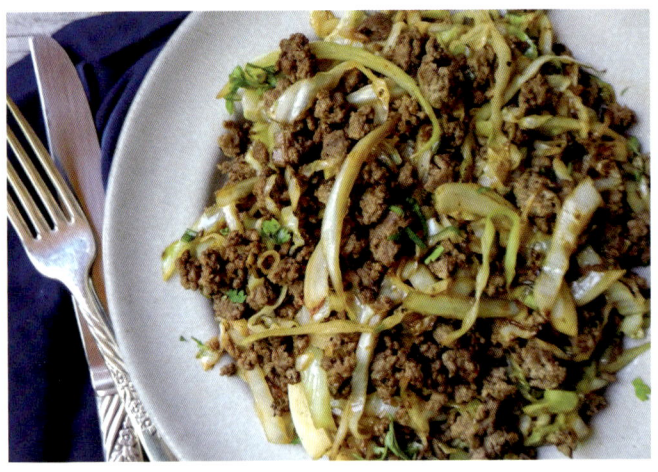

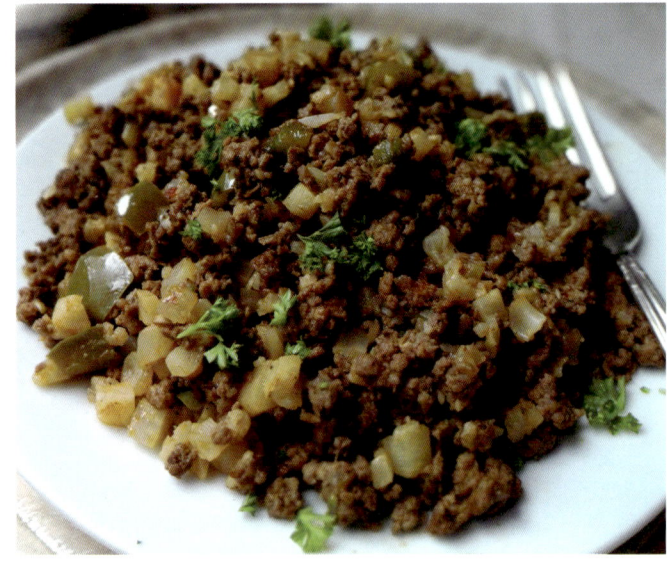

Crack Slaw

INGREDIENTS (SAUCE)
1 tsp. sugar free sweetener, granular
½ tsp. ground ginger
2 tsp. white vinegar
¼ C. soy sauce
1 tsp. garlic chili sauce (I use Sambal Oelek®)

INGREDIENTS (CRACK SLAW)
18 oz. lean ground beef, chicken, or turkey
Salt & pepper, to taste
2 T. olive oil
5 C. shredded cabbage
1 C. chopped green onion
2 tsp. minced garlic

DIRECTIONS
1. Add all sauce ingredients to a small bowl; stir to combine. Set aside.
2. In a large skillet, season the ground beef with salt and pepper. Brown over medium heat; stir to break up the meat.
3. Drain any fat and transfer beef to a bowl. Cover to keep warm; set aside.
4. In same skillet, heat oil over medium/medium high heat. When oil is hot, add cabbage, green onion, and garlic. Stir fry until cabbage is slightly wilted and tender.
5. Add the beef and sauce to the skillet. Stir to combine; heat through and serve.

SERVINGS
Entire recipe yield = 18 oz. lean protein + 6 C. veggies + 2 T. oil
⅓ recipe yield = 6 oz. lean protein + 2 C. veggies + 2 tsp. oil

Dirty Rice

INGREDIENTS
20 oz. frozen riced cauliflower
12 oz. lean ground beef
2 T. Sausage Seasoning, pg. 147
1 tsp. Cajun seasoning
¼ tsp. rubbed sage
1 T. + 1 tsp. olive oil
⅔ C. diced green pepper
½ C. diced celery
1 tsp. minced garlic
⅓ C. chopped green onion

DIRECTIONS
1. Cook riced cauliflower according to package directions; drain and set aside.
2. In a large skillet, season the ground beef with Sausage Seasoning, Cajun seasoning, and rubbed sage. Brown over medium heat; stir to break up the meat.
3. Transfer beef to a bowl; cover to keep warm.
4. Add oil to same skillet and heat over medium/medium high heat. Add green pepper, celery, and garlic; stir fry 4 minutes. Add green onion; stir fry an additional 4 minutes.
5. Add riced cauliflower and ground beef to skillet; fold to combine. Heat through and serve.

SERVINGS
Entire recipe yield = 12 oz. lean protein + 4 C. veggies + 4 tsp. oil
½ recipe = 6 oz. lean protein + 2 C. veggies + 2 tsp. oil

Fiesta Beef Nachos

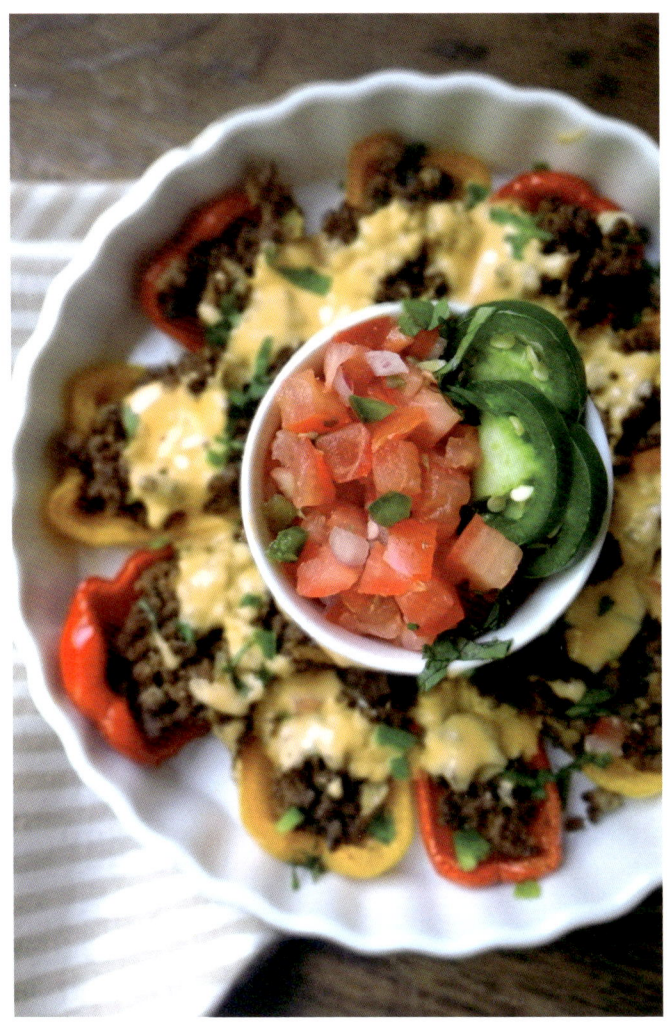

INGREDIENTS (NACHOS)
16 oz. lean ground beef
2 T. Taco Seasoning, pg. 149
1 tsp. Ideal Protein salt
1 ½ C. chopped fresh mushrooms (any variety)
½ C. chopped green onion
Olive oil cooking spray
1 ½ lb. bag mini sweet peppers (halved tip to root and seeded)
2 large eggs, lightly beaten

INGREDIENTS (TOPPINGS, OPTIONAL)
Minced jalapeno
Pico de Gallo, pg. 145
Chopped fresh cilantro
Ideal Protein cheese sauce mix, to taste*

DIRECTIONS
1. Preheat oven to 425°F degrees.
2. Add ground beef, taco seasoning, salt, mushrooms, and green onion to a large skillet. Cook over medium/medium high heat until ground beef is browned; stir to break up the meat.
3. Transfer beef to a bowl and place in fridge to cool.
4. Lightly coat a large, rimmed baking sheet with olive oil cooking spray. Place pepper halves on baking sheet in a single layer, cut side up. Lightly spray peppers with cooking spray; bake 10 minutes.
5. Add beaten eggs to cooled meat mixture; stir well to mix.
6. Evenly fill the pepper halves with the meat mixture; bake 10 minutes.
7. Taste and season with additional salt, if desired; add toppings of choice.

SERVINGS
Entire recipe yield = 18 oz. lean protein (beef + egg) + 6 C. veggies
⅓ recipe yield = 6 oz. lean protein (beef + egg) + 2 C. veggies

TIP: *Using 2 T. Ideal Protein cheese sauce mix, stir in enough water for desired consistency. Heat cheese in the microwave before topping nachos.

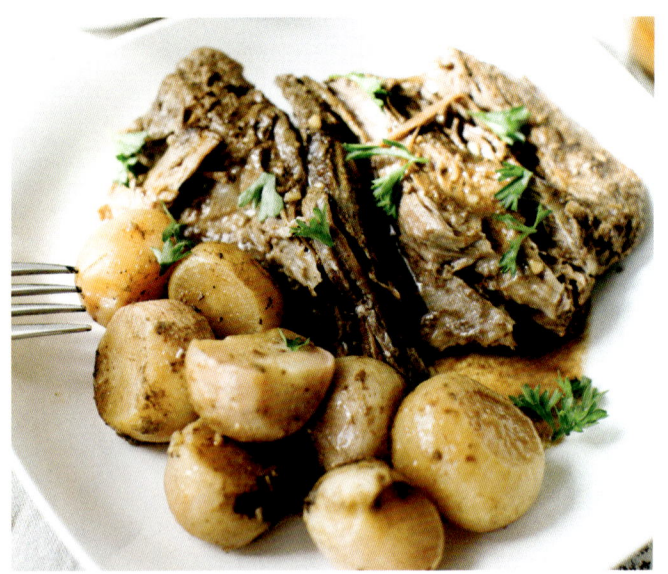

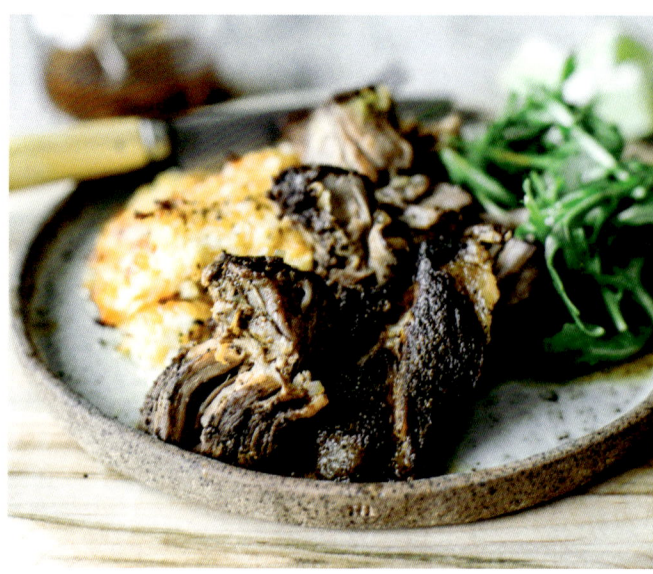

French Dip Beef
With baby fauxtatoes, Slow cooker recipe

INGREDIENTS (AU JUS)
¼ C. soy sauce
2 C. beef broth
1 T. Dijon mustard
2 tsp. onion powder
1 tsp. Ideal Protein salt
1 tsp. black pepper
1 tsp. minced garlic

INGREDIENTS (BEEF AND FAUXTATOES)
3 lb. boneless chuck roast
4 C. (1 lb.) radishes, ends trimmed

DIRECTIONS
1. Place all au jus ingredients in slow cooker; stir to mix.
2. Add roast to slow cooker; add radishes around roast.
3. Cover and cook on low 8 hours.

SERVINGS
Entire recipe yield = 48 oz. lean protein + 4 C. veggies
⅛ recipe yield = 6 oz. lean protein + ½ C. veggies

Green Chile Beef
Slow cooker recipe

INGREDIENTS
½ C. beef broth
¼ C. lime juice
2 T. dried minced onions
1 T. chili powder
1 tsp. garlic powder
1 tsp. Ideal Protein salt
1 tsp. black pepper
1 tsp. cumin
½ tsp. cayenne pepper
3 lb. boneless chuck roast
8 oz. can green chiles

DIRECTIONS
1. Place broth, lime juice and minced onions in bottom of slow cooker.
2. In a small bowl, mix dry spices together.
3. Rub entire beef roast with spice mixture; place in slow cooker.
4. Top roast with the green chiles.
5. Cover and cook on low 7-8 hours.

SERVINGS
Entire recipe yield = 48 oz. lean protein + 1 C. veggies (dried onion + chiles)
⅙ recipe yield = 8 oz. lean protein + 3 T. veggies (dried onion + chiles)

Italian Sausage Meatloaf

Makes two mini loaves

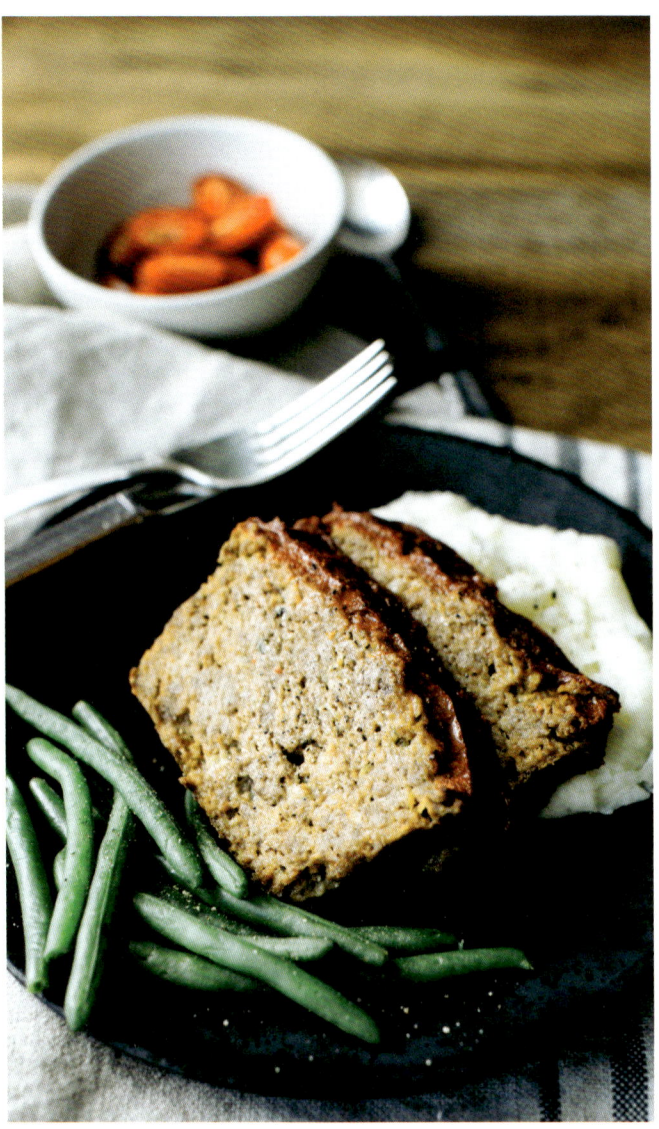

INGREDIENTS

1 C. shredded zucchini
2 T. Sausage Seasoning, pg. 147
1 large egg
6 T. Spaghizza Sauce, pg. 148 (divided)
17 oz. lean ground beef, turkey, or chicken
Cooking spray

DIRECTIONS

1. Preheat oven to 350˚F degrees.
2. Place shredded zucchini between several sheets of paper towels; squeeze as much liquid out as possible and place in a large mixing bowl.
3. To same bowl, add sausage seasoning, egg, and 2 T. of the Spaghizza Sauce; whisk to mix. Add ground beef and mix with hands until combined. (Avoid over working the mixture.)
4. Spray two 5 3/8" x 3" x 2 ⅛" inch mini loaf pans; divide meat mixture in half and place halves in separate loaf pans, pressing down firmly and evenly. Bake 25-30 minutes.
5. Heat the remaining Spaghizza Sauce and spread over loaves; serve.

SERVINGS

Entire recipe yield = 18 oz. lean protein (beef + egg) + 1 ½ C. veggies
⅓ recipe yield = 6 oz. lean protein (beef + egg) + ½ C. veggies

TIP: Excellent served with Cauliflower Mash (pg. 112) and steamed green beans.

Korean Beef & Cabbage

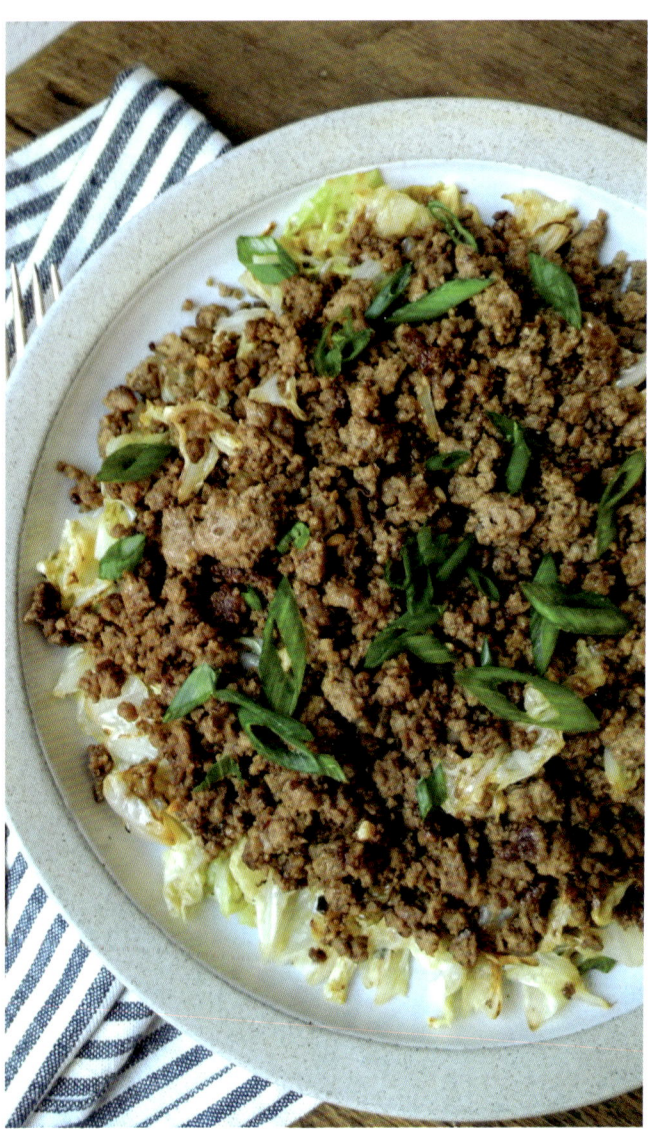

INGREDIENTS (SAUCE)
¼ C. soy sauce
¼ C. Ideal Protein maple syrup
1 tsp. garlic chili sauce (I use Sambal Oelek®)

INGREDIENTS (BEEF & CABBAGE)
5 ½ C. shredded napa cabbage
½ C. chopped green onion
2 T. toasted sesame oil, divided
18 oz. lean ground beef
1 ½ tsp. minced garlic
1 tsp. minced fresh ginger

DIRECTIONS
1. In a small bowl, mix all the sauce ingredients; set aside.
2. Place cabbage and green onion in a large resealable bag. Drizzle 1 T. of the sesame oil over the cabbage and onions; shake to coat. Set aside.
3. Heat the remaining 1 T. of the sesame oil in a large skillet over medium heat. Add ground beef, garlic, and ginger. Brown until hamburger has some bits of dark brown crusty texture. (Approximately ½ of the mixture should show this caramelized texture.)
4. Add soy sauce mixture to ground beef. Stir and cook until liquid is absorbed, and beef is glistening. Transfer beef mixture to a bowl; cover to keep warm.
5. Add cabbage and green onion to same skillet; stir fry over medium heat until cabbage is wilted and lightly browned.
6. Plate cabbage and layer beef over the top. Sprinkle with additional chopped green onion, if desired.

SERVINGS
Entire recipe yield = 18 oz. lean protein + 6 C. veggies + 2 T. oil
⅓ recipe yield = 6 oz. lean protein + 2 C. veggies + 2 tsp. oil

TIP: This recipe is also delicious using ground turkey in place of ground beef.

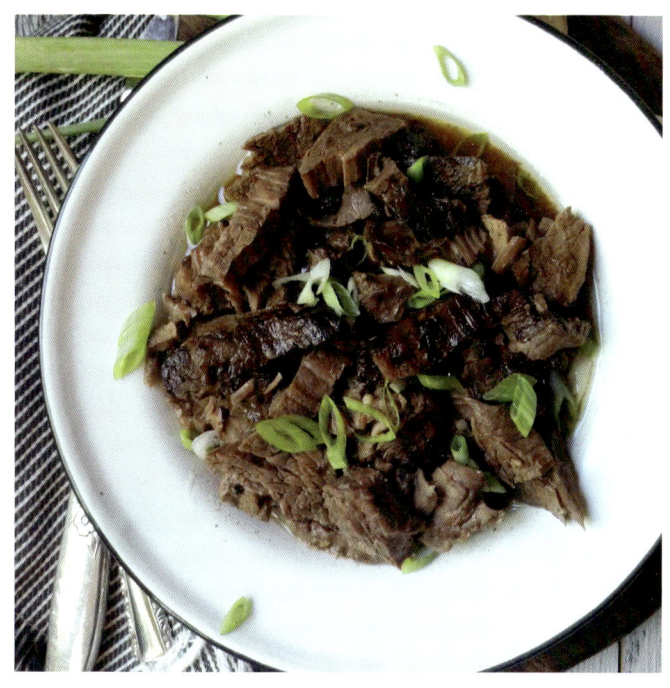

Mongolian Beef

Slow cooker recipe

INGREDIENTS

2 ¼ lbs. flank steak, sliced against the grain about
   ½" thick
½ C. low sodium soy sauce
½ C. water
¼ C. Ideal Protein maple syrup
1 T. toasted sesame oil
1 tsp. minced fresh ginger
1 tsp. minced garlic
⅔ C. chopped green onion

DIRECTIONS

1. Add the flank steak strips to the slow cooker.
2. In a medium bowl, stir together remaining
   ingredients (except green onion). Pour over
   flank steak.
3. Cover and cook on low 4-5 hours.
4. Stir in green onions and serve.

SERVINGS

Entire recipe yield = 36 oz. lean protein + ⅔ C.
veggies + 1 T. oil
⅙ recipe yield = 6 oz. lean protein + 2 T. veggies +
½ tsp. oil

NOTES: The Mongolian Beef is excellent served with
Thai Cucumber Salad, pg. 52.

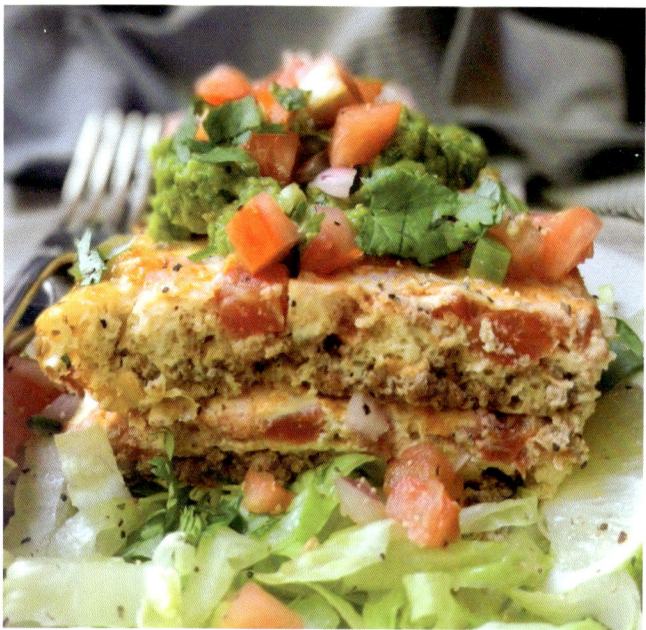

Naked Burrito Casserole

INGREDIENTS (CASSEROLE)

6 oz. lean ground beef, turkey, or chicken
1 T. Taco Seasoning, pg. 149
10 oz. can Rotel® diced tomatoes & green chilies,
   drained
4 eggs + 2 egg whites, lightly beaten

INGREDIENTS (TOPPINGS, OPTIONAL)

Shredded lettuce, unlimited
Chopped fresh cilantro
Mockamole, pg. 143
Pico de Gallo, pg. 145

DIRECTIONS

1. Preheat oven to 400° F degrees.
2. In a medium skillet, season the ground beef with
   taco seasoning. Brown over medium heat; stir to
   break up the meat.
3. Evenly spread ground beef in an 8 x 8-inch
   baking dish; spread the tomatoes and green
   chilies over the beef mixture. Pour beaten eggs
   over the top.
4. Bake 25 minutes or just until center of casserole
   is set, and eggs no longer jiggle. Do not over
   bake, or eggs will go from tender to tough.
5. Top with desired toppings.

SERVINGS

Entire recipe yield = 12 oz. lean protein + 2 C. veggies
½ recipe yield = 6 oz. lean protein + 1 C. veggies.

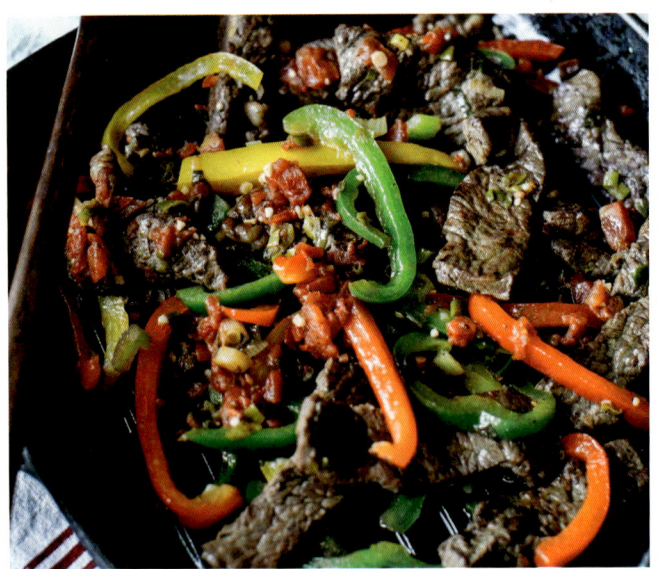

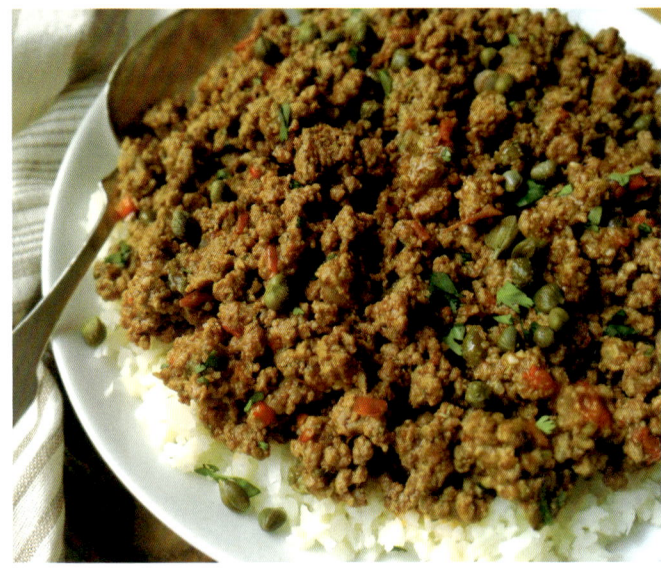

Pepper Steak

INGREDIENTS
1 ½ C. beef broth, divided
2 T. soy sauce
¼ tsp. sugar free sweetener, granular
½ tsp. black pepper
1 T. olive oil
18 oz. sirloin steak, sliced in ¼" strips
½ C. chopped green onion
1 tsp. minced garlic
2 C. sliced assorted bell peppers (green, yellow, and red)
½ C. sliced celery
1 C. canned diced tomatoes, drained

DIRECTIONS
1. In a small mixing bowl, mix 1 C. beef broth, soy sauce, sweetener, and black pepper. Set aside.
2. Heat oil in a large skillet over medium/medium high heat.
3. Add steak strips, green onion and garlic; cook till browned but not cooked through.
4. Add broth mixture to pan; simmer uncovered over low heat 20 minutes, stirring occasionally.
5. Add remaining ½ C. beef broth, peppers, celery, and tomatoes. Cover and simmer 10 minutes. Serve hot.

SERVINGS
Entire recipe yield = 18 oz. lean protein + 6 C. veggies + 1 T. oil
⅓ recipe yield = 6 oz. lean protein + 2 C. veggies + 1 tsp. oil

Picadillo
Instant Pot recipe

INGREDIENTS
2 ¼ lbs. (36 oz.) lean ground beef
1 tsp. kosher salt
¼ tsp. black pepper
1 ½ C. chopped Roma tomatoes
1 C. diced red bell pepper
2 T. dried minced onion
2 T. chopped fresh cilantro
1 tsp. minced garlic
3 T. water
2 oz. tomato sauce
2 bay leaves
3 T. capers + splash of juice
1 tsp. ground cumin

DIRECTIONS
1. Press sauté button on Instant Pot. Add ground beef; season with salt and pepper. Brown, stirring to break up meat.
2. Add tomatoes, bell pepper, dried minced onion, cilantro, and garlic. Stir 1 minute. Add remaining ingredients; stir to mix.
3. Cover, seal, and cook on high pressure 15 minutes. Quick release; remove bay leaves before serving.

SERVINGS
Entire recipe yield = 36 oz. lean protein + 3 C. veggies
⅙ recipe yield = 6 oz. lean protein + ½ C. veggies

TIP: Excellent served over cauliflower rice or Cauliflower Mash, pg. 112.

Pizza Burger Casserole

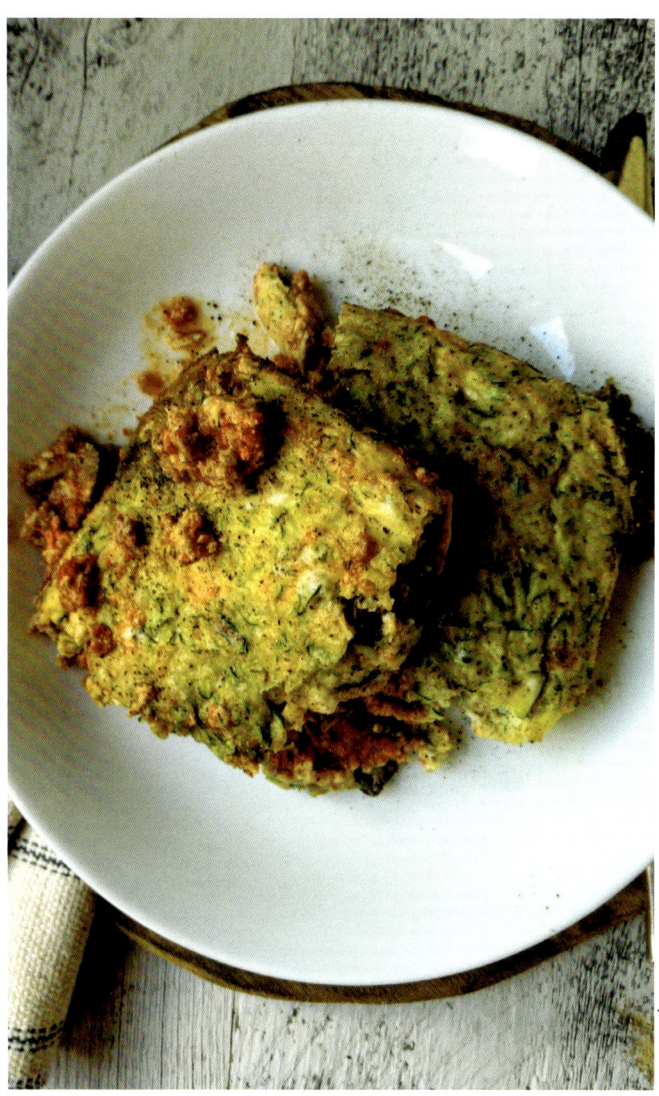

INGREDIENTS
1 ¾ C. shredded zucchini
6 oz. lean ground beef
¼ tsp. onion powder
¼ tsp. garlic powder
Salt and pepper, to taste
½ C. chopped bell pepper (any color)
½ C. sliced fresh mushrooms
¼ C. chopped green onion
4 eggs + 2 egg whites, lightly beaten
1 C. Spaghizza Sauce, pg. 148

DIRECTIONS
1. Preheat oven to 400°F degrees.
2. Place shredded zucchini in a strainer; lightly sprinkle with salt. Toss and set strainer in sink. (Salt will draw water out of zucchini.)
3. To a medium skillet, add ground beef; season with onion powder, garlic powder, salt, and pepper. Brown over medium heat; halfway through browning add bell pepper, mushrooms, and green onions. Set aside.
4. Place the shredded zucchini between several sheets of paper towels. Press to absorb the moisture out of the zucchini. Place in a bowl and stir in eggs.
5. In an 8 x 8-inch baking dish, evenly spread the ground beef mixture. Layer the Spaghizza Sauce over the beef and pour egg mixture over the top. Season with additional salt and pepper.
6. Bake 25 minutes or just until center of casserole is set, and eggs no longer jiggle. Do not over bake, or eggs will go from tender to tough.

SERVINGS
Entire recipe yield = 12 oz. lean protein + 6 C. veggies
½ recipe yield = 6 oz. lean protein + 3 C. veggies

TIP: Prepare the Spaghizza Sauce in advance and refrigerate or freeze for use in recipes like this.

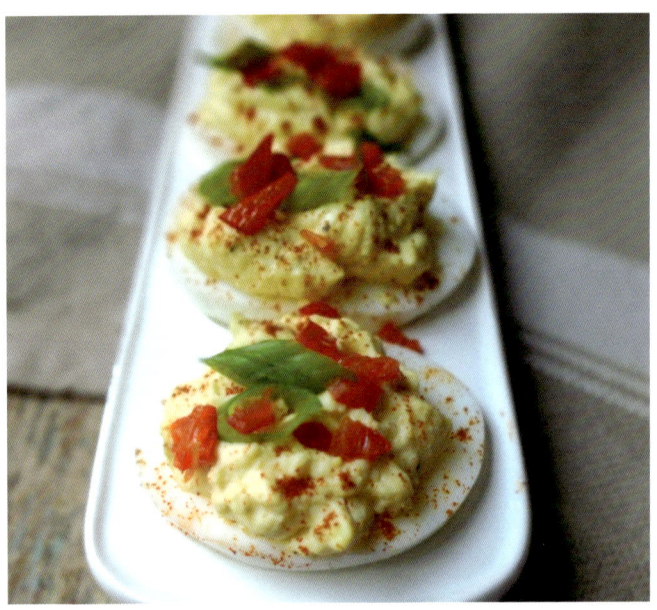

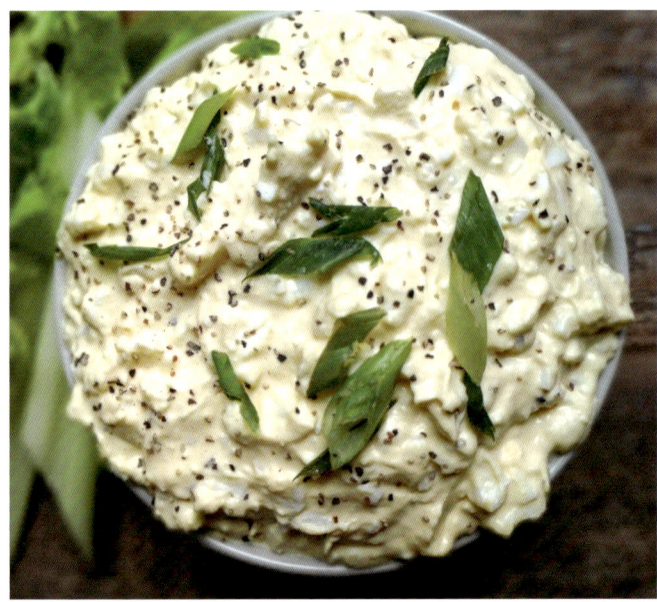

Deviled Eggs

INGREDIENTS (DEVILED EGGS)
6 hard-boiled eggs
2 T. Janeva's Mayonnaise, pg. 141
1 tsp. Dijon mustard
1 tsp. apple cider vinegar
Salt and pepper, to taste

INGREDIENTS (TOPPINGS, TO TASTE)
Smoked paprika
Chopped green onion (green part)
Chopped Fresno or jalapeno pepper, seeded

DIRECTIONS
1. Slice eggs in half lengthwise. Using a spoon, remove yolks and place in a shallow bowl; mash with a fork.
2. Add remaining deviled egg ingredients; stir until smooth.
3. Using two spoons, scoop egg mixture with one spoon; use the other spoon to scrape filling evenly into egg halves.
4. Sprinkle with paprika. Top with green onion and jalapeno, if desired.

SERVINGS
1 whole egg (2 Deviled Egg halves) = 1 oz. lean protein + 1 tsp. oil (mayo) + add for any veggies consumed

TIP: No more than 2 whole Deviled Eggs should be eaten in one day due to the maximum oil protocol of 2 tsp. per day.

Egg Salad

INGREDIENTS
6 hard-boiled eggs
3 T. Janeva's Mayonnaise, pg. 141
2 T. Walden Farms mayo or coleslaw dressing
1 tsp. yellow mustard
1 tsp. lemon juice
1 tsp. apple cider vinegar
¼ tsp. onion powder
Sea salt and black pepper, to taste

DIRECTIONS
1. Chop eggs and add to a medium size mixing bowl.
2. Add remaining ingredients; stir to combine.
3. Cover and store refrigerated.

SERVINGS
⅓ recipe yield = 2 oz. lean protein + 2 tsp. oil

TIP: Serve with celery stalks, Ideal Protein Dorados or Crisps, or serve on savory bread from recipes in this cookbook.

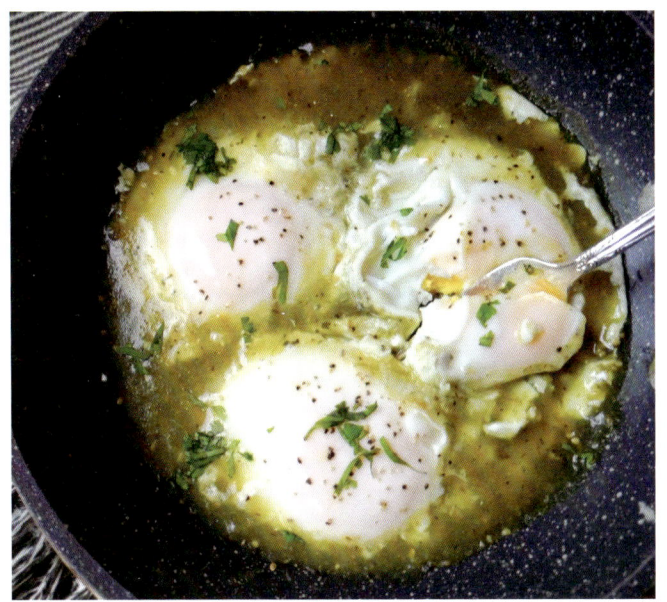

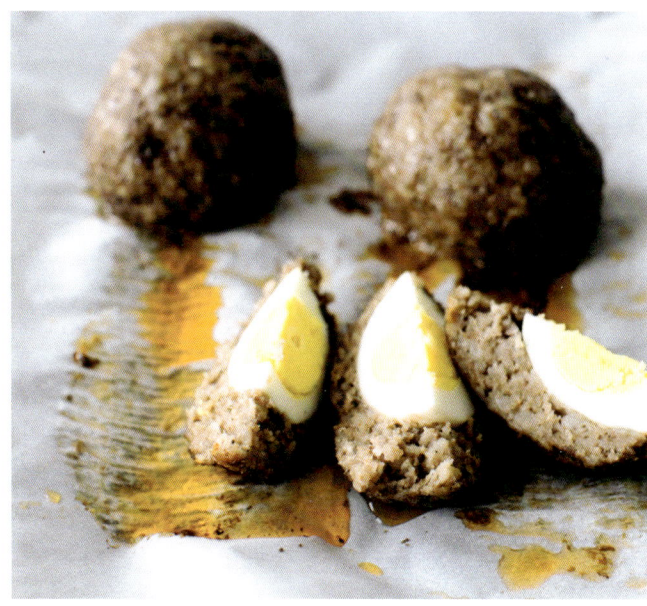

Salsa Verde Eggs

INGREDIENTS
¾ C. Tomatillo Salsa Verde, pg. 150
3 large eggs
Salt and pepper, to taste

DIRECTIONS
1. Add salsa to a medium skillet and heat on medium until hot and bubbly.
2. Make three divots in the salsa with the back of a spoon; crack an egg into each divot.
3. Reduce heat to low/medium low. Cover and cook about 2 ½ - 3 minutes for over-easy yolks (soft but not runny.)
4. Season with salt and pepper. For serving suggestions, see TIP.

SERVINGS
Entire recipe yield = 4–6 oz. lean protein + ¾ C. veggies

TIP: Serve over crushed Ideal Protein Dorado chips for a Mexican style meal. Also delicious served with toasted savory bread made from a recipe in this cookbook.

Scotch Eggs

INGREDIENTS
4 oz. lean ground chicken, turkey, or pork
1 tsp. Sausage Seasoning, pg. 147
2 hard-boiled eggs
Salt and pepper, to taste

DIRECTIONS
1. Preheat oven to 375°F degrees.
2. In a small bowl, combine ground chicken and Sausage Seasoning.
3. Make into two patties; wrap each egg with a patty and seal.
4. Place eggs on a rimmed baking sheet.
5. Bake 22-25 minutes or until deep golden brown.
6. Serve with salt and pepper. May be served hot or cold—keep refrigerated if storing.

SERVINGS
2 Scotch eggs = 6 oz. lean protein

TIP: Perfect for a meal on the go when prepared in advance.

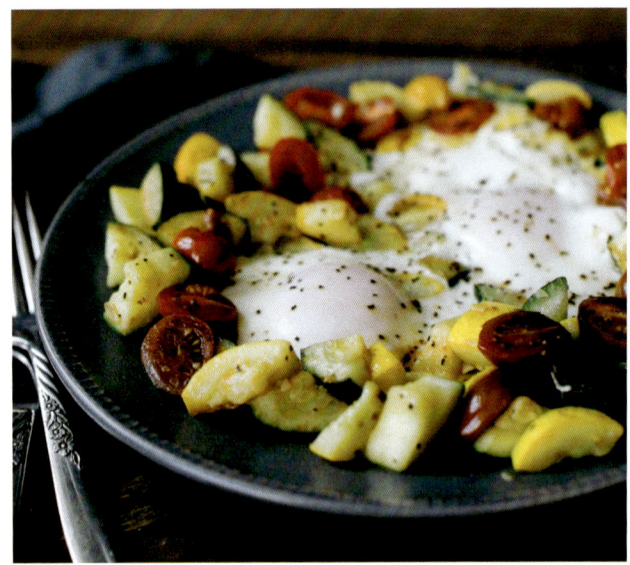

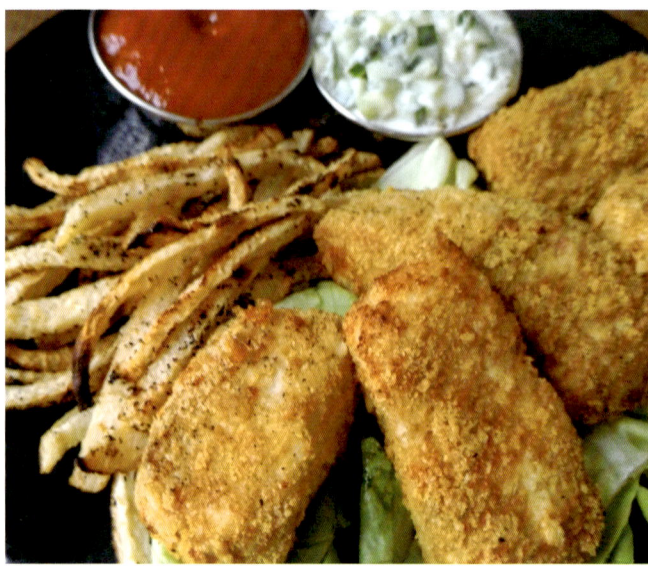

Skillet Garden Eggs

INGREDIENTS
1 T. + 1 tsp. olive oil
1 ½ C. zucchini (unpeeled), cut in bite size chunks
1 ½ C. summer squash (unpeeled), cut in bite size chunks
Garlic powder, to taste
1 C. grape or baby heirloom tomatoes, halved
6 large eggs
Salt and pepper, to taste
2 T. water
Chopped fresh basil, to taste

DIRECTIONS
1. Heat olive oil in a large skillet over medium heat. Add zucchini, summer squash, and garlic powder. Stir fry 5 minutes or until squash is lightly browned and caramelized.
2. Add tomatoes and cook 2 minutes; gently stir during cooking.
3. Clear 6 open spots in the skillet, and crack 1 egg into each spot. Season dish with salt and pepper. Add water to skillet and cover. Cook 2-3 minutes or until eggs whites are cooked over egg yolks, leaving the yolks runny.
4. Sprinkle with basil before serving.

SERVINGS
½ recipe yield = 4–6 oz. lean protein + 2 C. veggies + 2 tsp. oil

Fried Fish
Air fryer recipe

INGREDIENTS
1 pkg. Ideal Protein salt and vinegar chips (divided)
6 oz. fish fillet (tilapia, mahi mahi, walleye, or other white fish)
2 T. liquid egg whites
Olive oil cooking spray
Salt and pepper, to taste

DIRECTIONS
1. Using ¾ of the bag of chips, crush to fine crumbs. The remaining ¼ bag of chips may be served whole alongside the meal or for a later snack. Spread crumbs out on a small plate.
2. Cut fish fillet into 4 chunks or strips. Dredge fish in egg whites, then press into crumbs coating all sides. Lightly coat breaded fish with olive oil cooking spray.
3. Coat bottom of air fryer basket with cooking spray. Add breaded fish in one layer.
4. Bake 12 minutes at 400°F degrees or until fish flakes with a fork; flip fish once during baking.
5. Season with salt and pepper, if desired.

SERVINGS
Entire recipe yield = 6 oz. lean protein + 1 unrestricted (if eating the remaining ¼ bag of chips)

TIP: Total cook time will depend on thickness of fish fillet. I used mahi mahi which was about 1-inch thick. Thinner fillets will take less cook time.

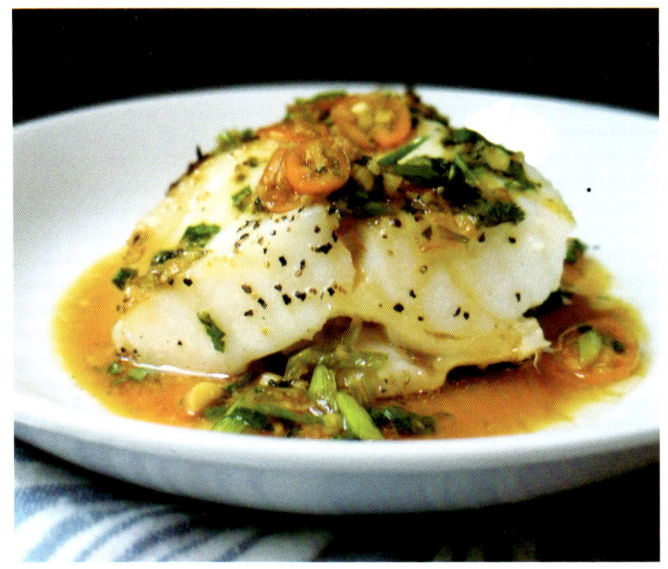

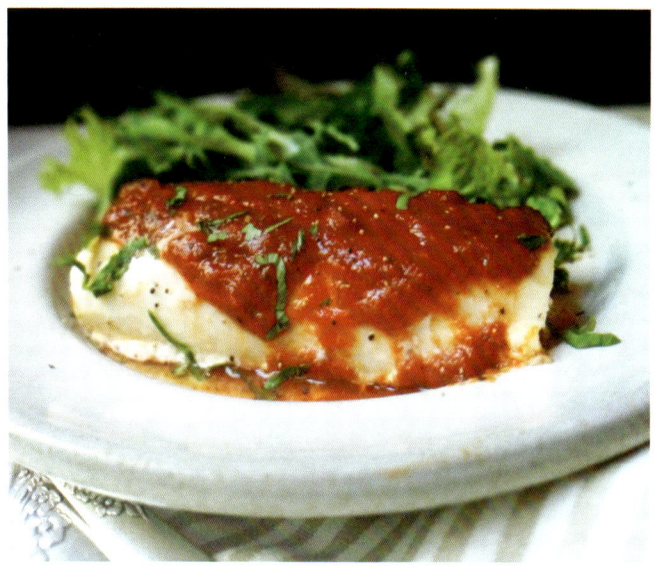

Ginger Soy Sea Bass

INGREDIENTS
2 T. chopped fresh cilantro
2 T. chopped green onion (white and green parts)
1 T. minced fresh ginger
2 T. lime juice
1 ½ T. soy sauce
1 serrano chili, thinly sliced
4 tsp. mild olive oil, divided
2 – 6 oz. sea bass fillets (about 1-inch thick)

DIRECTIONS
1. Preheat the oven to 500°F degrees.
2. To a small bowl, add the cilantro, green onion, ginger, lime juice, soy sauce, serrano chili and 2 tsp. of the olive oil. Stir to mix.
3. Brush the sea bass fillets on both sides with remaining 2 tsp. oil and place skin side down (if fillets have skin) in an 8 x 8-inch baking pan.
4. Spoon ½ the sauce over fillets, reserving the other half.
5. Bake 20-25 minutes or until fish is opaque in the center and flakes easily with a fork.
6. Plate fillets and drizzle remaining sauce on top.

SERVINGS
Entire recipe yield = 12 oz. lean protein + ¼ C. veggies + 4 tsp. oil
½ recipe yield = 6 oz. lean protein + 2 T. veggies + 2 tsp. oil

NOTE: Skin of sea bass should not be eaten in this recipe.

Italian Fish Fillets

INGREDIENTS
½ recipe Spaghizza Sauce (pg. 148), divided
2 – 6 oz. mahi mahi, sea bass, or tilapia fish fillets
Chopped fresh basil, to taste

DIRECTIONS
1. Preheat oven to 375°F degrees.
2. Spread a few spoonfuls of the Spaghizza Sauce on the bottom of an 8 x 8-inch baking dish or pie plate.
3. Arrange fish over sauce. Top fish with remaining sauce.
4. Bake uncovered 20 minutes or until fish flakes easily with a fork. Sprinkle with fresh basil.

SERVINGS
Entire recipe yield = 12 oz. lean protein + 2 ½ C. veggies + 1 ½ tsp. oil
½ recipe yield = 6 oz. lean protein + 1 ¼ C. veggies + ¾ tsp. oil

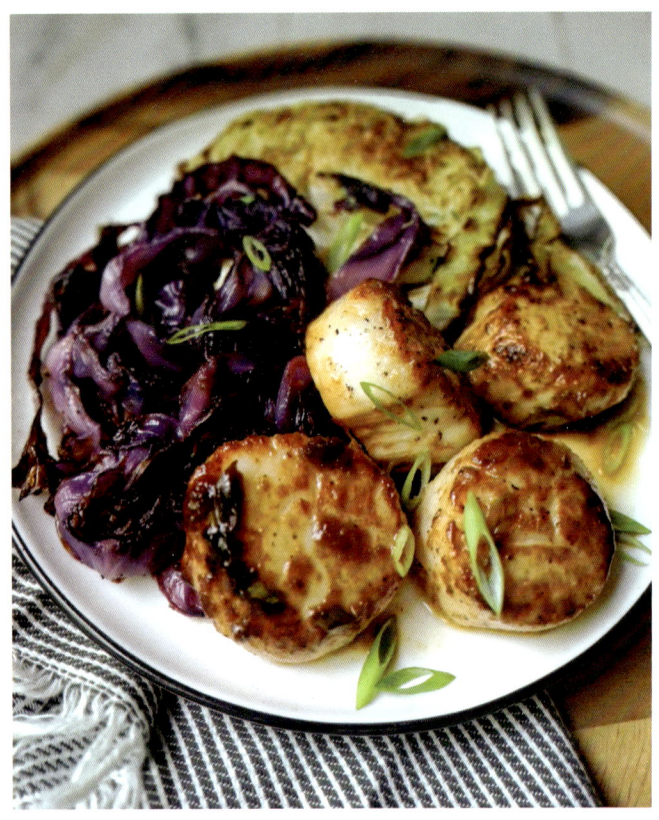

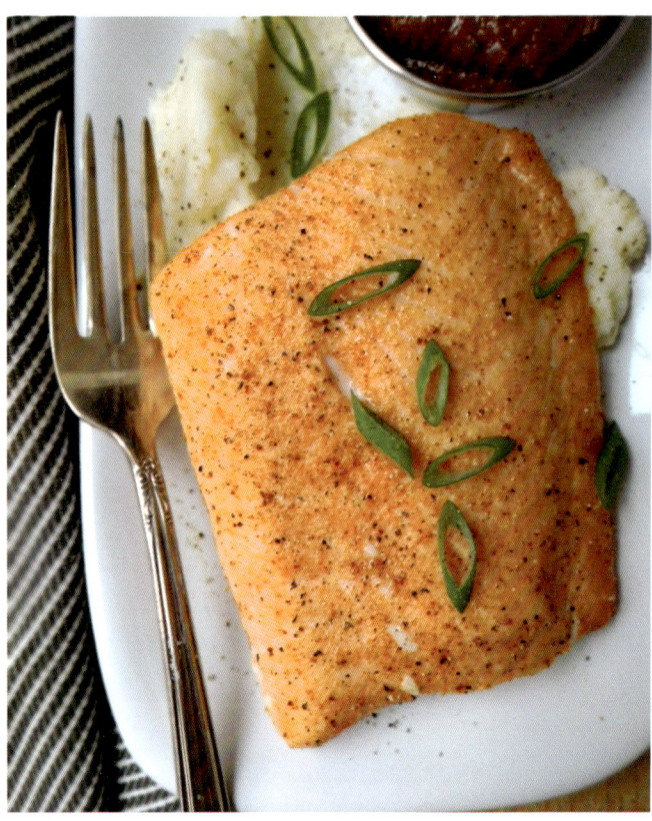

Lemon Garlic Seared Scallops

Just 3 minutes cooking time

INGREDIENTS

12 oz. sea scallops (medium to large size)
Sea salt and black pepper, to taste
Garlic powder, to taste
1 T. + 1 tsp. olive oil
Fresh lemon zest and juice, to taste

DIRECTIONS

1. Rinse scallops with cold water; pat dry with paper towels. Season with salt, pepper, and garlic powder on each side.
2. Heat oil in a skillet over medium high/high heat. When oil begins to lightly smoke, add scallops making sure they are not touching.
3. Sear scallops 1 ½ minutes on each side; do not touch them while searing.
4. To serve, squeeze lemon juice over scallops and sprinkle with lemon zest. Season with additional salt and pepper, if necessary.

SERVINGS

Entire recipe yield = 12 oz. lean protein
½ recipe yield = 6 oz. lean protein

Perfect Salmon Every Time

A no-fail method

INGREDIENTS

6 oz. skinless salmon fillet
½ tsp. olive oil
Salt and pepper, to taste
Cajun seasoning, to taste (or other favorite seasoning)

DIRECTIONS

1. Line a rimmed baking sheet with parchment paper and place salmon fillet on pan.
2. Brush salmon with olive oil; season with remaining ingredients.
3. Place salmon in a cold oven. Turn oven to 400° F degrees; bake 25 minutes.

SERVINGS

Entire recipe yield = 6 oz. lean protein + ½ tsp. oil

TIP: This recipe may easily be doubled or more to accommodate additional meals.

Shrimp & Noodle Stir Fry

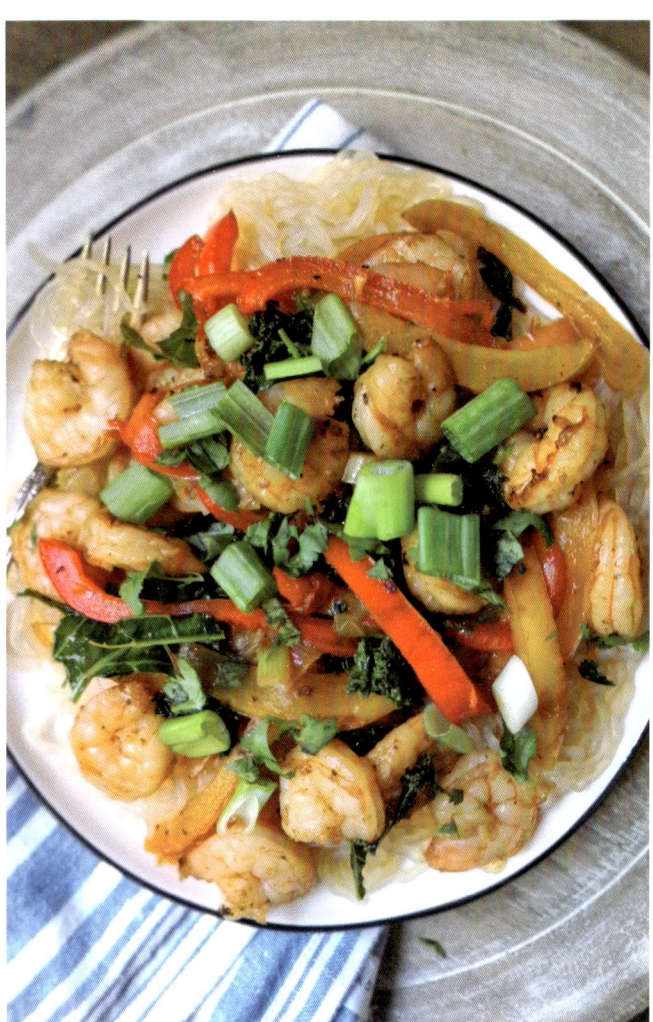

INGREDIENTS (STIR FRY SAUCE)
¼ C. soy sauce
1 T. sugar free sweetener, granular
1 T. white vinegar
2 tsp. minced fresh ginger

INGREDIENTS (STIR FRY)
2 pkgs. Ideal Protein konjac spaghetti (drained and rinsed)
2 tsp. olive oil
2 ½ C. julienned bell peppers (yellow, red, and orange)
½ C. chopped green onion
2 tsp. toasted sesame oil
12 oz. large raw shrimp (deveined, peeled, no tails)
1 Fresno pepper, seeded and minced
1 C. packed curly kale, stemmed and hand torn
2 T. chopped fresh cilantro

DIRECTIONS
1. In a small mixing bowl, combine sauce ingredients; set aside.
2. Add konjac noodles and 2 T. stir fry sauce to a medium bowl. Toss to coat noodles; set aside.
3. Heat the olive oil in a large skillet over medium/medium high heat. When oil is hot, add bell peppers and stir fry until lightly browned. Add green onion and stir.
4. Move peppers and onion mixture to outside edges of skillet; add sesame oil to center and heat. Add shrimp to hot oil and cook 2-3 minutes or until opaque. Add Fresno pepper and remaining sauce; stir fry to combine shrimp and veggies.
5. Add kale; stir fry until wilted and sauce is reduced.
6. Heat noodles in microwave until hot; serve stir fry over noodles. Sprinkle with cilantro and additional chopped green onions, if desired.

SERVINGS
Entire recipe yield = 12 oz. lean protein + 4 C. veggies + 4 tsp. oil + 2 C. konjac spaghetti
½ recipe yield = 6 oz. lean protein + 2 C. veggies + 2 tsp. oil + 1 C. konjac spaghetti

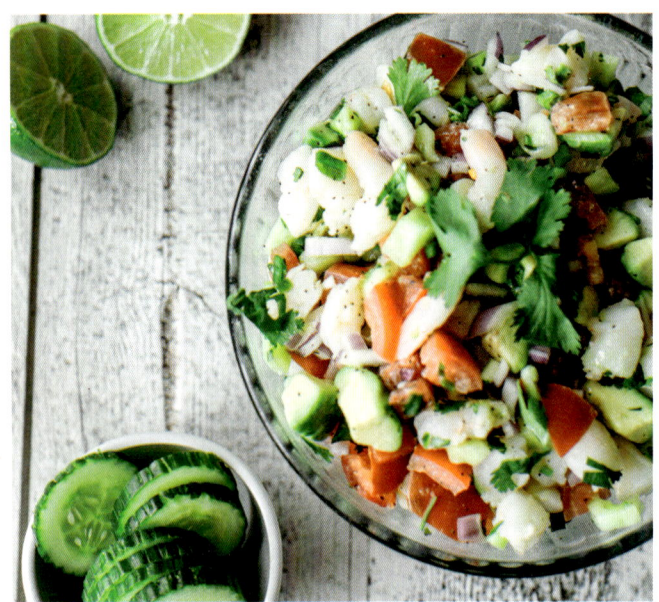

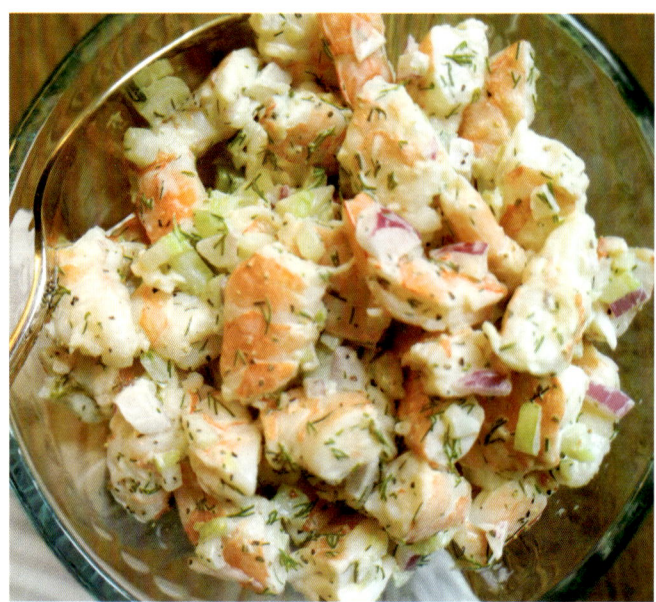

Shrimp Ceviche

INGREDIENTS
6 oz. cooked shrimp (deveined, tails off)
¾ C. diced tomato
¾ C. diced cucumber
¼ C. diced yellow onion
2 T. chopped green onion
2 T. chopped fresh cilantro
1-2 tsp. minced jalapeno pepper
1 T. lime or lemon juice
Sea salt, to taste
Black pepper, to taste

DIRECTIONS
1. Cut shrimp in small chunks and place in a medium size mixing bowl.
2. Add remaining ingredients; gently fold to mix.
3. Keep ceviche refrigerated until ready to serve.

SERVINGS
Entire recipe yield = 6 oz. lean protein + 2 C. veggies

TIP: Perfect for cold snacking or bringing to an event; excellent served with any of the Ideal Protein Dorados or chips.

Shrimp Salad

INGREDIENTS (SALAD)
12 oz. cooked large shrimp (deveined, tails off)
2 T. minced red onion
¼ C. finely chopped celery
1 ½ T. finely chopped fresh dill
Salt and pepper, to taste

INGREDIENTS (DRESSING)
2 T. + 1 tsp. Janeva's Mayonnaise, pg. 141
½ tsp. lemon juice
¼ tsp. Dijon mustard

DIRECTIONS
1. Cut shrimp into small bite size pieces and place in a large mixing bowl. Add remaining salad ingredients to shrimp; gently fold to mix. Season with salt and pepper.
2. In a small mixing bowl, whisk all dressing ingredients. Pour over salad, and gently fold to mix. Cover and store in fridge until ready to serve.
3. Fold salad before serving.

SERVINGS
Entire recipe yield = 12 oz. lean protein + ¼ C & 2 T. veggies + 2 tsp. oil (mayonnaise)
½ recipe yield = 6 oz. lean protein + 3 T. veggies + 1 tsp. oil (mayonnaise)

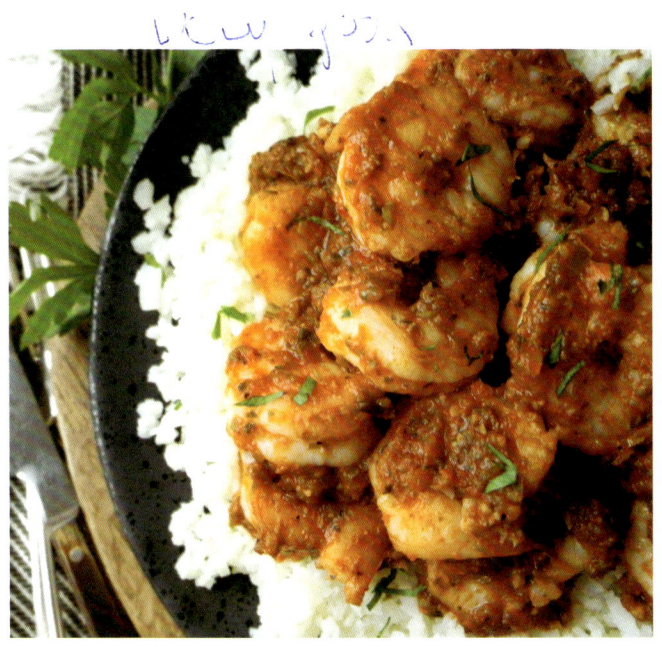

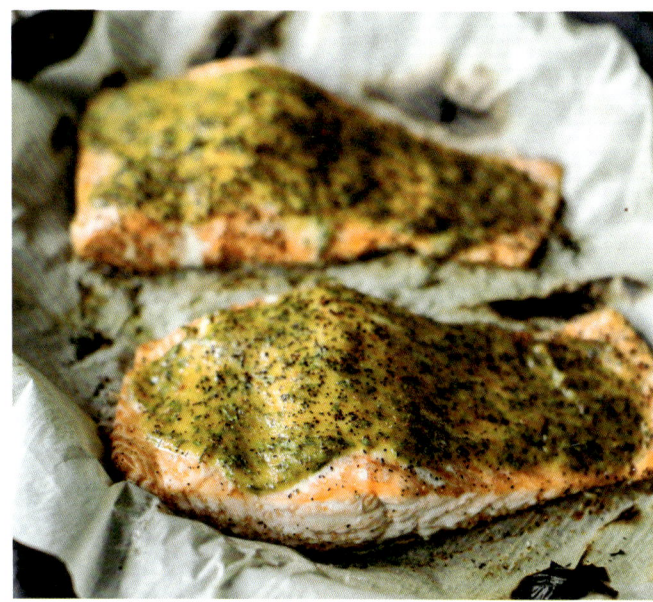

Sofrito Shrimp

A popular Puerto Rican dish

INGREDIENTS

½ C. Sofrito, pg. 148
½ C. tomato sauce
1 T. olive oil
12 oz. raw medium size shrimp (deveined, tails off)
½ tsp. garlic powder
Salt & pepper, to taste
Chopped fresh cilantro or green onion,
   to taste (optional)

DIRECTIONS

1. In a medium bowl, stir together the sofrito and tomato sauce; set aside.
2. Heat olive oil in a large skillet over medium high heat. Add shrimp and season with garlic powder, salt and pepper; stir fry 3-4 minutes or until shrimp is pink all the way through.
3. Reduce heat to medium/medium low; add sofrito mixture and continue to simmer 3-4 minutes, stirring often.
4. Plate and sprinkle with cilantro or green onion, if desired.

SERVINGS

Entire recipe yield = 12 oz. lean protein + 1 ½ C. veggies
½ recipe yield = 6 oz. lean protein + ¾ C. veggies

TIP: Delicious served over cauliflower rice or Ideal Protein konjac spaghetti.

Tarragon Dijon Glazed Salmon

INGREDIENTS

2 – 6 oz. salmon fillets (skin on or off)
Sea salt and pepper, to taste
Creole or Cajun seasoning, to taste
1 T. + 1 tsp. Dijon mustard
2 T. Ideal Protein maple syrup
1 tsp. olive oil
¼ tsp. onion powder
1 T. chopped fresh tarragon leaves

DIRECTIONS

1. Place salmon skin side down on a parchment paper lined baking sheet; season with salt, pepper, and Creole seasoning.
2. Add the Dijon, syrup, oil, onion powder, and tarragon to a small bowl; stir to mix. Spread mixture evenly over salmon fillets.
3. Place salmon in a cold oven. Turn oven to 400°F degrees; bake 25 minutes.

SERVINGS

Entire recipe yield = 12 oz. lean protein + 1 tsp. oil
½ recipe yield = 6 oz. lean protein + ½ tsp. oil

Teriyaki Tuna Steak

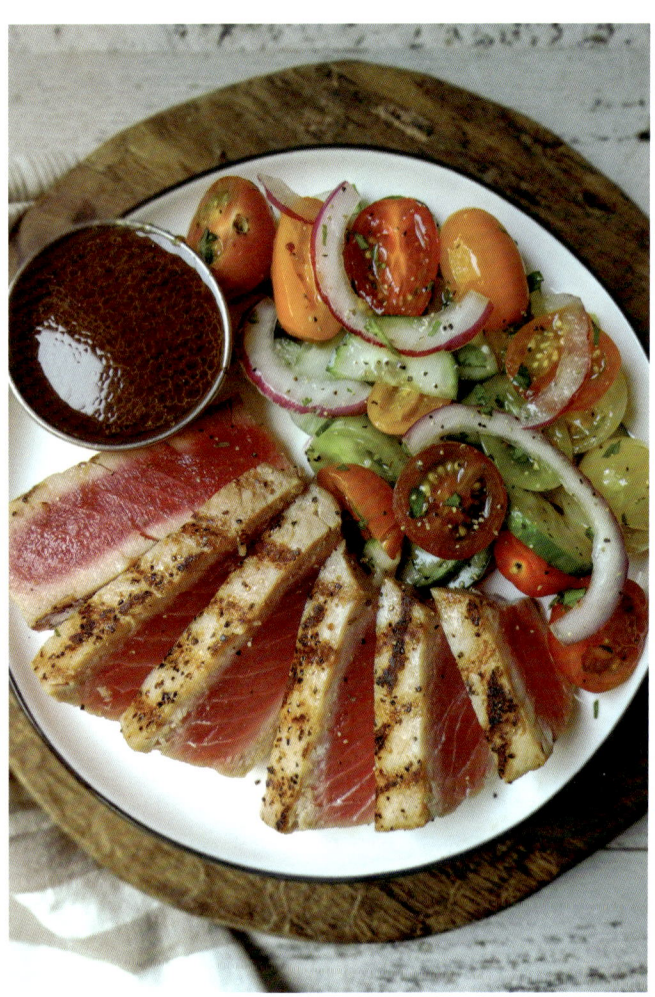

INGREDIENTS
1 – 6 oz. tuna steak
3 T. Teriyaki Sauce, pg. 150
1 tsp. olive oil

DIRECTIONS
1. Add tuna steak to a resealable plastic bag and pour sauce over tuna. Seal and toss bag back and forth to coat tuna. Marinate in fridge 1 hour. Remove tuna steak from bag; plate and set aside. Discard marinade.
2. Brush a grill pan or skillet with oil; heat over medium high heat. When oil is hot, add tuna steak to pan.
3. Cook 1 minute. Lift steak with tongs and turn clockwise (about a 1-inch turn); cook an additional minute on same side. (Cook time will yield a medium rare tuna steak. For a medium steak, cook 1 minute longer on each side.)
4. Flip steak and repeat direction #3. Plate and slice to serve. Drizzle additional Teriyaki Sauce over steak, if desired.

SERVINGS
Entire recipe yield = 6 oz. lean protein + 1 ½ tsp. oil

'Apple' Pork Roast

Slow cooker recipe

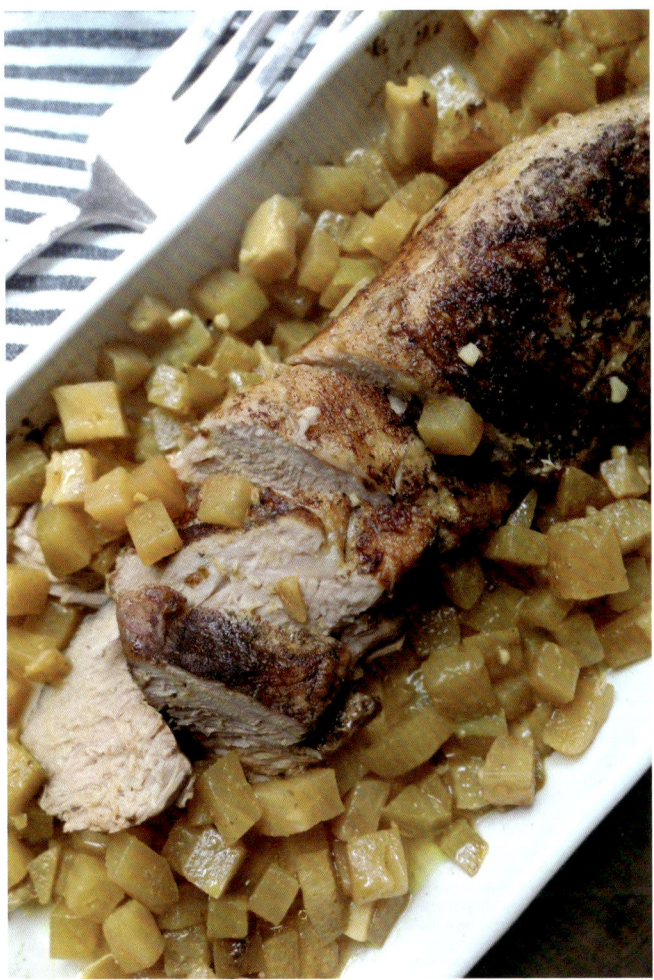

INGREDIENTS (SEASONINGS)
1 tsp. yellow curry powder
1 tsp. onion powder
1 tsp. ground mustard
½ tsp. garlic powder
½ tsp. salt
¼ tsp. black pepper
¼ tsp. cinnamon

INGREDIENTS (PORK)
1 ½ lb. pork tenderloin
2 T. + 2 tsp. olive oil, divided
1 C. chicken broth
1 T. apple cider vinegar
4 C. diced chayote squash

DIRECTIONS
1. Combine seasonings in a small bowl. Rub seasoning over entire pork tenderloin.
2. Heat 1 T. + 1 tsp. oil in a large skillet over medium/medium high heat; brown pork tenderloin 10 minutes turning once during browning.
3. Transfer tenderloin to slow cooker; pour chicken broth and apple cider vinegar over tenderloin.
4. Heat the remaining 1 T. + 1 tsp. oil in same large skillet over medium/medium high heat. Add chayote squash and stir fry 5 minutes; add squash to slow cooker.
5. Cover and cook on low 3-4 hours or until internal temp reaches 145°F degrees.

SERVINGS
Entire recipe yield = 24 oz. lean protein + 4 C. veggies + 8 tsp. oil
¼ recipe yield = 6 oz. lean protein + 1 C. veggies + 2 tsp. oil

TIP: Chayote squash will take on the flavor and texture of apples in this recipe – a classic combination with pork.

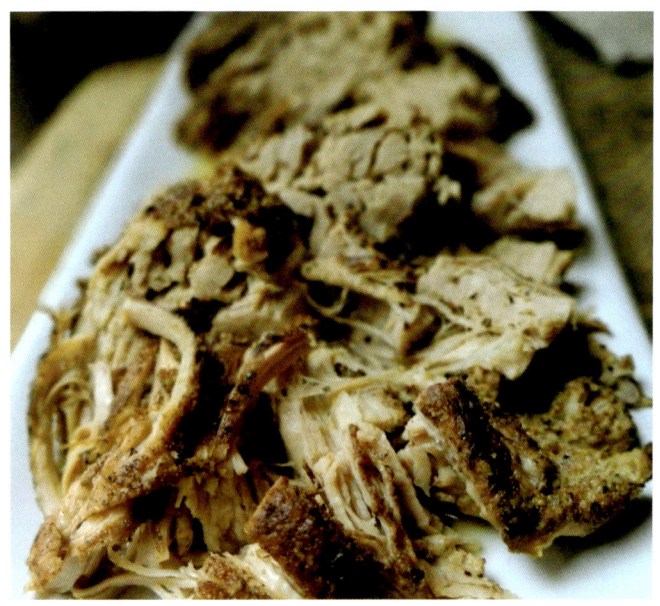

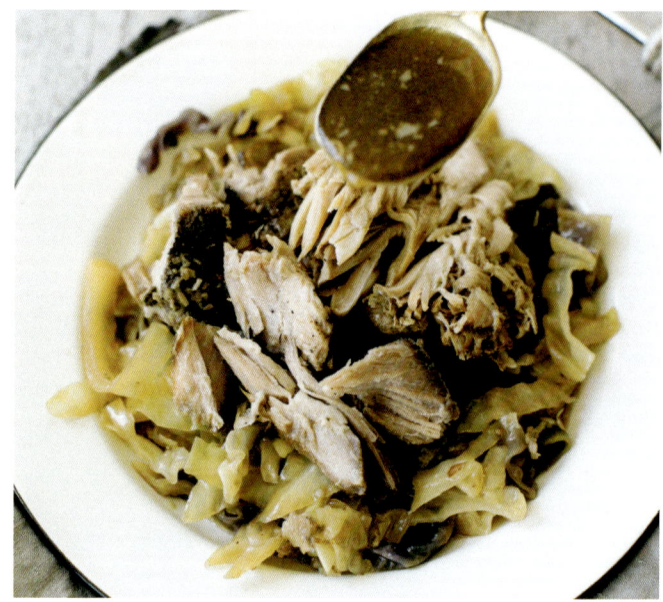

Jerk Pork Tenderloin
Slow cooker recipe

INGREDIENTS
1 ½ lb. pork tenderloin
2 T. Jerk Seasoning, pg. 142
1 T. + 1 tsp. olive oil
1 C. beef broth

DIRECTIONS
1. Rub entire pork tenderloin with the jerk seasoning.
2. Heat oil in a large skillet over medium/medium high heat. Brown pork tenderloin 10 minutes turning once during browning.
3. Add beef broth and tenderloin to slow cooker.
4. Cover and cook on low 3-4 hours or until internal temp reaches 145°F degrees.

SERVINGS
Entire recipe yield = 24 oz. lean protein + 4 tsp. oil
¼ recipe yield = 6 oz. lean protein + 1 tsp. oil

TIP: As a serving option, the meat may be chopped or pulled and mixed with the Sassy BBQ Sauce (pg. 147) for a BBQ Pulled Pork meal.

Kalua Pork & Cabbage
Slow cooker recipe

INGREDIENTS
4 C. sliced green cabbage (¼-inch slices)
4 C. sliced red cabbage (¼-inch slices)
1 tsp. kosher salt
1 tsp. black pepper
1 tsp. garlic powder
2 tsp. dried minced onion
1 tsp. ground ginger
3 lbs. boneless center cut pork loin roast
⅓ C. chicken broth
3 T. soy sauce
1 tsp. liquid smoke flavoring

DIRECTIONS
1. Place cabbage on the bottom of a large slow cooker.
2. Combine dry spices in a small bowl; rub over entire pork roast. Place roast in slow cooker on top of cabbage.
3. In a small bowl, combine chicken broth, soy sauce, and liquid smoke flavoring. Pour over pork roast.
4. Cover and cook 4-5 hours on low or until internal temp reaches 145°F degrees.
5. Serve by slicing into steaks and top with cabbage. Drizzle with juice from slow cooker.

SERVINGS
Entire recipe yield = 48 oz. lean protein + 8 C. veggies
⅛ recipe yield = 6 oz. lean protein + 1 C. veggies

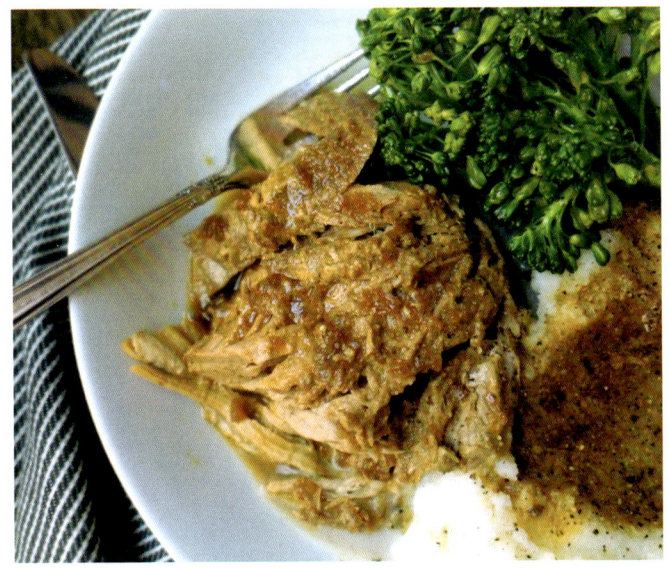

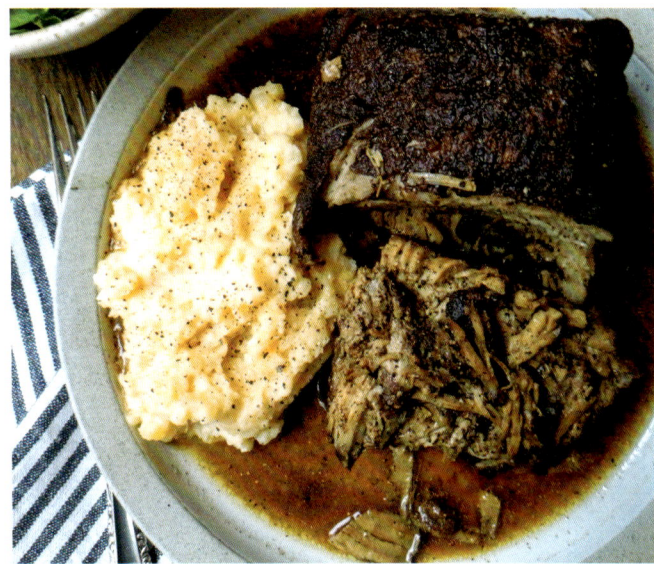

Melt-In-Your-Mouth Pork Tenderloin
Slow cooker recipe

INGREDIENTS
1 ½ lbs. pork tenderloin
¼ C. soy sauce
3 T. Ideal Protein maple syrup
1 ½ T. Dijon mustard
1 T. + 1 tsp. olive oil
1 T. + 1 ½ tsp. dried minced onions
1 ½ tsp. garlic powder
1 tsp. onion powder

DIRECTIONS
1. Place tenderloin in slow cooker.
2. Combine remaining ingredients and pour over tenderloin.
3. Cook on low 3-4 hours or until internal temp reaches 145°F degrees.
4. Turn tenderloin once during cooking.
5. Slice and serve, pouring desired amount of au jus marinade over the pork.

SERVINGS
Entire recipe yield = 24 oz. lean protein + ⅓ C. veggies (dried onions)
¼ recipe yield = 6 oz. lean protein + 1½ T. veggies (dried onions)

Pumpkin Spice Pork Roast
Slow cooker recipe

INGREDIENTS (SPICE RUB)
1 T. pumpkin pie spice, pg. 145
2 tsp. ground mustard
1 tsp. ground ginger
1 T. kosher salt
1 tsp. onion powder
½ tsp. smoked paprika
½ tsp. garlic powder
¼ tsp. black pepper

INGREDIENTS (PORK ROAST)
1 ½ lbs. pork tenderloin
2 T. olive oil
1 C. beef broth

DIRECTIONS
1. Combine seasonings in a small bowl. Rub entire pork tenderloin with the spice rub.
2. Heat the oil in a large skillet over medium/ medium high heat. Brown pork tenderloin 10 minutes turning once during browning.
3. Add beef broth and tenderloin to slow cooker.
4. Cover and cook on low 3-4 hours or until internal temp reaches 145°F degrees.

SERVINGS
Entire recipe yield = 24 oz. lean protein
¼ recipe yield = 6 oz. lean protein

TIP: Delicious served with Garlic Rutabaga Mash, pg. 117, or Cauliflower Mash, pg. 112.

Sausage Zucchini Lasagna

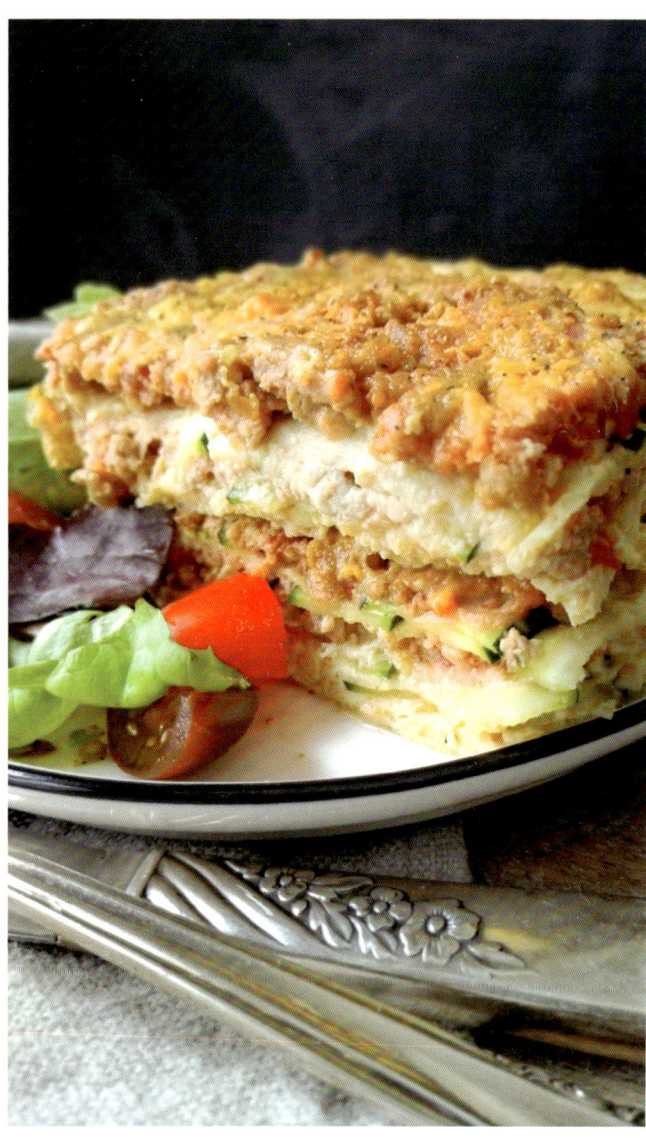

INGREDIENTS

2 C. (10.6 oz) zucchini, thinly sliced lengthwise into planks
Ideal Protein salt
1 T. olive oil
6 oz. lean ground pork
1 T. Sausage Seasoning, pg. 147
10 oz. can Rotel® diced tomatoes and chilies (undrained)
¼ tsp. garlic powder
¼ tsp. Italian seasoning
Pinch cayenne pepper
4 large eggs
2 large egg whites
Cooking spray

DIRECTIONS

1. Preheat oven to 350°F degrees.
2. Place zucchini planks in a large colander in the sink. Sprinkle strips lightly with salt and toss so salt covers most of the zucchini. Let rest while preparing remaining recipe. (This will take the moisture out of the zucchini, so the lasagna won't be watery.)
3. Heat oil in a medium skillet over medium heat; brown ground pork seasoned with sausage seasoning. Set aside.
4. Place the diced tomatoes and chiles, garlic powder, Italian seasoning, and cayenne pepper in a blender; blend until smooth. Set aside.
5. In a medium bowl, lightly beat together the eggs + egg whites. Set aside.
6. Spray an 8" x 8" square baking pan with cooking spray.
7. Remove zucchini strips from colander, blot with paper towels to remove excess moisture. Layer ½ the zucchini strips, covering the bottom of the baking pan.
8. Layer ½ the seasoned meat, spreading evenly.
9. Pour ½ the tomato mixture evenly over the meat.
10. Pour ½ the eggs evenly over the tomato mixture.
11. Repeat these layers, in order.
12. Bake 40 minutes.

SERVINGS

Entire recipe yield = 12 oz. lean protein + 4 C. veggies
½ recipe yield = 6 oz. lean protein + 2 C. veggies

Asian-Style Spaghetti & Meatballs
Air Fryer recipe

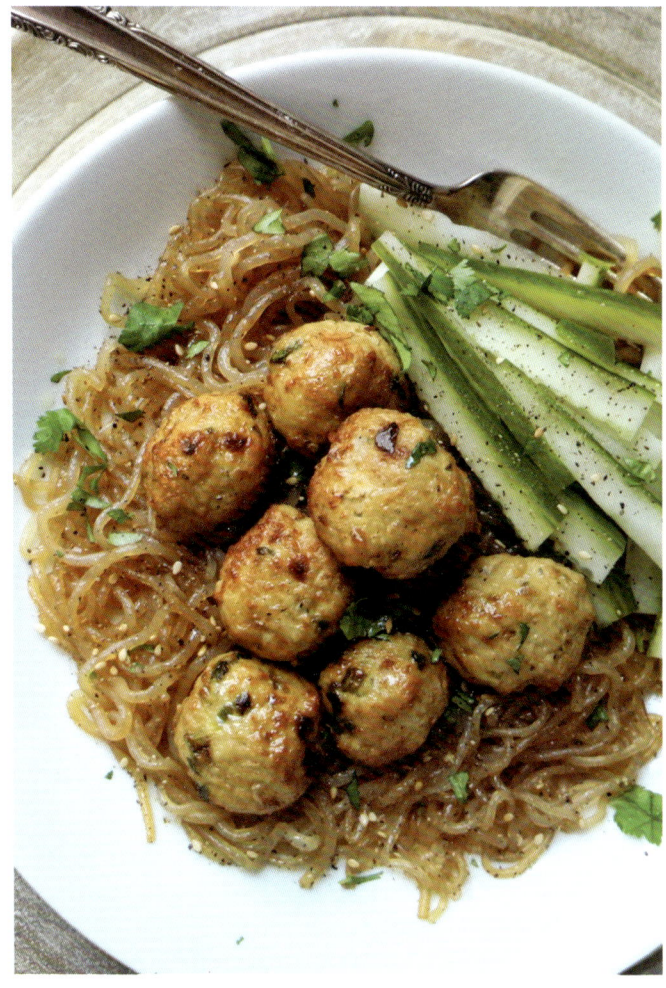

INGREDIENTS (MEATBALLS)
1 pkg. Ideal Protein garlic parmesan croutons, crushed to crumbs
1 large egg
2 T. lime juice
1 T. Ideal Protein maple syrup
1 tsp. soy sauce
1 T. grated fresh ginger
1 T. minced jalapeno pepper (seeded)
¼ C. fresh cilantro, finely chopped
2 T. finely chopped green onion
17 oz. ground chicken

INGREDIENTS (SPAGHETTI)
3 packages Ideal Protein konjac spaghetti
1 T. toasted sesame oil
3 T. soy sauce
Pinch of red pepper flakes

DIRECTIONS
1. Add all meatball ingredients (except chicken) to a medium mixing bowl, whisk to blend.
2. Add ground chicken and mix with hands until blended. Shape into tablespoon size meatballs (using a small cookie dough scoop works great.)
3. Place meatballs in air fryer basket; meatballs can be touching but not stacked. (Bake in batches if necessary.)
4. Bake at 400°F degrees for 10-12 minutes turning meatballs once during baking.
5. Meanwhile, drain and rinse konjac spaghetti noodles; pat dry. Add to a skillet with oil, soy sauce, and red pepper flakes. Stir fry 3 minutes over medium heat.
6. Plate konjac spaghetti noodles and top with meatballs. Sprinkle with additional chopped cilantro, if desired.

SERVINGS
Entire recipe yield = 18 oz. lean protein (ground chicken + egg) + 3 T. veggies + 1 T. oil + 3 C. konjac spaghetti
⅓ recipe yield = 6 oz. lean protein (ground chicken + egg) + 1 T. veggies + 1 tsp. oil + 1 C. konjac spaghetti

TIP: Delicious served with julienned fresh cucumber.

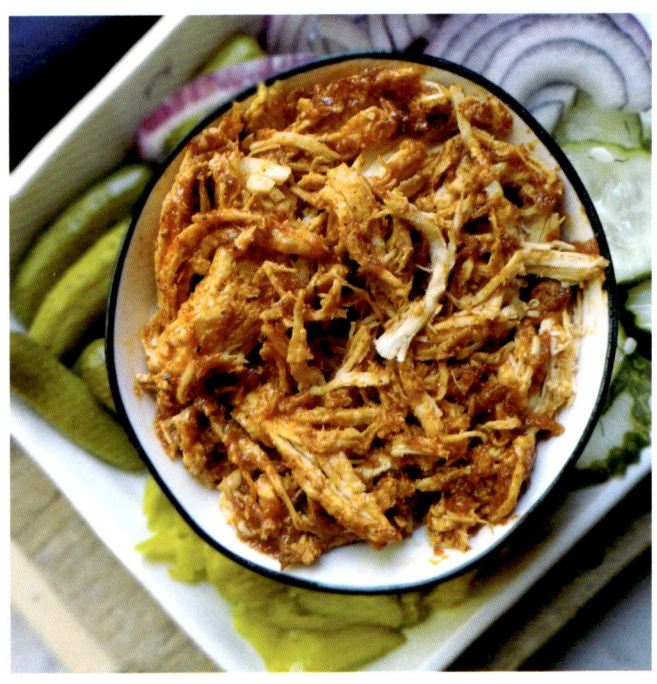

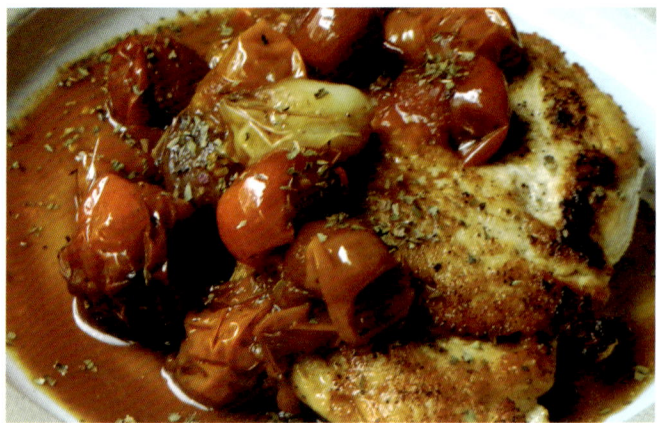

BBQ Pulled Chicken

Slow cooker recipe – juicy and tender chicken!

INGREDIENTS

42 oz. (2 lbs. 10 oz.) chicken breasts, boneless and
   skinless
Sassy BBQ Sauce, pg. 147 (use entire recipe)

DIRECTIONS

1. Place chicken breasts in slow cooker.
2. Pour BBQ sauce over chicken; spread sauce to
   completely coat chicken.
3. Cover and cook on high 3 hours; chicken is done
   when cooked through and easy to shred.
4. Transfer chicken breasts to a work surface; using
   two forks, shred chicken meat.
5. Return shredded chicken to slow cooker;
   stir into juices.

SERVINGS

Entire recipe yield = 42 oz. lean protein + BBQ
Sauce (2 C. veggies + 1 T. oil)
½ recipe yield = 6 oz. lean protein + BBQ Sauce (¼
C. veggies + ¼ tsp. oil)

TIP: BBQ Pulled Chicken freezes nicely when stored
in an airtight container.

Bruschetta Chicken

INGREDIENTS

2 - 6 oz. chicken breasts, boneless and skinless
¾ tsp. sea salt
½ tsp. black pepper
¾ tsp. garlic powder
4 tsp. olive oil, divided
¼ C. Ideal Protein balsamic dressing
1 ½ tsp. minced garlic
4 C. cherry tomatoes (or baby heirloom tomatoes)
2 T. chopped fresh basil

DIRECTIONS

1. Place chicken breasts in a large resealable plastic
   bag. Using a meat mallet, pound chicken evenly
   to ½-inch thickness. Season both sides of the
   breasts with salt, pepper, and garlic powder.
2. Heat 2 tsp. oil in a large skillet over medium/medium
   high heat. When oil is hot, add chicken breasts and
   cook 3 minutes each side. Once cooked, transfer
   chicken to a plate and cover to keep warm.
3. Meanwhile, heat the balsamic dressing over
   medium heat to bubbling in a small saucepan.
   Reduce heat to medium low and simmer 6
   minutes to thicken; stir often.
4. Add the remaining oil, dressing, garlic, and
   tomatoes to the hot skillet. Cover and cook on
   medium/medium low 8 minutes or until tomatoes start to blister.
5. Top chicken with tomato and dressing mixture.
   Sprinkle with basil.

SERVINGS

Entire recipe yield = 12 oz. lean protein + 4 C.
veggies + 4 tsp. oil
½ recipe yield = 6 oz. lean protein + 2 C. veggies +
2 tsp. oil

Buffalo Chicken Meatballs

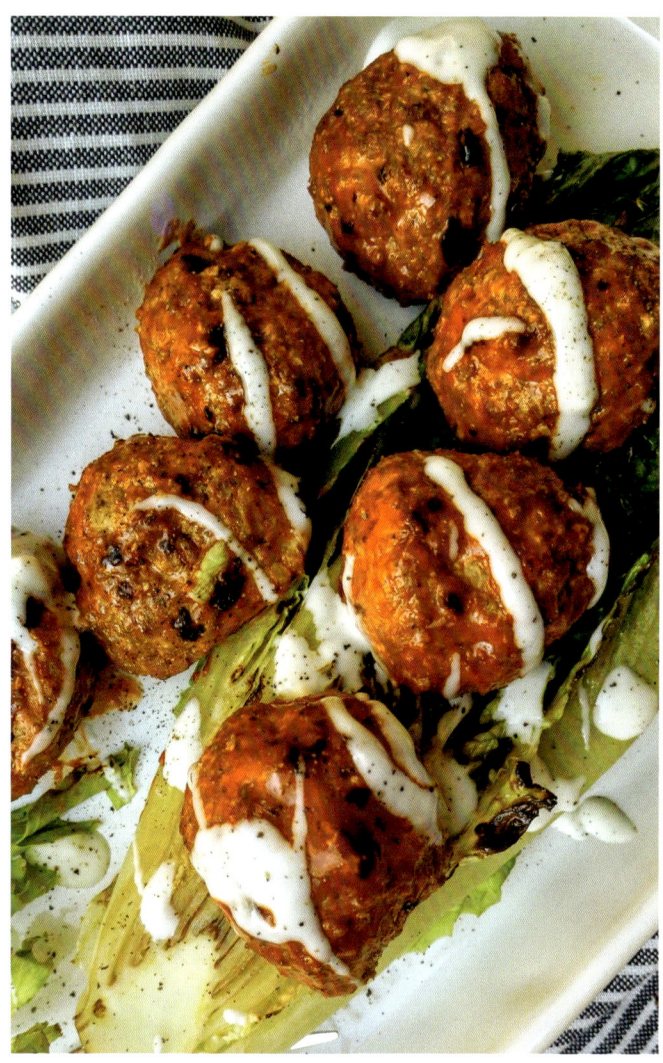

INGREDIENTS

2 C. (7 oz.) cauliflower florets
½ C. chopped green onion
½ C. chopped zucchini
18 oz. ground chicken or turkey
1 tsp. garlic powder
1 tsp. onion powder
1 ¼ tsp. Ideal Protein salt
3 T. liquid egg whites
½ C. Buffalo wing hot sauce
Walden Farms blue cheese dressing, for dipping
Celery sticks, optional

DIRECTIONS

1. Preheat oven to 350°F degrees.
2. Place cauliflower, green onion, and zucchini in a food processor; pulse to consistency of rice. Blot mixture with paper towels to absorb excess moisture.
3. In a large bowl, combine ground chicken, riced veggie mixture, garlic powder, onion powder, salt, and liquid egg whites. Gently mix with hands until combined. Avoid over-working the mix.
4. Line a baking sheet with parchment paper. Scoop meat mixture (about 1 scant ice cream scoop for each meatball) and gently roll portions between palms to form a smooth ball. Place meatballs on baking sheet, spaced apart.
5. Bake meatballs 20 minutes. Remove meatballs from oven.
6. Pour Buffalo wing sauce into a bowl and transfer meatballs to the bowl; toss to coat. Let the meatballs sit in the sauce; raise the oven temperature to 450°F degrees and replace parchment paper with a new sheet.
7. When oven has reached 450°F degrees, give meatballs another toss in the bowl, transfer meatballs to baking sheet and bake an additional 15 - 20 minutes or until lightly browned and done.
8. Serve with additional Buffalo wing sauce, dressing, and celery sticks, if desired.

SERVINGS

Entire recipe yield = 18 oz. lean protein + 3 C. veggies
⅓ recipe yield = 6 oz. lean protein + 1 C. veggies

TIP: Serve meatballs over grilled romaine lettuce topped with dressing, salt, and pepper.

Chicken & Asparagus Stir Fry

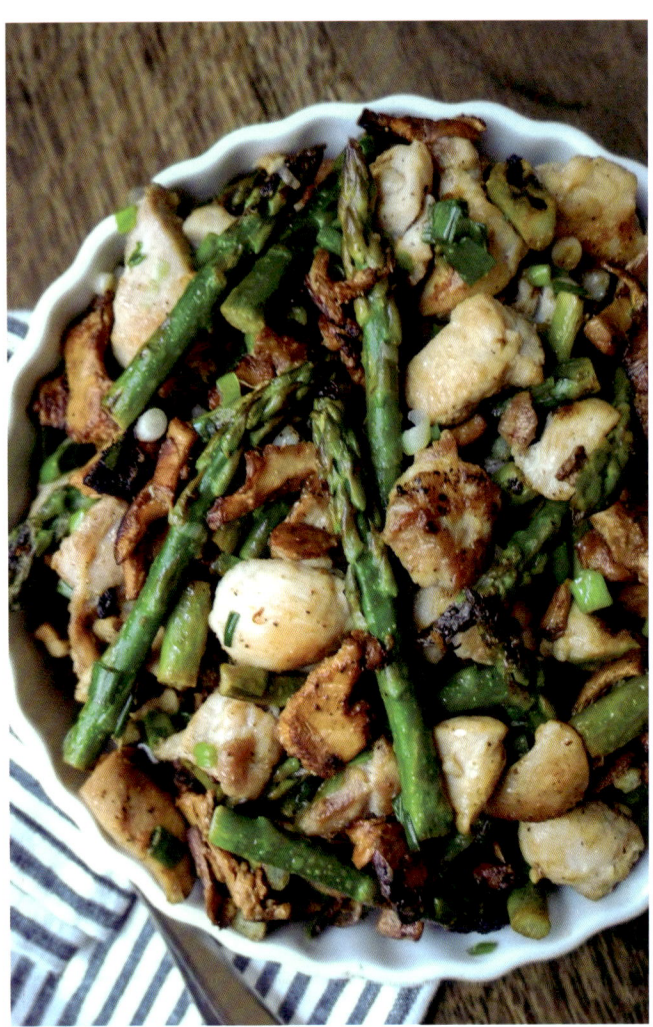

INGREDIENTS

2 T. + 2 tsp. olive oil, divided
24 oz. chicken breast, boneless and skinless
  (cut into bite size pieces)
Salt and pepper, to taste
4 C. sliced baby bella mushrooms
1 C. chopped green onion
3 C. fresh asparagus tips (cut 2" from tip)
3 T. lemon juice
3 T. soy sauce
1 tsp. garlic powder

DIRECTIONS

1. Heat 1 T. + 1 tsp. oil in a large skillet over medium heat. Add chicken in one layer and season with salt and pepper.
2. Cook chicken 4 minutes undisturbed; flip and cook another 4 minutes undisturbed, until golden brown.
3. Transfer chicken to a plate using a slotted spoon (reserving any oil in pan). Cover chicken with aluminum foil to keep warm; set aside.
4. Add remaining 1 T. + 1 tsp. oil to pan and heat over medium heat. When oil is hot, add mushrooms and stir fry 3-4 minutes or until lightly browned.
5. Add remaining ingredients (except chicken); fold to mix. Cover and cook 3-4 minutes until asparagus is tender crisp, folding occasionally.
6. Add chicken and heat through. Serve with additional soy sauce, if desired.

SERVINGS

Entire recipe yield = 24 oz. lean protein + 8 C. veggies + 8 tsp. oil
¼ recipe yield = 6 oz. lean protein + 2 C. veggies + 2 tsp. oil

Chicken Cacciatore Spaghetti & Meatballs

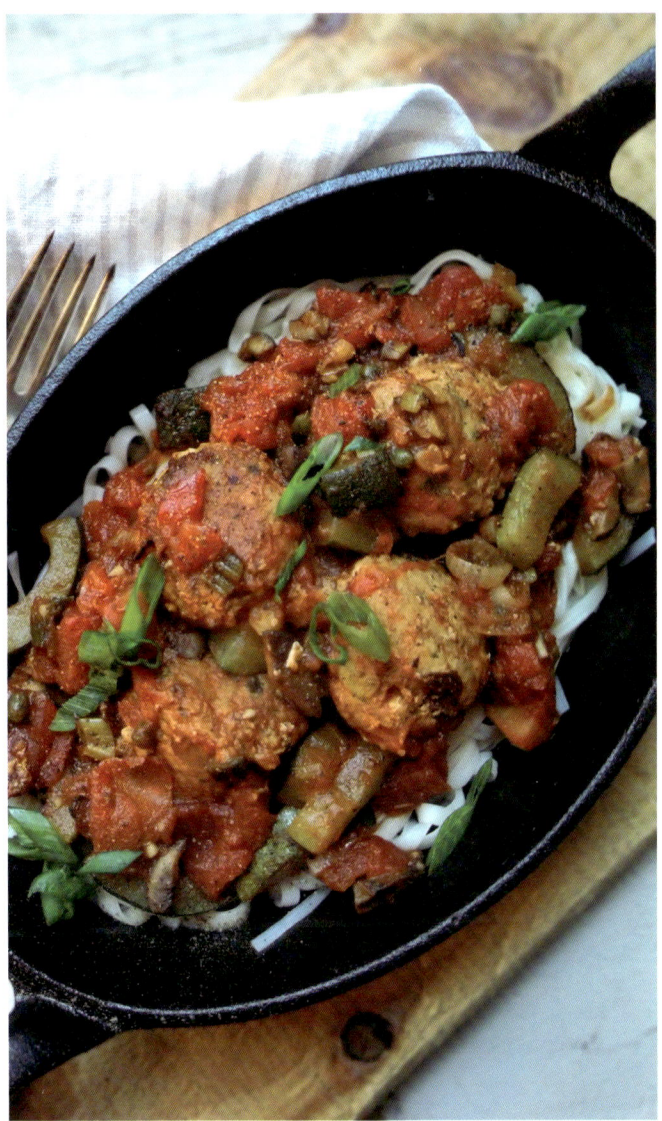

INGREDIENTS (MEATBALLS)
17 oz. ground chicken or turkey
1 large egg, lightly beaten
2 T. chopped fresh Italian parsley
1 tsp. kosher salt
½ tsp. garlic powder
¼ tsp. black pepper
1 T. olive oil

INGREDIENTS (SAUCE)
1 T. olive oil
1 C. chopped baby bella mushrooms
½ C. chopped green onion
1 ½ C. chopped zucchini, skin on (pith removed)
1 - 14.5 oz. can diced tomatoes, undrained
1 C. chicken broth
1 tsp. minced garlic
1 T. capers, drained
1 tsp. dried oregano
¼ tsp. red pepper flakes
3 packages Ideal Protein konjac spaghetti, optional

DIRECTIONS
1. Combine all meatball ingredients (except oil) in a medium bowl and mix well. Make 12 meatballs.
2. Brush a large skillet with the oil and heat over medium heat. Add meatballs and brown all sides. Transfer meatballs to a plate; cover to keep warm while preparing sauce.
3. Prepare sauce by adding oil to same skillet; heat over medium heat. Add mushrooms, green onion, and zucchini. Sauté 2-3 minutes or until lightly browned.
4. Add remaining sauce ingredients to skillet (except konjac spaghetti); stir. Return meatballs to skillet; cover and simmer 8-10 minutes. Remove cover and cook a few minutes longer for a thicker sauce.
5. Serve over warmed konjac spaghetti, if desired.

SERVINGS
Entire recipe yield = 18 oz. lean protein + 6 C. veggies + 6 tsp. oil + 3 C. konjac spaghetti
⅓ recipe yield = 6 oz. lean protein + 2 C. veggies + 2 tsp. oil + 1 C. konjac spaghetti

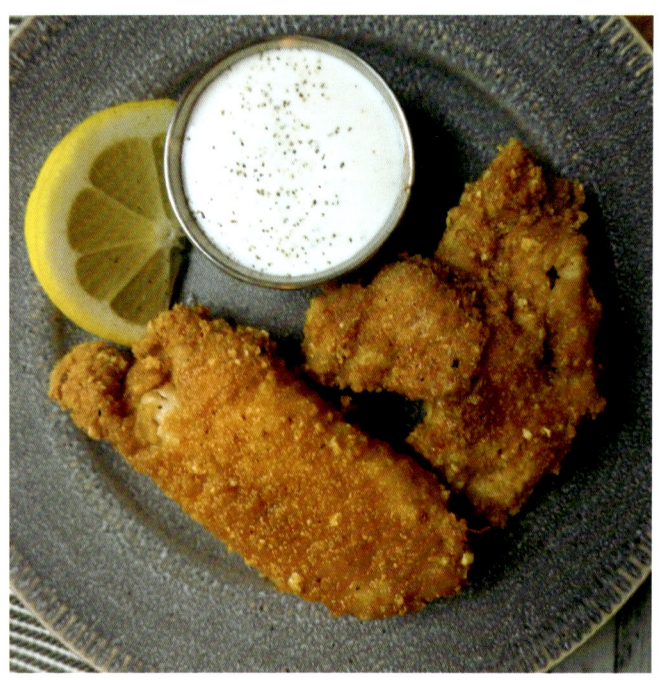

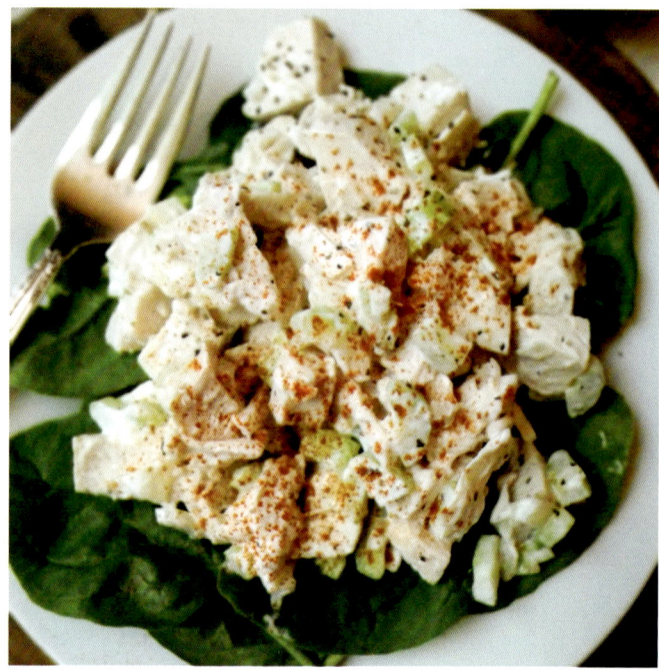

Chicken Fingers
Air Fryer recipe

INGREDIENTS
1 pkg. Ideal Protein chips or Dorados (any flavor),
   crushed to fine crumbs
1 T. liquid egg whites
6 oz. chicken tenders
Olive oil spray
Ideal Protein salt, to taste

DIRECTIONS
1. Place crumbs and egg whites on two separate small plates.
2. Dredge tenders in egg whites; press into crumbs coating both sides.
3. Spray olive oil on both sides of breaded tenders; season with salt. Place tenders in air fryer basket in one layer.
4. Cook 10-12 minutes at 400°F flipping once during cooking.

SERVINGS
Entire recipe yield = 6 oz. lean protein + 1 unrestricted + ⅛ tsp. oil

Chicken Salad

INGREDIENTS
6 oz. cooked chicken breast, cut in bite size pieces
¼ C. chopped celery
2 T. chopped yellow onion
1 T. Janeva's mayonnaise, pg. 141
Salt and pepper, to taste
Smoked paprika, to taste

DIRECTIONS
1. Place all ingredients in a medium bowl; gently fold to mix.

SERVINGS
Entire recipe yield = 6 oz. lean protein + 2 T. veggies + 2 tsp. oil (mayonnaise)

NOTE: Celery is unlimited and not considered toward veggie count.

TIP: Delicious served with Carolina Cabbage Slaw, pg. 46

Chicken Shawarma

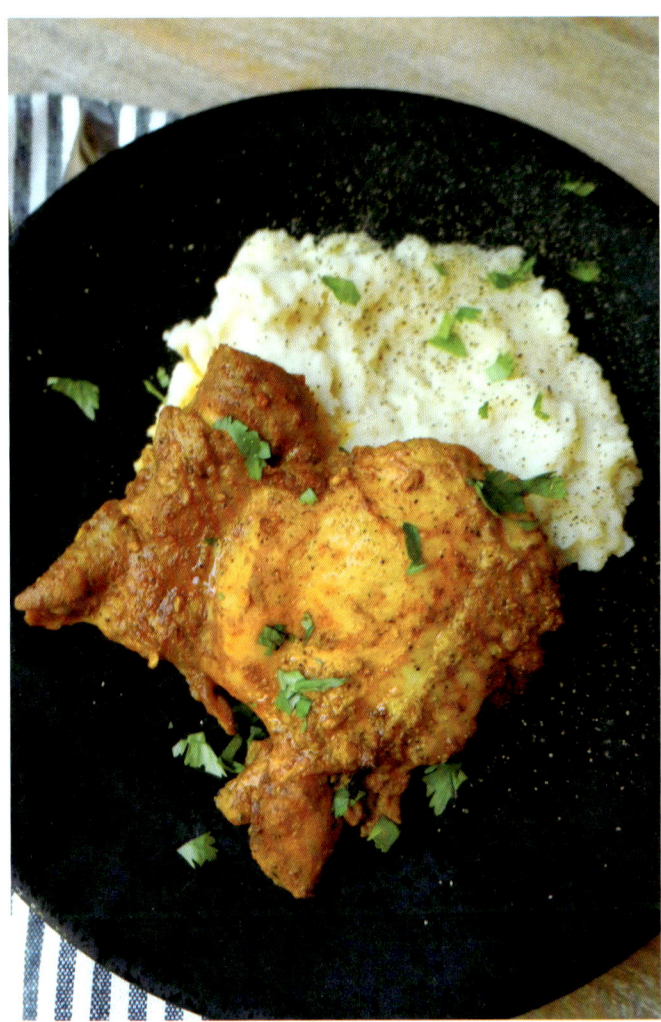

INGREDIENTS

30 oz. chicken thighs, boneless and skinless*
¼ C. lemon juice
1 T. + 2 tsp. olive oil
2 tsp. minced garlic
2 tsp. smoked paprika
2 tsp. ground cumin
1 tsp. turmeric
½ tsp. cinnamon
1 tsp. Ideal Protein salt
1 tsp. black pepper
Chopped fresh cilantro, to taste

DIRECTIONS

1. Trim any fat from the chicken thighs and discard. Place chicken in a large resealable plastic bag; set aside.
2. In a medium mixing bowl, add remaining ingredients (except cilantro); stir to blend.
3. Pour marinade over chicken; remove as much air as possible and seal the bag. Toss or massage bag to coat chicken and place in refrigerator to marinate at least 2 hours or up to 14 hours.
4. Preheat oven to 425° F degrees.
5. Line a baking sheet with aluminum foil. Lay chicken thighs on baking sheet at least 2 inches apart (discard marinade). Bake 20 minutes.
6. Turn oven heat to broil. Move oven rack to highest rung and broil chicken approximately 2 minutes or until browned. Serve topped with cilantro.

SERVINGS

Entire recipe yield = 30 oz. lean protein + 5 tsp. oil
⅕ recipe yield = 6 oz. lean protein + 1 tsp. oil

TIP: *Boneless and skinless chicken breast may be used in place of the chicken thighs; however, the breasts must be pounded to ½-inch thickness, or they will not cook properly. This meal is delicious served with Celery Root Puree (pg. 114), or Cauliflower Mash (pg. 112).

Chinese 5 Spice Chicken

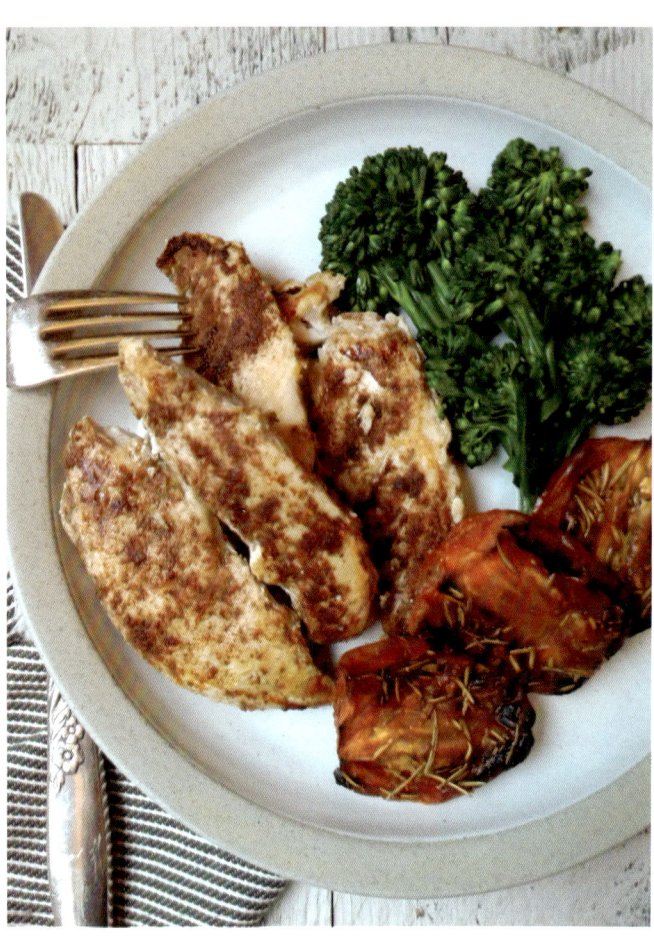

INGREDIENTS

18 oz. chicken tenders, boneless and skinless
1 T. white vinegar
1 T. soy sauce
1 ½ tsp. Chinese five spice powder
1 tsp. minced garlic
1 tsp. minced fresh ginger
½ tsp. sea salt
1 T. olive oil

DIRECTIONS

1. Place chicken tenders in a large resealable plastic bag. Using a meat mallet, pound tenders to ½-inch thickness. Leave in bag (for marinating) and set aside.
2. Whisk remaining ingredients (except oil) in a small bowl. Pour over chicken; remove as much air from the bag as possible and seal bag. Toss to coat chicken and marinate chicken in fridge at least 4 hours or overnight.
3. Brush a grill pan or skillet with olive oil; heat over medium/medium high heat. When oil is hot, add chicken and cook 6-8 minutes flipping once during cooking. Discard marinade.

SERVINGS

Entire recipe yield = 18 oz. lean protein + 1 T. oil
⅓ recipe yield = 6 oz. lean protein + 1 tsp. oil

TIP: Delicious served with roasted spaghetti squash, tomatoes, broccolini and/or Bok choy.

Gyros

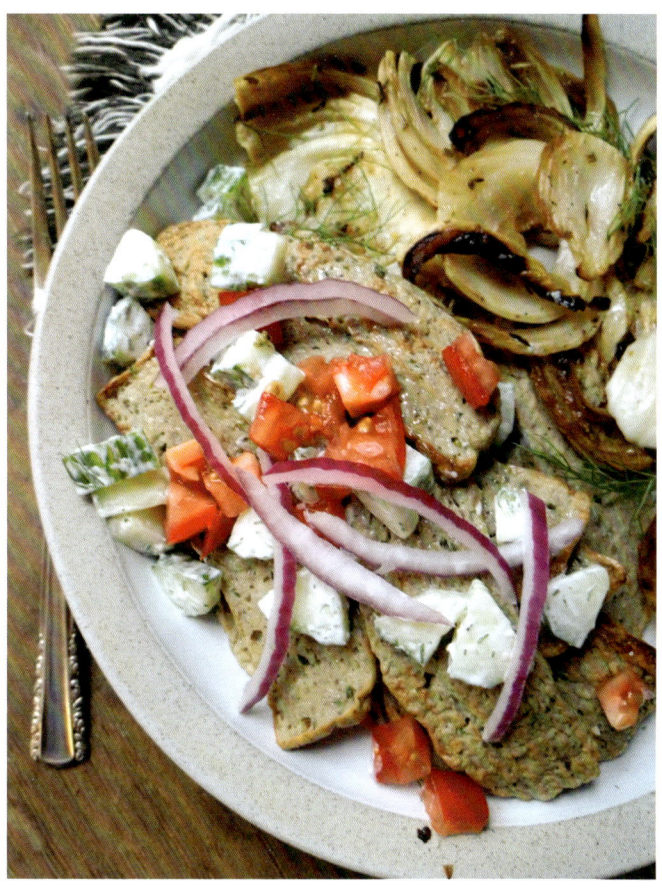

INGREDIENTS
17 oz. ground chicken or lamb
2 tsp. kosher salt
½ tsp. freshly ground black pepper
¼ C. chopped green onions
2 T. fresh oregano leaves
½ tsp. minced garlic
1 large egg

DIRECTIONS
1. Preheat oven to 300°F degrees.
2. Place all gyro ingredients in the bowl of a food processor. Process until a smooth puree is formed, scraping down sides of bowl as necessary.
3. Line a rimmed baking sheet with aluminum foil. With moistened hands, shape the gyro mixture into a rectangle about 7-inches long x 4-inches wide. Bake 30-35 minutes or until the center of loaf reaches at least 160°F degrees on an instant-read thermometer. Remove from oven and allow to rest for 15 minutes.
4. Adjust oven rack to highest position below broiler element and preheat broiler. Slice the loaf of chicken meat crosswise into 4-inch strips about ¼-inch thick.
5. Lay the strips in a single layer on rimmed baking sheet. Broil gyro strips until edges are browned (about 2 minutes); flip strips and brown other side (about 2 minutes). Watch closely as the broiler works quickly and meat can dry out if over cooked.

SERVINGS
Entire recipe yield = 18 oz. lean protein (lean protein + egg)
⅓ recipe yield = 6 oz. lean protein (lean protein + egg)

TIP: Gyro meat is delicious served over a salad,or alongside the Apple Cider Roasted Fennel, pg. 108.

Italian Chicken & Spinach Skillet

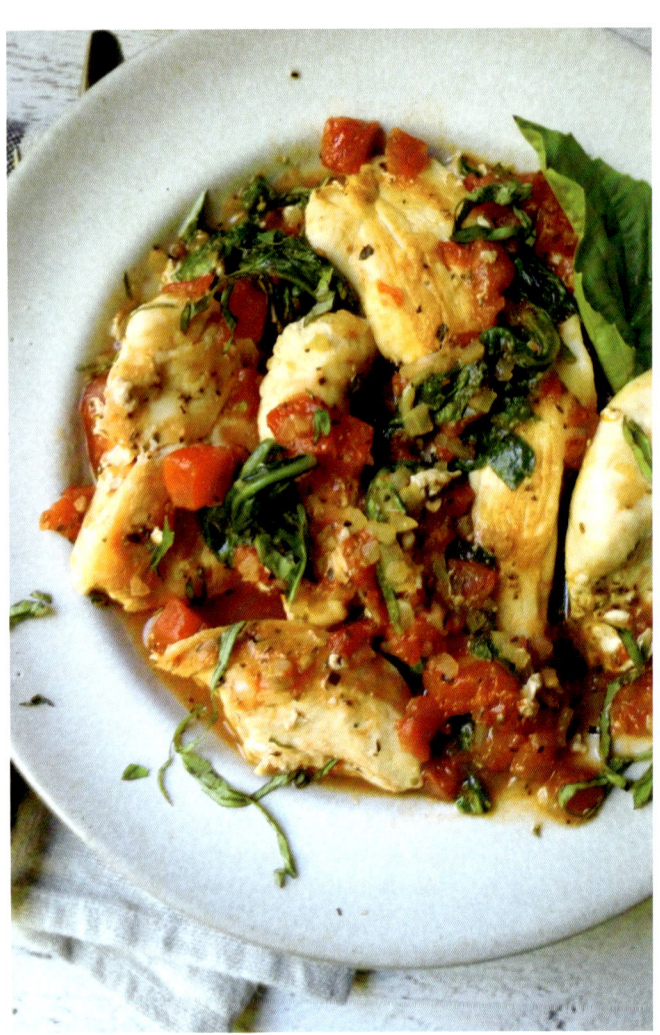

INGREDIENTS

½ C. chicken broth
2 T. dried minced onion
2 T. olive oil
30 oz. chicken tenders, boneless & skinless
1 tsp. dried basil leaves
1 tsp. Ideal Protein salt
½ tsp. black pepper
½ tsp. garlic powder
½ tsp. oregano leaves
14.5 oz. can petite diced tomatoes, undrained
4 C. fresh baby spinach, firmly packed

DIRECTIONS

1. Combine chicken broth and minced onion in a small bowl (to hydrate onions); set aside.
2. Heat oil in a large skillet on medium heat. Add chicken; cook 5 minutes or until lightly browned.
3. Flip and pour broth mixture over the chicken; sprinkle with dry seasonings and cook an additional 5 minutes.
4. Add tomatoes to skillet and reduce heat to medium low; cover and simmer 3 minutes.
5. Add spinach to skillet; cover and cook 2 minutes or until spinach begins to wilt. Stir wilted spinach into skillet mixture.

SERVINGS

Entire recipe yield = 30 oz. lean protein + 7 ½ C. veggies + 2 T. oil
⅕ recipe yield = 6 oz. lean protein + 1 ¼ C. veggies + 1 ¼ tsp. oil

Jamaican Curry Chicken
Instant Pot recipe

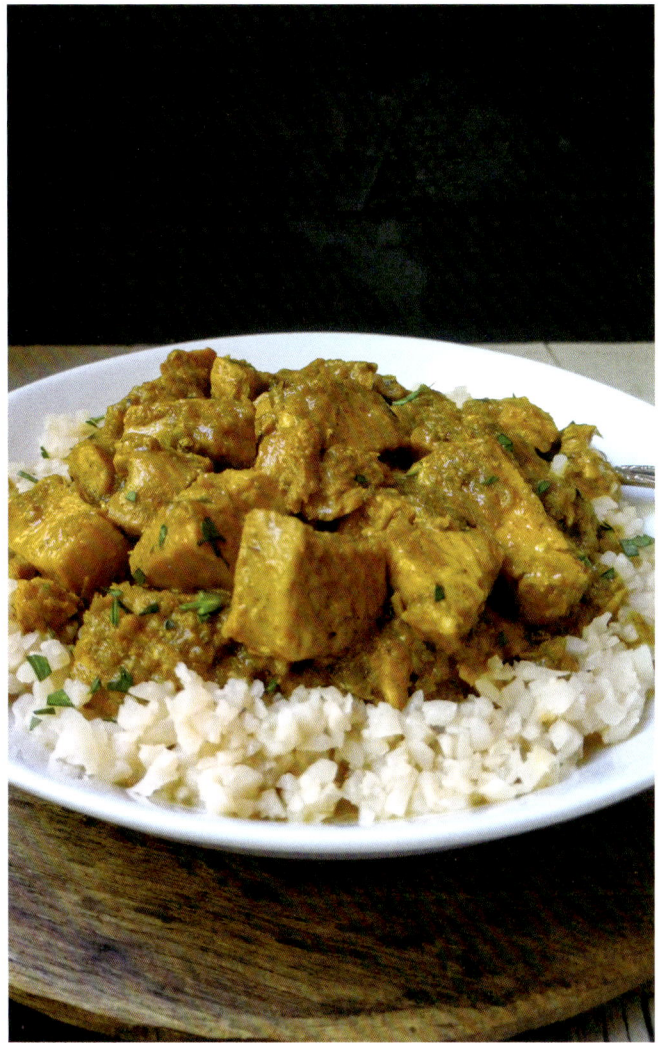

INGREDIENTS

2 T. olive oil
1 T. minced garlic
1 T. minced fresh ginger
¼ C. dried minced onion
1 serrano pepper (split, seeded and chopped)
1 tsp. sea salt
1 T. + 1 ½ tsp. Jamaican curry powder
½ tsp. dried thyme
½ tsp. ground allspice
½ C. water, divided
18 oz. chicken breasts (boneless & skinless), cut in 1-inch chunks

DIRECTIONS

1. Add oil to the instant pot and heat on sauté mode. When oil is hot, add garlic, ginger, and dried minced onion; cook 1 minute, stirring constantly.
2. Add serrano pepper and remaining spices. Cook 1 minute stirring constantly. (Add up to ¼ C. of the water as necessary to deglaze the pot and scrape off any spices that have stuck to the bottom.)
3. Add chicken and remaining ¼ C. water; stir to coat chicken with spice mixture.
4. Cover instant pot with lid and seal. Cook on high pressure 6 minutes; let naturally release 10 minutes, then quick release pressure.

SERVINGS

Entire recipe yield = 18 oz. lean protein + 1 C. veggies (dried onion) + 2 T. oil
⅓ recipe yield = 6 oz. lean protein + ⅓ C. veggies (dried onion) + 2 tsp. oil

NOTE: The serrano pepper is nominal and not counted in the veggie total.

TIP: Excellent served over cauliflower rice.

Lemon Garlic Chicken

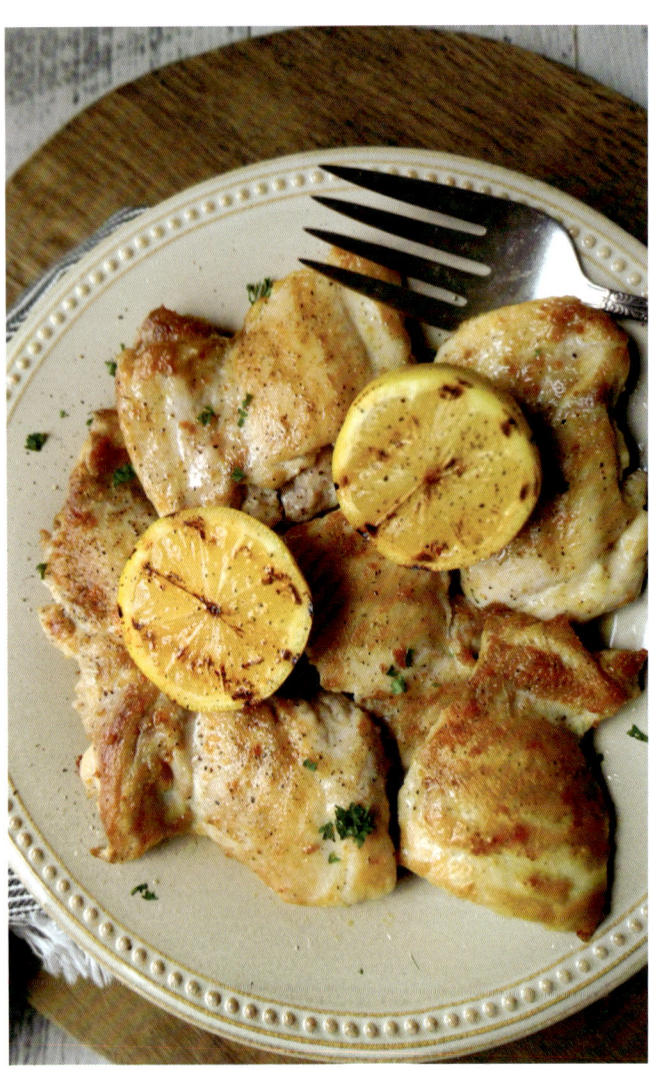

INGREDIENTS

1 lemon
½ C. chicken broth
3 T. olive oil, divided
2 tsp. Dijon mustard
1 tsp. minced garlic
1 tsp. dried oregano
½ tsp. dried thyme leaves
½ tsp. salt
¼ tsp. black pepper
36 oz. chicken thighs, boneless and skinless*

DIRECTIONS

1. Zest and juice the lemon; add to a medium mixing bowl. Discard lemon.
2. To same bowl, add 2 T. of the olive oil and remaining ingredients (except chicken); whisk to blend.
3. Pour marinade mixture into a large plastic resealable bag. Add chicken, remove air, and seal. Marinate chicken 2 hours to overnight, turning bag occasionally. Keep stored in fridge.
4. Remove chicken from marinade shaking off excess liquid. Plate, set aside, and discard marinade.
5. Brush a stove top grill pan with remaining olive oil. Heat over medium heat. When oil is hot, add chicken thighs and cook both sides 4-5 minutes.

SERVINGS

Entire recipe yield = 36 oz. lean protein + 3 T. oil
⅙ recipe yield = 6 oz. lean protein + 1 ½ tsp. oil

TIP: *Chicken breasts may be subbed for the chicken thighs in this recipe. To prepare, place breasts in a large resealable bag and pound to ½-inch thickness before marinating. Follow same recipe directions for cooking.

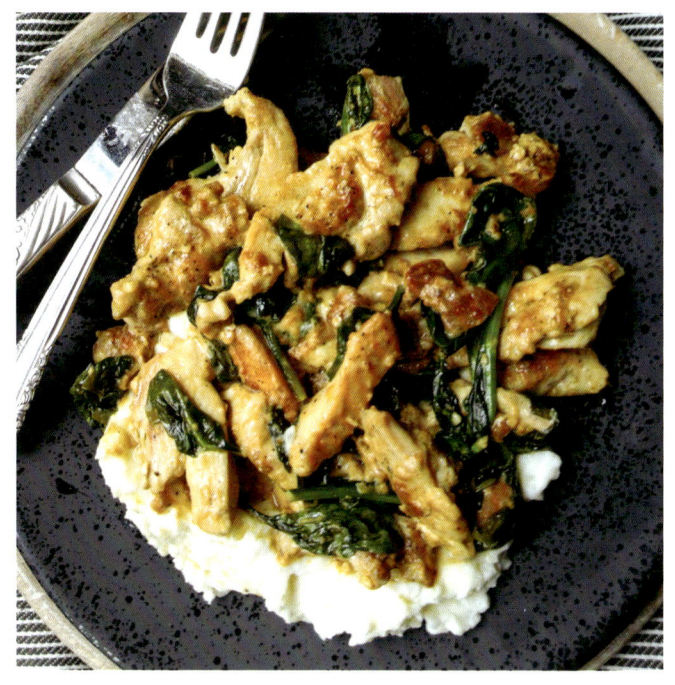

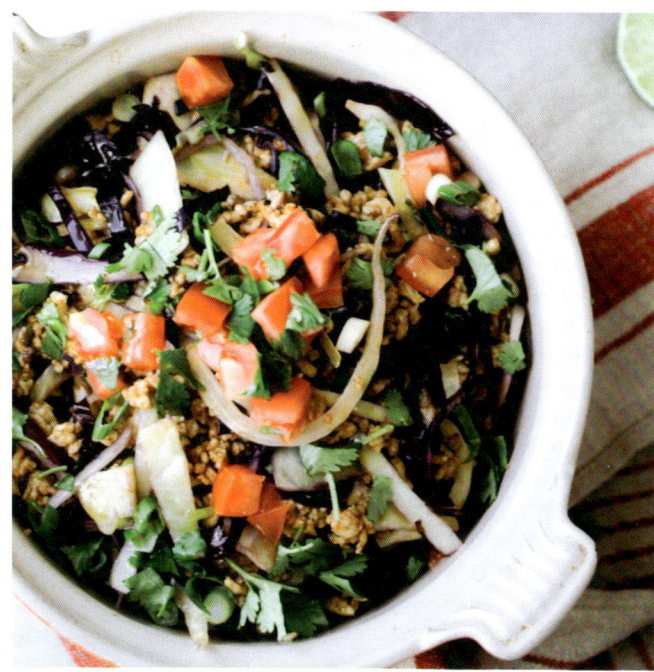

Maple Dijon Chicken Skillet

INGREDIENTS
¼ C. Ideal Protein maple syrup
¼ C. Dijon mustard
1 T. apple cider vinegar
1 tsp. minced garlic
1 T. olive oil
18 oz. chicken thighs, boneless and skinless
   (cut in ½" inch strips)
Salt & pepper, to taste
3 C. fresh spinach, firmly packed

DIRECTIONS
1. Add the syrup, mustard, vinegar, and garlic to a small bowl; stir to mix. Set aside.
2. Heat oil in a large skillet over medium heat. When oil is hot, add chicken and spread in one layer. Season with salt and pepper. Cook 6 minutes flipping once during cooking, until lightly browned and crispy.
3. Stir in mustard mixture. Add spinach; cover and cook 1 minute or until spinach is wilted. Stir spinach into chicken mixture. Season with additional salt and pepper if desired.

SERVINGS
Entire recipe yield = 18 oz. lean protein + 1 T. oil
⅓ recipe yield = 6 oz. lean protein + 1 tsp. oil

Mexican Crack Slaw

INGREDIENTS
12 oz. ground turkey, chicken, or beef
1 T. Taco Seasoning, pg. 149
1 T + 1 tsp. avocado oil or olive oil
1 ¾ C. thinly sliced green cabbage
1 ¾ C. thinly sliced red cabbage
½ C. chopped green onion
Chopped fresh cilantro, to taste
Pico de Gallo, pg. 145 (for topping, optional)

DIRECTIONS
1. Add ground turkey and taco seasoning to a large skillet; brown over medium heat. Transfer turkey to a bowl; set aside.
2. To same skillet, add oil and heat over medium heat. When oil is hot, add cabbage and green onion. Stir fry until cabbage is softened and wilted, approximately 10-12 minutes.
3. Add ground turkey; heat through.
4. Serve topped with cilantro and Pico de Gallo, if desired.

SERVINGS
Entire recipe yield = 12 oz. lean protein + 4 C. veggies + 4 tsp. oil
½ recipe yield = 6 oz. lean protein + 2 C. veggies + 2 tsp. oil

Moroccan Chicken
With curry cauliflower puree

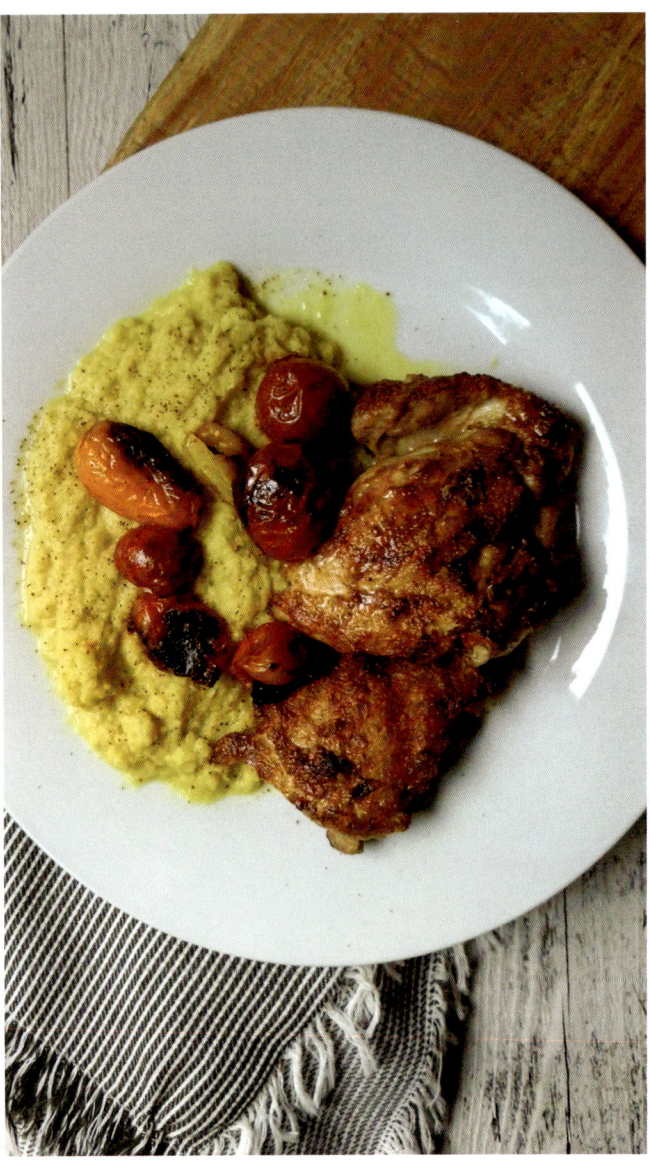

INGREDIENTS (CHICKEN)
1 tsp. ground ginger
½ tsp. ground coriander
½ tsp. ground cumin
½ tsp. kosher salt
¼ tsp. cayenne pepper
¼ tsp. black pepper
1 T. + 1 tsp. olive oil
12 oz. chicken thighs, boneless and skinless
1 C. cherry or baby heirloom tomatoes

INGREDIENTS (CAULIFLOWER PUREE)
3 C. fresh or frozen cauliflower florets
⅔ C. chicken broth
¾ tsp. curry powder
2 T. half and half cream
Kosher salt and black pepper, to taste

DIRECTIONS
1. In a large bowl mix the ginger, coriander, cumin, salt, cayenne pepper and black pepper.
2. Add chicken thighs to bowl and toss with seasonings to coat; set aside.
3. Add cauliflower florets, chicken broth and curry powder to a medium saucepan. Heat to a low boil over high heat. Reduce heat; cover and simmer 10 minutes. Remove from heat.
4. Meanwhile, heat oil in a large skillet over medium/medium high heat. Add chicken thighs and tomatoes; cook chicken thighs 5 minutes each side while occasionally stirring the tomatoes until blistered. Plate and cover to keep warm while finishing cauliflower puree.
5. To the cooked cauliflower, add half and half cream, salt, and pepper. Using a stick blender, puree cauliflower mixture.
6. Plate puree and top with chicken and tomatoes. Season with additional salt and pepper, if necessary.

SERVINGS
Entire recipe yield = 12 oz. lean protein + 4 C. veggies + 4 tsp. oil + 1 oz. half and half cream
½ recipe yield = 6 oz. lean protein + 2 C. veggies + 2 tsp. oil + 0.5 oz. half and half cream

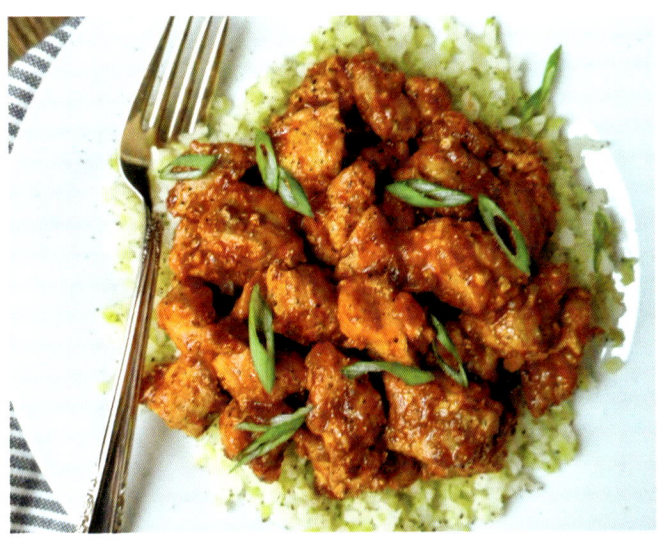

Orange Chicken

INGREDIENTS (ORANGE SAUCE)
½ C. Walden Farms orange marmalade
½ C. Sassy BBQ sauce, pg. 147
2 T. soy sauce
½ tsp. onion powder
1 tsp. minced garlic
¼ tsp. red pepper flakes

INGREDIENTS (CHICKEN)
24 oz. chicken breast or thighs, boneless and
   skinless (cut in 1" inch chunks)
Salt and pepper, to taste
1 T. + 1 tsp. olive oil

DIRECTIONS
1. In a medium bowl, whisk orange sauce ingredients until blended; set aside.
2. Season chicken with salt and pepper.
3. Brush the bottom of a large skillet with oil; heat over medium/medium high heat. When oil is hot, add chicken and stir fry 6-8 minutes or until lightly browned and cooked through.
4. Stir orange sauce into chicken to coat and reduce heat to medium/medium low. Cook 4 minutes, stirring constantly. Cover pan, turn off burner, let rest on burner 3-4 minutes.
5. Stir to coat and serve.

SERVINGS
Entire recipe yield = 24 oz. lean protein + ½ C. veggies (BBQ sauce) + 4 tsp. oil
¼ recipe yield = 6 oz. lean protein + 2 T. veggies (BBQ sauce) + 1 tsp. oil

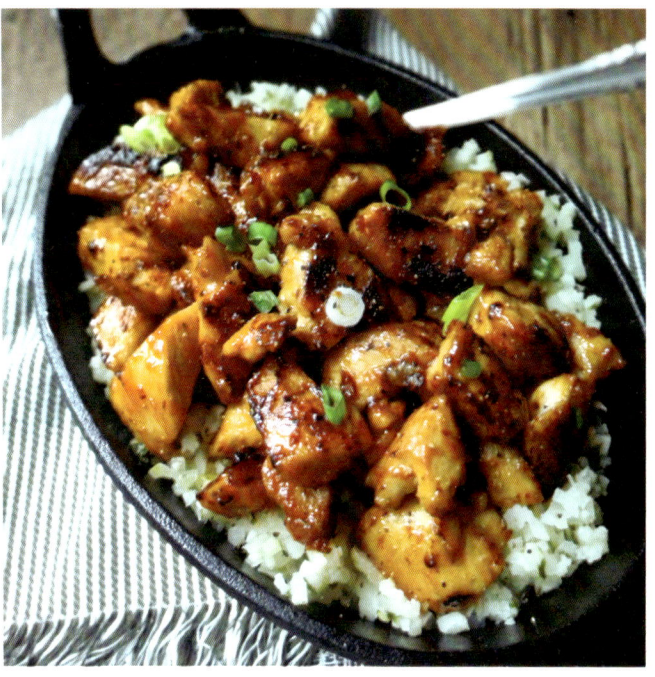

Sweet & Sour Chicken

INGREDIENTS
12 oz. chicken breasts, skinless and boneless
   (cut in 1" chunks)
Salt and pepper, to taste
1 T. + 1 tsp. olive oil
¼ C. Sweet & Sour Sauce, pg. 149

DIRECTIONS
1. Season chicken with salt and pepper.
2. Brush the bottom of a skillet with oil; heat over medium/medium high heat.
3. Add chicken; stir fry for 10 minutes or until lightly browned.
4. Reduce heat to just under medium; add sweet & sour sauce. Stir fry until sauce reduces and thickens.

SERVINGS
Entire recipe yield = 12 oz. lean protein + ½ C. veggies (sauce)
½ recipe yield = 6 oz. lean protein + ¼ C. veggies (sauce)

TIP: Excellent served over cauliflower rice – I use Green Giant® steamer bags of the cauliflower rice making this recipe quick and easy.

Tikka Masala

A popular Indian chicken dish full of flavor, spice and heat!

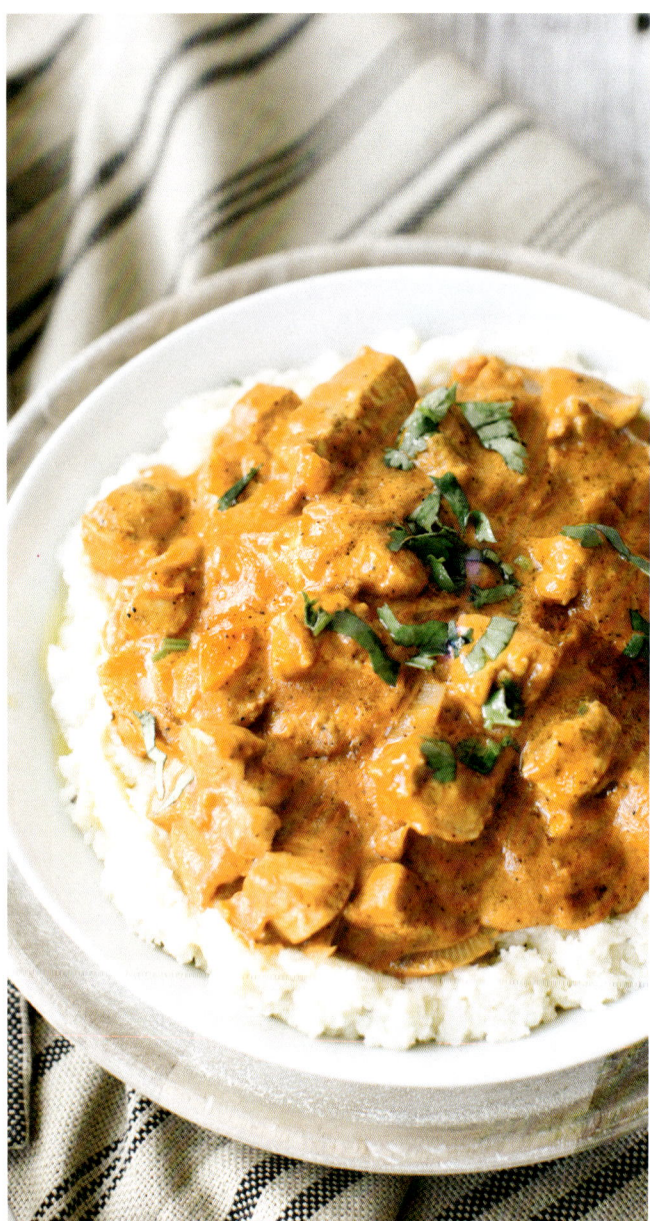

INGREDIENTS

2 T. olive oil
18 oz. chicken breasts, boneless and skinless
  (cut in bite size chunks)
½ C. chopped green onion
2 tsp. minced garlic
1 tsp. sea salt
½ tsp. black pepper
2 tsp. coriander
2 tsp. cumin
1 ½ tsp. paprika
½ tsp. cardamom
¼ tsp. nutmeg
¼ tsp. ground ginger
¼ tsp. cayenne pepper (optional)
¼ C. tomato paste
3 oz. half and half cream
½ C. chopped fresh cilantro, for topping

DIRECTIONS

1. Heat olive oil in a large skillet over medium/medium high heat.
2. Add chicken, green onion, and garlic; season with salt and pepper. Brown chicken approximately 10 minutes or until cooked through, stirring occasionally.
3. Add remaining seasonings; reduce heat to medium/medium low. Stir fry approximately 1-2 minutes to toast spices.
4. Add tomato paste and half and half cream to skillet; stir until thoroughly mixed. Simmer and stir until sauce thickens.
5. Serve topped with cilantro.

SERVINGS

Entire recipe yield = 18 oz. lean protein + 1 C. veggies + 3 oz. half and half cream
⅓ recipe yield = 6 oz. lean protein + ⅓ C. veggies + 1 oz. half and half cream

TIP: Excellent served over cauliflower rice.

Turkey Zoodle Crustless Quiche

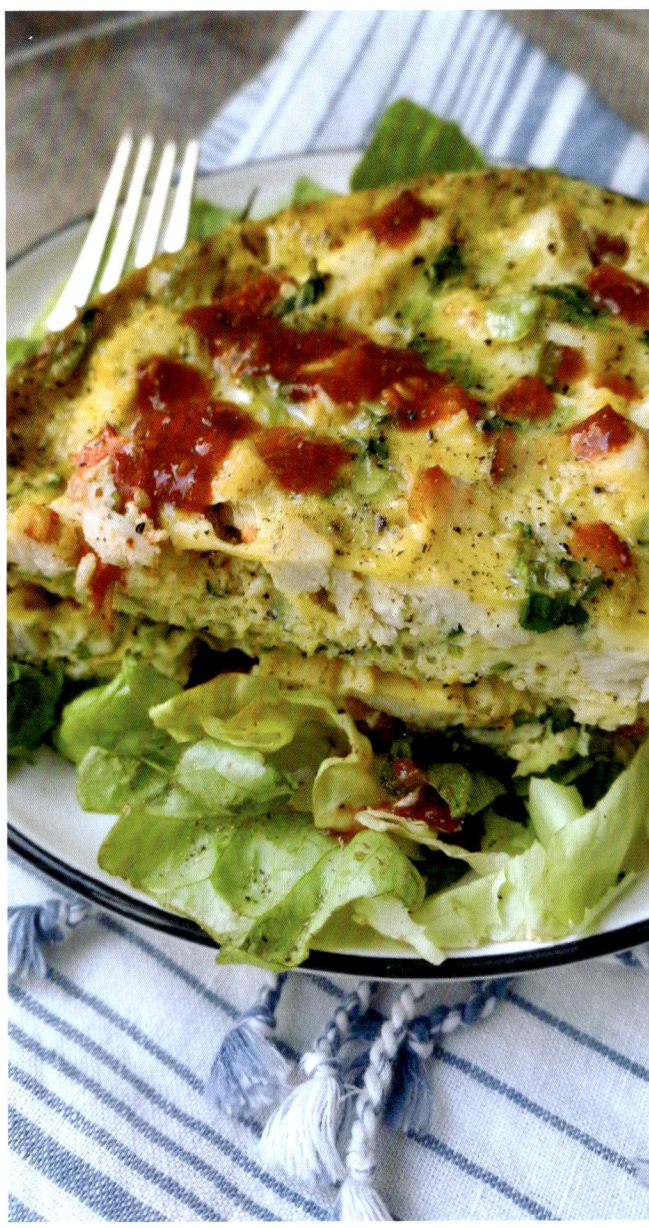

INGREDIENTS

2 C. spiralized zucchini (zoodles)
Salt for zoodles
6 oz. lean ground turkey
4 large eggs + 2 egg whites
2 T. half and half cream
1 tsp. Ideal Protein salt
½ tsp. black pepper
¼ tsp. nutmeg
¾ C. diced fresh tomatoes
¼ C. chopped green onion
Hot sauce, to taste (optional)

DIRECTIONS

1. Preheat oven to 350° F degrees.
2. Place a double layer of paper towels on a work surface. Spread zoodles on towels in a single layer; lightly sprinkle with salt. Roll up zoodles in the paper towels; set aside.
3. In a small skillet, brown the turkey over medium heat. Stir to break up the meat. Remove from heat.
4. In a large mixing bowl, whisk eggs and egg whites until blended but not frothy. Stir in cream, salt, pepper, and nutmeg.
5. Gently press zoodles in paper towels to absorb moisture. Remove zoodles and place in a single layer in a 9-inch pie pan.
6. Evenly sprinkle tomatoes and cooked turkey over zoodles. Pour egg mixture over the top and sprinkle with green onion.
7. Bake 30-35 minutes or until eggs are just set in the middle. Serve with hot sauce, if desired.

SERVINGS

Entire recipe yield = 12 oz. lean protein + 3 C. veggies + 1 oz. half and half cream
½ recipe yield = 6 oz. lean protein + 1 ½ C. veggies + 0.5 oz. half and half cream

TIP: To serve, slice into 4 pieces and stack 2 for ½ recipe yield.

veggies

RAW VEGGIE WEIGHT CHART

SIZE	SELECT VEGGIE	GRAMS	OUNCES
1 cup	Asparagus	34	4.7
1 cup	Bean Sprouts	100	4
1 cup	Bell Peppers	149	5.3
1 cup	Broccoli	91	3.2
1 cup	Cabbage (all)	89	3.1
1 cup	Cauliflower	100	3.5
1 cup	Celery	100	3.5
1 cup	Chayote	160	5.6
1 cup	Collards	36	1.27
1 cup	Cucumber	104	3.7
1 cup	Fennel	87	3.1
1 cup	Green Onions	100	3.5
1 cup	Jicama	130	4.59
1 cup	Kale	67	2.4
1 cup	Kohlrabi	135	4.76
1 cup	Mushrooms	96	3.4
1 cup	Okra	100	3.5
1 cup	Onions	160	5.6
1 cup	Hot Peppers	150	5.3
1 cup	Radishes	116	4.1
1 cup	Rhubarb	122	4.3
1 cup	Sauerkraut	142	5
1 cup	Spinach	30	1.1
1 cup	Swiss Chard	36	1.3
1 cup	Turnip	150	5.3
1 cup	Yellow Squash	124	4.4
1 cup	Zucchini	150	5.3
SIZE	OCCASIONAL VEGGIE	GRAMS	OUNCES
1 cup	Beans (Green & Wax)	150	5.3
1 cup	Brussel Sprouts	88	3.1
1 cup	Eggplant	82	2.9
1 cup	Rutabaga	140	4.9
1 cup	Snow Peas	98	3.5
1 cup	Tomatoes	180	6.3

ROASTED VEGGIE CHART

TIME AND TEMP: 400°F to 450°F is typically the perfect temperature for roasting most vegetables. It allows for a golden brown and caramelized exterior with a fork-tender interior; however, cooking times will vary depending on the veggie. Always preheat the oven and roast veggies on a rimmed baking sheet on the center oven rack unless a recipe states otherwise. If your veggies are not browning enough, move baking sheet to the bottom rack of the oven and/or slightly increase time and temp.

PREPARING VEGGIES: Always use fresh veggies—frozen veggies will steam in the oven rather than roast.

Uniformly cut the veggies so they cook evenly (see chart for cut/prep suggestions); toss prepared veggies in olive oil—**use ½ to 1 tsp. olive oil for every 1 C. of veggies.** Sprinkle with desired seasonings (see chart for simple suggestions.)

ROASTING: Place veggies in one layer on a rimmed baking sheet—give the veggies space! If the pan is too crowded, roast in batches or use two baking sheets and rotate in oven during roasting. Total roasting time is listed in the chart—**always flip the veggies halfway through roasting time.**

VEGGIE	CUT/PREP	TEMP/TIME	SEASONINGS
Asparagus	Whole spears, snap off woody ends	425°F / 15-20 min	Salt/pepper, Lemon zest (after roasting)
Bell Peppers	Bite size pieces	450°F / 25-30 min	Salt/pepper, Italian seasoning, oregano
Broccoli	Bite size pieces (1" florets)	425°F / 20-25 min	Salt/pepper, lemon juice, red pepper flakes
Brussel Sprouts	Halved or quartered	425°F / 20-25 min	Salt/pepper, garlic powder
Cabbage	2" slices, toss to loosen	425°F / 18-20 min	Salt/pepper, garlic powder, Cajun or Creole seasoning
Cauliflower	Bite size pieces (1" florets)	450°F / 25-30 min	Salt, garlic powder, cumin
Chayote Squash	Diced (½" cubes)	425°F / 18-22 min	Smoked salt or sea salt, garlic powder
Fennel	Sliced (¼" slices)	425°F / 20-25 min	Sea salt, black pepper, garlic powder
Green Beans	Whole, ends trimmed	425°F / 15-20 min	Salt/pepper, garlic powder
Mushrooms (button)	Halved	450°F / 15-20 min	Salt/pepper, garlic powder
Okra	Halved (tip to root)	400°F / 18 min (Roast cut side down for 15 min; flip and bake 3 min more)	Salt/pepper, garlic powder
Radishes	Halved or quartered	400°F / 12-15 min	Salt/pepper, garlic powder
Tomatoes (cherry)	Halved	425°F / 22-25 min	Minced garlic, black pepper
Zucchini/ Summer Squash	Cut into ½" rounds, then quartered	425°F / 30 min	Sea salt, black pepper, garlic powder

Apple Cider Roasted Fennel

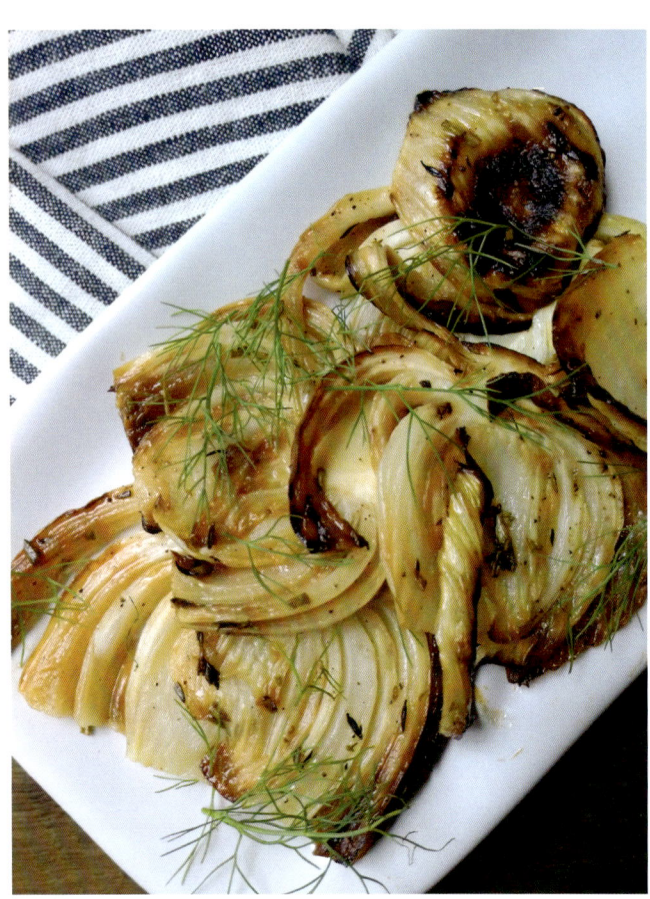

INGREDIENTS
1 C. apple cider vinegar
2 C. sliced fennel (see step 4)
2 tsp. extra virgin olive oil
1 tsp. chopped fresh thyme leaves
1 tsp. chopped fresh rosemary leaves
Kosher salt, to taste
Black pepper, to taste

DIRECTIONS
1. In a small saucepan, heat vinegar over medium/medium high heat. Bring to a low boil; reduce heat and simmer approximately 15 minutes or until reduced by two thirds (to about ⅓ C.). Set aside to cool.
2. Preheat oven to 425°F degrees.
3. Meanwhile, prep fennel head by cutting off tops reserving 3-4 frond sprigs (delicate leaves) for a flavorful garnish; discard long green stems.
4. When slicing fennel bulb, keep the root intact by resting root end on cutting board and vertically slice fennel into ¼" slices.
5. To a large plastic resealable bag, add 2 T. of the reduced apple cider vinegar, fennel slices, olive oil, thyme, and rosemary. Seal bag and gently toss to coat.
6. Spread fennel in one layer on a rimmed baking sheet. Season with salt and pepper. Roast 20-25 minutes or until browned and caramelized; flip once halfway through roasting.
7. Serve hot drizzled with the remaining apple cider vinegar. Tear frond sprigs and sprinkle over roasted fennel.

SERVINGS
Entire recipe yield = 2 C. veggies + 2 tsp. oil

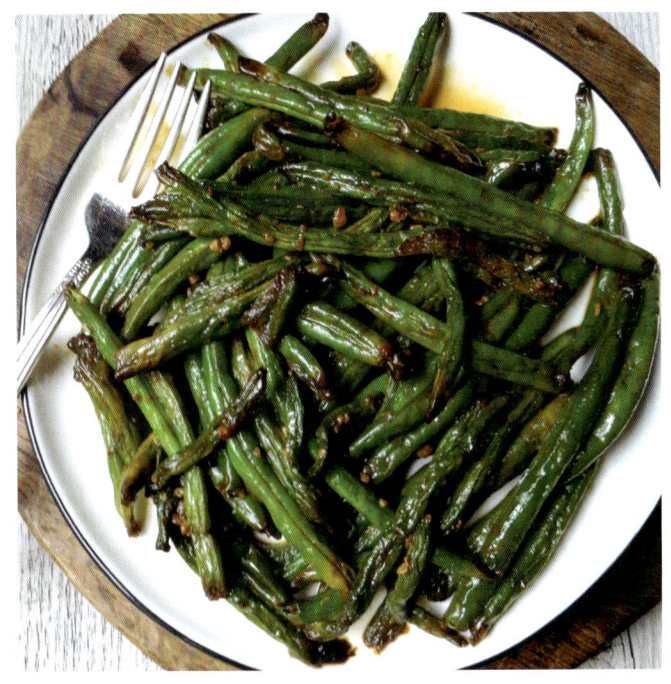

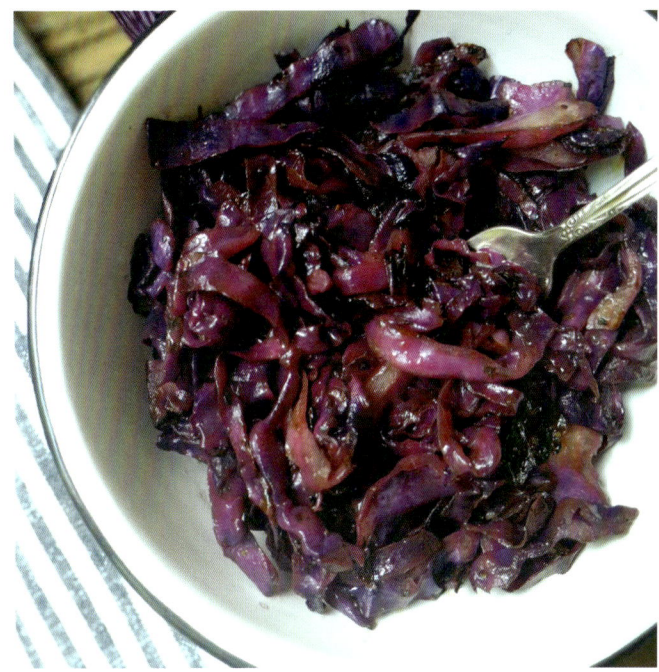

Asian Green Beans

INGREDIENTS
2 C. fresh green beans
2 tsp. olive oil
1 tsp. chopped garlic
½ tsp. minced ginger (or ⅛ tsp. ground ginger)
2 T. soy sauce
Water

DIRECTIONS
1. Steam the green beans by adding 1-inch water to a medium saucepan. Add the steamer basket; place green beans into the basket. Bring water to a boil over high heat. When water starts to boil, cover, reduce heat and simmer. Steam approximately 8-10 minutes or until fork tender, checking occasionally. Drain.
2. In a skillet, heat olive oil on medium/medium high heat. Add the garlic, ginger, and soy sauce. Stir to mix.
3. Add the green beans; sauté until heated through and slightly wilted.

SERVINGS
Entire recipe yield = 2 C. veggies + 2 tsp. oil

Braised Red Cabbage

INGREDIENTS
1 tsp. sugar free sweetener, granular
1 T. + 2 tsp. Ideal Protein balsamic dressing
2 tsp. olive oil
2 C. thinly sliced red cabbage
Ideal Protein salt, to taste
Pepper, to taste
¼ C. chicken broth

DIRECTIONS
1. In a small bowl, mix the sweetener and balsamic dressing; set aside.
2. In a medium skillet, heat the olive oil on medium/medium high heat. When oil is hot, add cabbage and season with salt and pepper. Stir fry 5 minutes.
3. Add balsamic mixture; stir fry an additional 3 minutes.
4. Reduce heat to medium/medium low and add chicken broth to cabbage. Cover and cook 3-5 minutes, stirring occasionally. Serve hot.

SERVINGS
Entire recipe yield = 2 C. veggies + 2 tsp. oil

TIP: An excellent side dish, especially when served with pork. Recipe may easily be doubled.

Buffalo Cauliflower Au Gratin

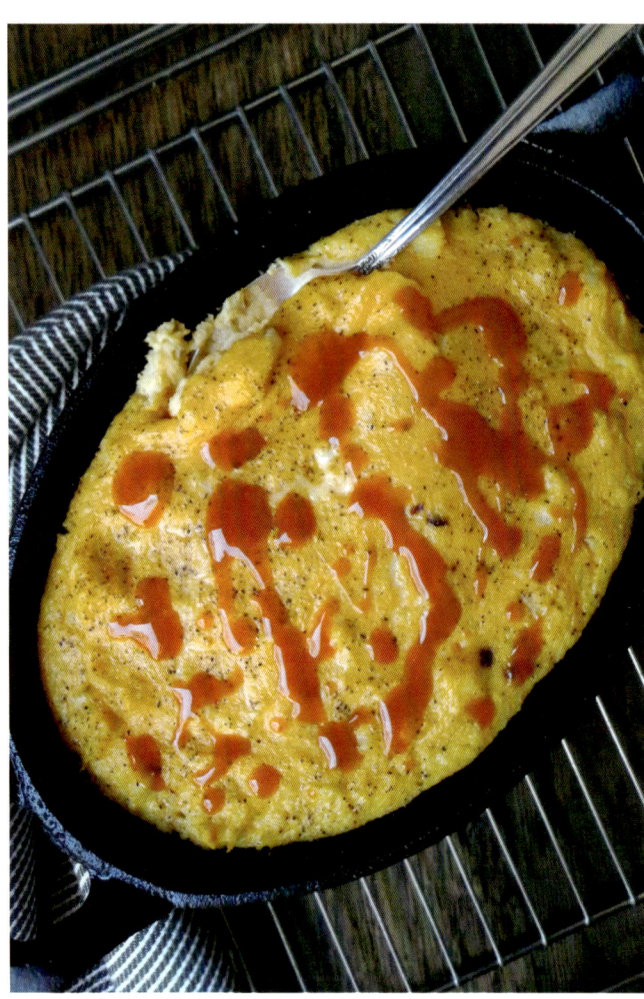

INGREDIENTS

4 C. (14 oz.) cauliflower florets, cut in bite size
 pieces
1 Ideal Protein cheddar cheese sauce mix
½ tsp. ground mustard
¼ tsp. salt
⅛ tsp. black pepper
⅛ tsp. onion powder
⅛ tsp. garlic powder
Two pinches red pepper flakes
1 large egg
¼ C. water
2 T. half and half cream
Cooking spray
Buffalo wing sauce, to taste (for topping)
Chopped green onions, to taste (optional for topping)

DIRECTIONS

1. Preheat oven to 350°F degrees.
2. Place florets in a large microwave proof bowl;
   add 1-inch water. Cover and microwave on high
   8-10 minutes or until fork tender. Drain and place
   cauliflower back in bowl.
3. Place half of the steamed florets in a food
   processor and blend until creamy. Add blended
   cauliflower to the whole florets and fold to mix.
   Set aside.
4. To a mixing bowl, add remaining ingredients and
   whisk to blend. Add cauliflower mixture to the
   sauce and fold to coat.
5. Add cheesy cauliflower mixture to a small
   sprayed casserole dish (about 5-6" diameter);
   bake 25-30 minutes. (Do not overbake or cheese
   will become grainy.)
6. Top with buffalo wing sauce and green onions, if
   desired. Season with additional salt and pepper,
   if necessary.

SERVINGS

Entire recipe yield = 1 unrestricted + 4 C. veggies
+ 1 oz. lean protein (egg) + 1 oz. half and half cream
½ recipe yield = ½ unrestricted + 2 C. veggies +
0.5 oz. lean protein (egg) + 0.5 oz. half and half cream

Cabbage Hashbrowns

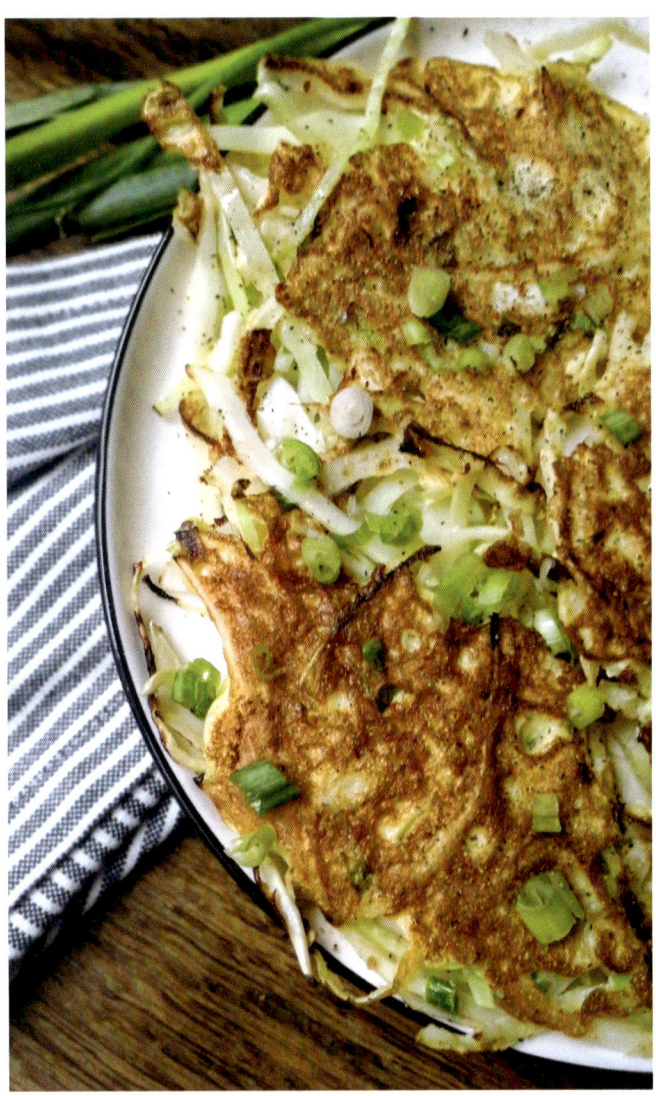

INGREDIENTS
2 C. thinly sliced cabbage
1 large egg
¼ tsp. garlic powder
¼ tsp. sea salt
Black pepper, to taste
2 T. chopped green onion
2 tsp. olive oil

DIRECTIONS
1. Place cabbage in a microwave proof bowl; add 1-inch water. Cover and cook in microwave on high 6 minutes. Drain and pat dry.
2. In a medium mixing bowl, whisk egg, garlic powder, salt, and pepper until combined. Stir in cabbage and green onion.
3. Heat oil in a large skillet over medium/medium high heat. Divide hashbrown mixture into 4 patties; place in skillet and press down with spatula to flatten.
4. Cook until golden brown, about 3 minutes each side. Season with additional salt and pepper, if desired.

SERVINGS
Entire recipe yield (4 hashbrown patties) = 2 C. and 2 T. veggies + 1 oz. lean protein (egg) + 2 tsp. oil
½ recipe yield (2 hashbrown patties) = 1 C. and 1 T. veggies + 0.5 oz. lean protein (egg) + 1 tsp. oil

TIP: Delicious drizzled with hot sauce.

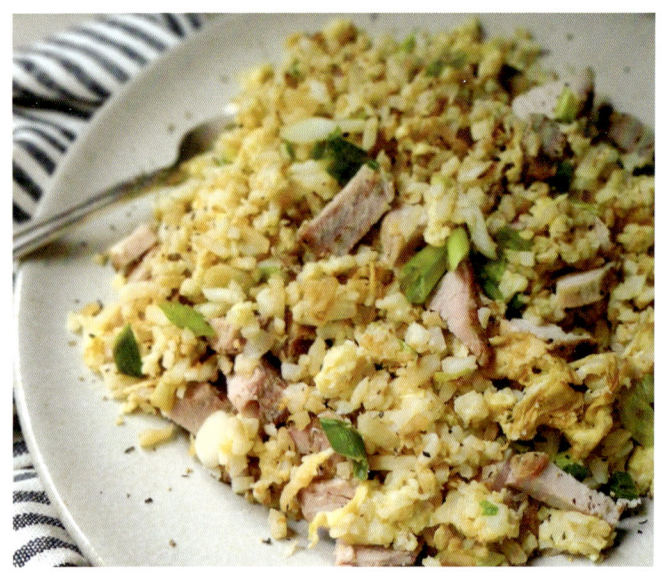

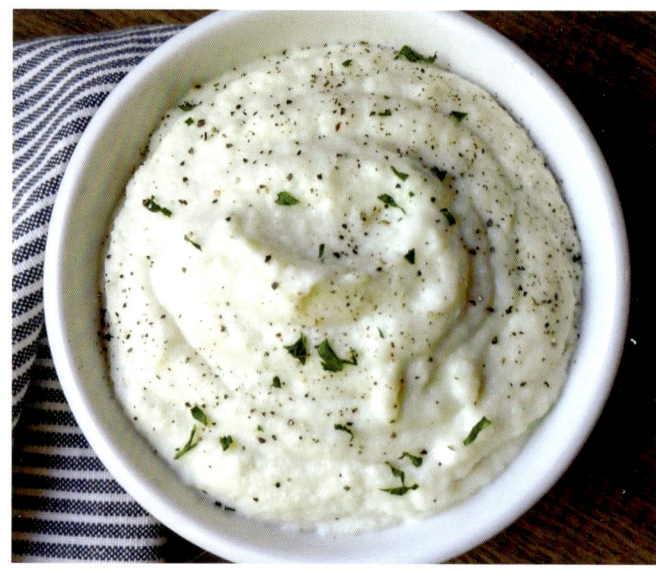

Cauliflower Fried Rice

INGREDIENTS

2 tsp. olive oil
10 oz. frozen riced cauliflower
¼ C. chopped green onion
¼ tsp. garlic powder
1 egg, lightly beaten
1 T. soy sauce
Black pepper, to taste
5 oz. cooked and diced pork, chicken, steak, or shrimp (optional)

DIRECTIONS

1. Heat oil in a skillet over medium heat. When the oil is hot, add the frozen riced cauliflower, green onion, and garlic powder. Stir fry 10-12 minutes or until cauliflower begins to lightly brown.
2. Drizzle beaten egg into the pan with the cauliflower mixture; stir fry until egg is cooked. Season with soy sauce and black pepper.
3. Add cooked pork, chicken, steak, or shrimp if desired. Heat through.

SERVINGS

Entire recipe yield = 3 ¼ C. veggies + 1 oz. lean protein (egg) + 2 tsp. oil
½ recipe yield = 1 ½ C. and 2 T. veggies + 0.5 lean protein (egg) + 1 tsp. oil

NOTE: If adding cooked lean animal protein (pork, etc.), include the lean protein ounces when calculating lean protein serving(s). The addition of pork is shown in photo.

Cauliflower Mash

INGREDIENTS

14 oz. (4 C.) cauliflower florets (bite size pieces)
Water^
Garlic powder, to taste
Salt and pepper, to taste

DIRECTIONS

1. Place the cauliflower in a medium saucepan and cover with water.
2. Bring to a boil. Reduce heat and cover; simmer 15 minutes or until fork tender. Drain.
3. Blot cauliflower with paper towels to absorb excess moisture.
4. Place cauliflower in a food processor. Add garlic powder, salt and pepper; puree.

SERVINGS

Entire recipe yield = 4 C. veggies
½ recipe yield = 2 C. veggies

TIP: *Chicken broth may be substituted for the water to give the mash more flavor.

Cauliflower Stuffing

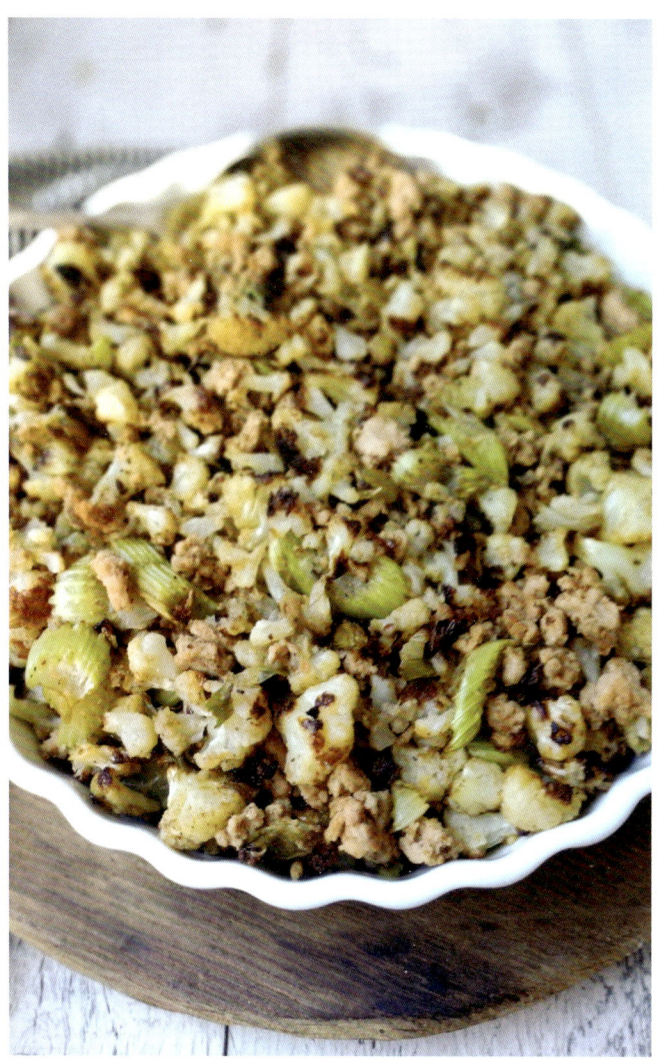

INGREDIENTS

2 T. + 2 tsp. olive oil
¼ tsp. butter extract
6 C. cauliflower florets (cut in small bite size pieces)
1 C. thinly sliced celery
1 C. chopped green onion
½ tsp. salt
¼ tsp. pepper
¾ tsp. poultry seasoning, divided
4 oz. lean ground turkey
¾ tsp. Sausage Seasoning, pg. 147

DIRECTIONS

1. Preheat oven to 425°F degrees.
2. In a small bowl, mix olive oil and butter extract; set aside.
3. Place cauliflower, celery, and green onion in a large resealable plastic bag. Add olive oil mixture; sprinkle in salt, pepper, and ½ tsp. poultry seasoning. Seal bag and toss to coat.
4. Spread cauliflower mixture evenly onto a large, rimmed baking sheet. Roast 30 minutes flipping cauliflower halfway through roasting time.
5. Meanwhile, add ground turkey, ¼ tsp. poultry seasoning, and Sausage Seasoning to a small skillet; brown over medium heat.
6. Place roasted cauliflower and turkey sausage mixture in a mixing bowl and toss. Taste and season with additional seasoning if necessary. Serve hot.

SERVINGS

Entire recipe yield = 8 C. veggies + 4 oz. lean protein + 8 tsp. oil
¼ recipe yield = 2 C. veggies + 1 oz. lean protein + 2 tsp. oil

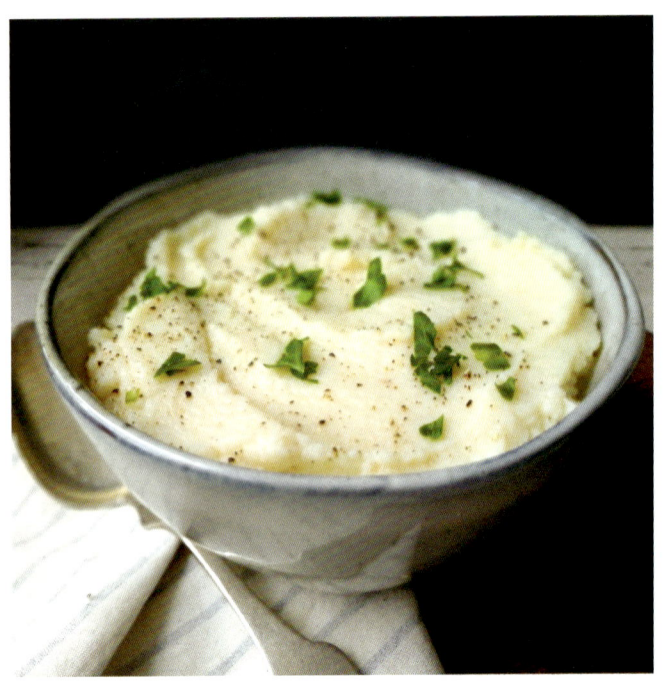

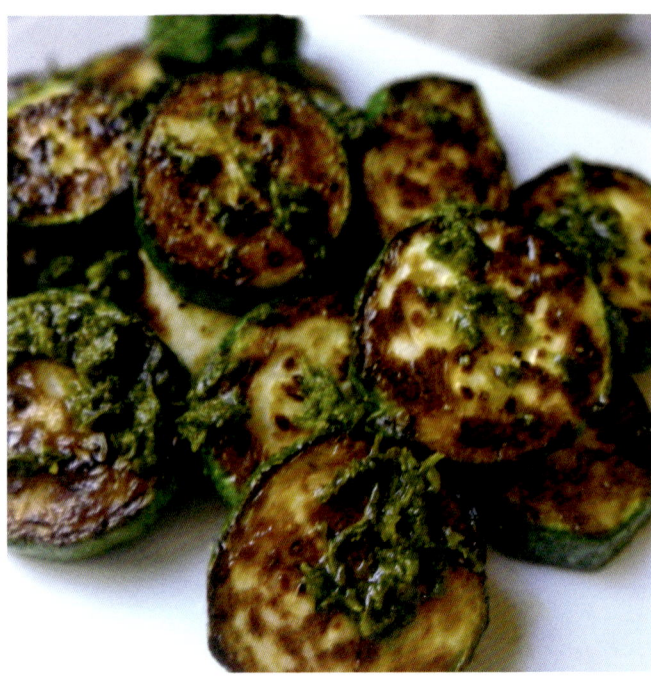

Celery Root Puree

Served as a side dish

INGREDIENTS

4 C. diced celery root
¼ C. half and half cream
1 T. chicken broth (or more for desired texture)
¼ tsp. sea salt
¼ tsp. garlic powder
Black pepper, to taste

DIRECTIONS

1. Place celery root in a medium saucepan and add water to cover. Bring to a boil; reduce heat and simmer 10 minutes or until fork tender. Drain.
2. Add celery root and remaining ingredients to a food processor; puree.
3. Season with additional salt and pepper if desired.

SERVINGS

Entire recipe yield = 4 C. veggies + 2 oz. half and half cream
½ recipe yield = 2 C. veggies + 1 oz. half and half cream

Chimichurri Zucchini

INGREDIENTS

3 C. zucchini slices, sliced ½" thick (unpeeled)
Ideal Protein salt
2 tsp. olive oil, divided
Garlic powder, to taste
Black pepper, to taste
1 T. Chimichurri Sauce, pg. 138

DIRECTIONS

1. Lightly sprinkle zucchini rounds on both sides with salt and place in a colander; let rest 30 minutes. Blot zucchini rounds with paper towels to absorb moisture.
2. Brush a large skillet with 1 tsp. olive oil and heat over medium/medium high heat. When oil is hot, add zucchini rounds in a single layer and brush tops with remaining 1 tsp. of olive oil. Season lightly with garlic powder and black pepper.
3. Cook 2 ½ minutes each side until golden brown. Plate and brush chimichurri sauce on zucchini.

SERVINGS

Entire recipe yield = 3 C. veggies + 1 T. oil*
⅓ recipe yield = 1 C. veggies + 1 tsp. oil*

NOTE: *Total oil includes the oil from the recipe and the Chimichurri Sauce.

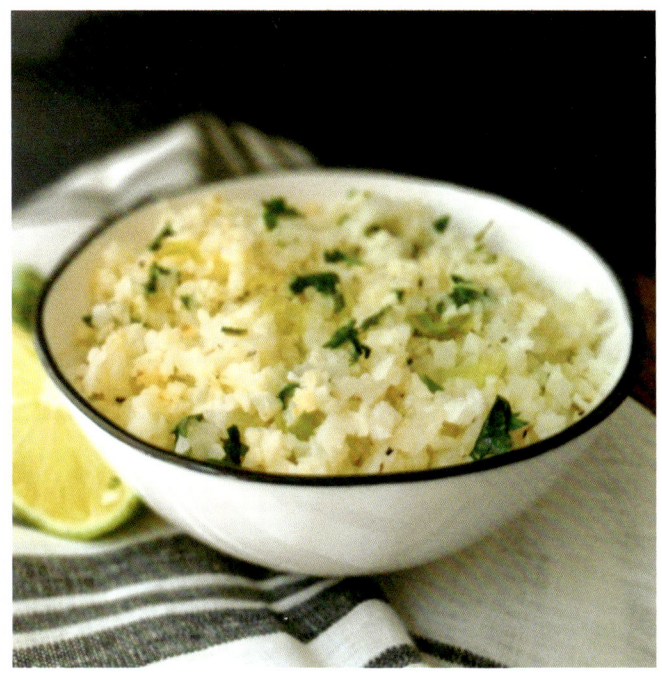

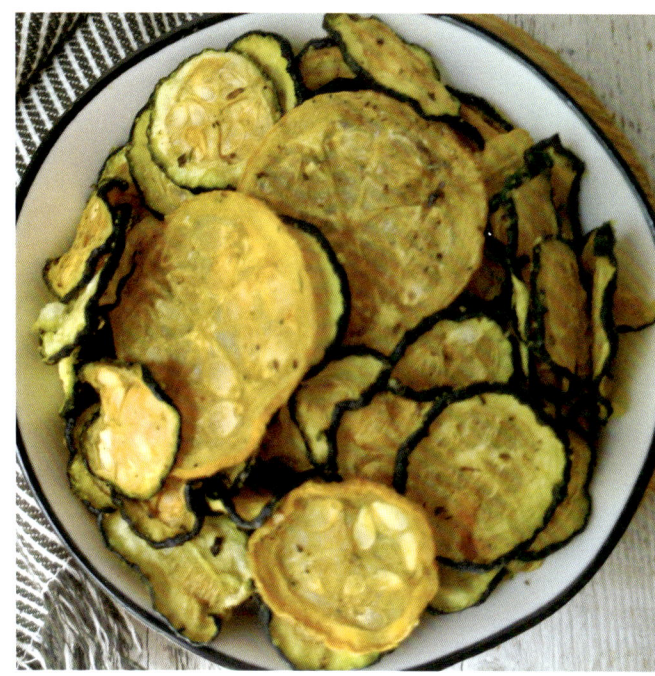

Cilantro Lime Cauliflower Rice

INGREDIENTS
¼ C. chicken broth
1 T. lime juice
¼ tsp. coconut extract (optional)
1 T. olive oil
10 oz. frozen riced cauliflower
¼ C. chopped green onion
2 T. chopped fresh cilantro
Salt & pepper, to taste

DIRECTIONS
1. In a small bowl, combine the chicken broth, lime juice and coconut extract; set aside.
2. Brush the bottom of a large skillet with oil; heat on medium/medium high heat. When skillet is hot, add frozen riced cauliflower and green onion; stir fry until rice is lightly browned and tender, approximately 10-12 minutes.
3. Add chicken broth mixture; stir until heated through. Fold in cilantro and season with salt and pepper.

SERVINGS
Entire recipe yield = 3 ¼ C. veggies + 1 T. oil
½ recipe yield = 1 ½ C. and 2 T. veggies + 1 ½ tsp. oil

Crispy Squash Chips

INGREDIENTS
2 C. thinly sliced zucchini or yellow squash (sliced ⅛ inch thick)
Salt
Olive oil spray
Garlic powder, to taste

DIRECTIONS
1. Preheat oven to 200°F degrees.
2. Place squash slices in one layer on a few layers of paper towels. Sprinkle lightly with salt. Place an additional layer of paper towels on top and let rest 15 minutes. Press down on paper towel to absorb moisture from squash chips.
3. Lightly spray a large rimmed baking sheet with olive oil. Place squash chips in one layer on baking sheet. Lightly spray with olive oil and season with garlic powder.
4. Bake 2 hours or until lightly golden brown. Serve immediately.

SERVINGS
Entire recipe yield = 2 C. veggies + 1 tsp. oil (approximately)

TIP: Watch chips closely near end of bake time as they can quickly over bake. Remove chips from baking sheet with a metal spatula to prevent breaking.

Crispy Veggie Fries
Oven or air fryer method

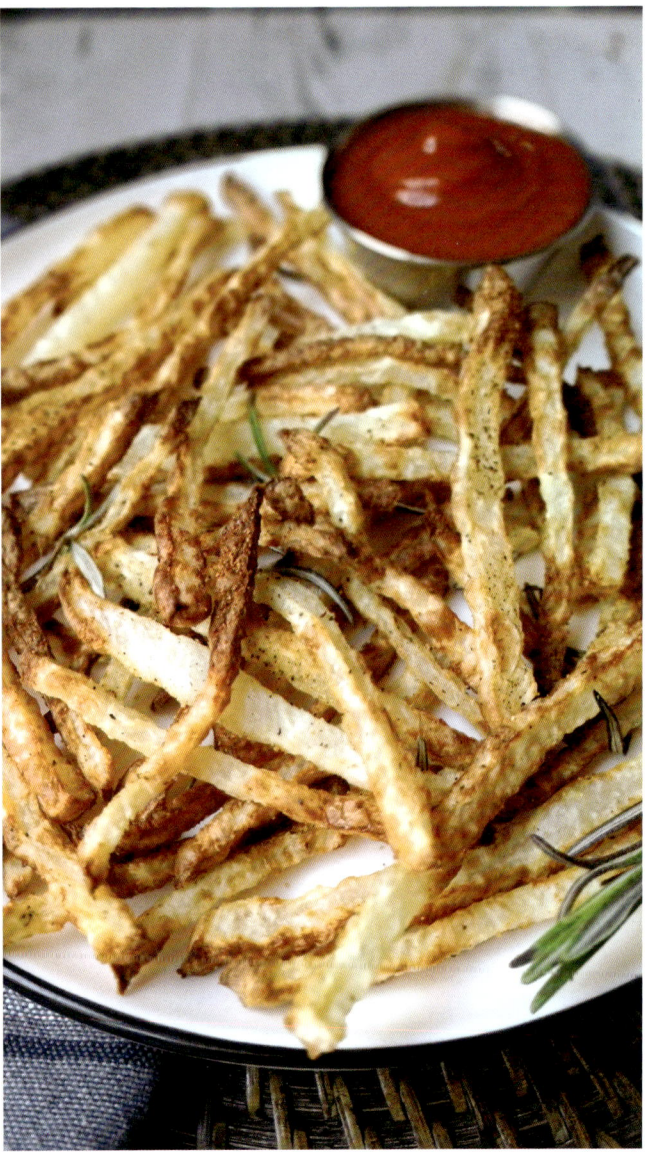

INGREDIENTS
2 C. rutabaga, celery root, turnip or jicama
  (cut into fries)
1 egg white
Salt and pepper, to taste
Garlic powder, to taste
Paprika, to taste
Olive oil cooking spray

DIRECTIONS
1. Preheat oven to 425°F degrees.
2. Place fries in a microwave safe bowl; add 1 inch water. Cover and microwave 8 minutes on high or until fork tender.
3. Drain in a colander, pat dry and cool. Set aside.
4. Meanwhile, place egg white in a small bowl and whisk about 30 seconds till frothy.
5. Place cooled fries in a large resealable plastic bag, pour in egg whites and shake to coat.
6. Place fries on a sprayed, rimmed baking sheet; spread fries so they aren't touching each other. Lightly spray fries with cooking spray and sprinkle with salt, pepper, garlic powder and paprika.
7. Bake 20–30 minutes (or until lightly browned), flipping once halfway through baking time. Baking time varies slightly based on veggie choice.

SERVINGS
Entire recipe yield = 2 C. veggies + ½ tsp. oil (approximately)

TIP: Recipe includes optional seasoning ideas; however, seasonings of choice may be subbed.

Air fryer method: Follow directions #1-5 above. Place one layer of fries in air fryer basket (this may have to be done in batches.) Bake 15-20 minutes at 350°F degrees turning fries once during cooking.

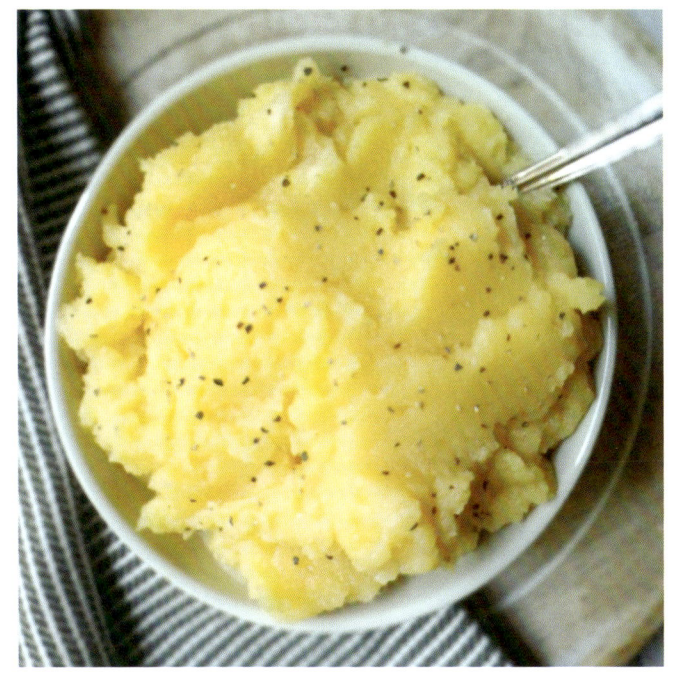

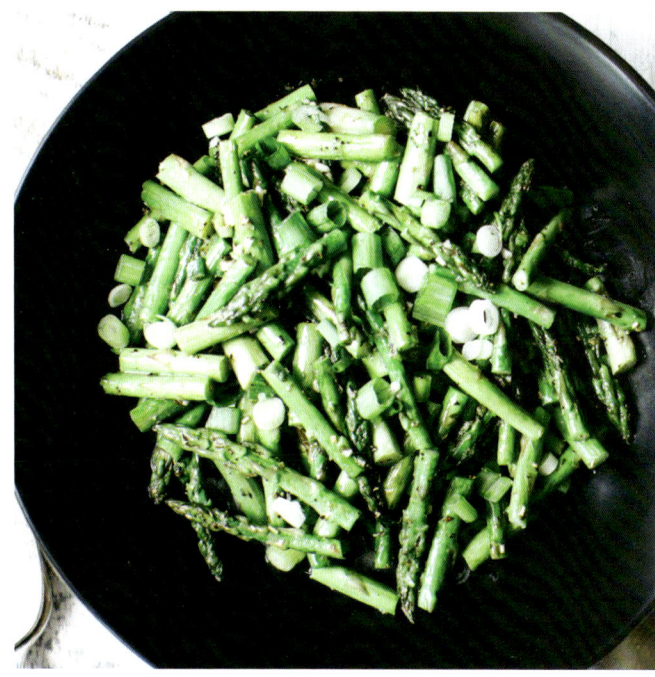

Garlic Rutabaga Mash

INGREDIENTS
2 C. diced rutabaga
1 C. chicken broth
Water
Garlic powder, to taste
Onion powder, to taste
Salt and pepper, to taste
1 T. half and half cream

DIRECTIONS
1. Place rutabaga in a medium saucepan; add chicken broth and enough water to cover rutabaga.
2. Bring to a boil over high heat. Reduce heat; simmer until rutabaga is fork tender, about 15 minutes.
3. Drain and blot rutabaga with paper towels to absorb excess moisture.
4. Place rutabaga, garlic powder, onion powder, salt, pepper, and half and half cream in a food processor; puree.

SERVINGS
Entire recipe yield = 2 C. veggies + 0.5 oz. half and half cream

TIP: Turnips may be substituted for the rutabagas in this dish.

Italian Asparagus

INGREDIENTS
4 C. (about 1 bunch) asparagus
1 T. + 1 tsp. olive oil
1 tsp. dried Italian seasoning
1 tsp. minced garlic
¼ tsp. kosher salt
⅛ tsp. black pepper
2 T. chopped green onion, divided

DIRECTIONS
1. Prepare the asparagus by cutting off about 1-1 ½" of the bottom ends of the stalks (woody part); discard ends. Cut asparagus spears into 2" pieces.
2. Brush the bottom of a large skillet with oil. Heat over medium/medium high heat until hot.
3. Add asparagus and gently stir fry 5-7 minutes or until fork tender.
4. Add remaining ingredients using only 1 T. of the green onion. Reduce heat to medium and stir fry an additional 2 minutes.
5. Sprinkle with remaining 1 T. green onion before serving. Season with additional salt and pepper, if desired.

SERVINGS
Entire recipe yield = 4 C. + 2 T. veggies + 4 tsp. oil
½ recipe yield = 2 C. + 1 T. veggies + 2 tsp. oil

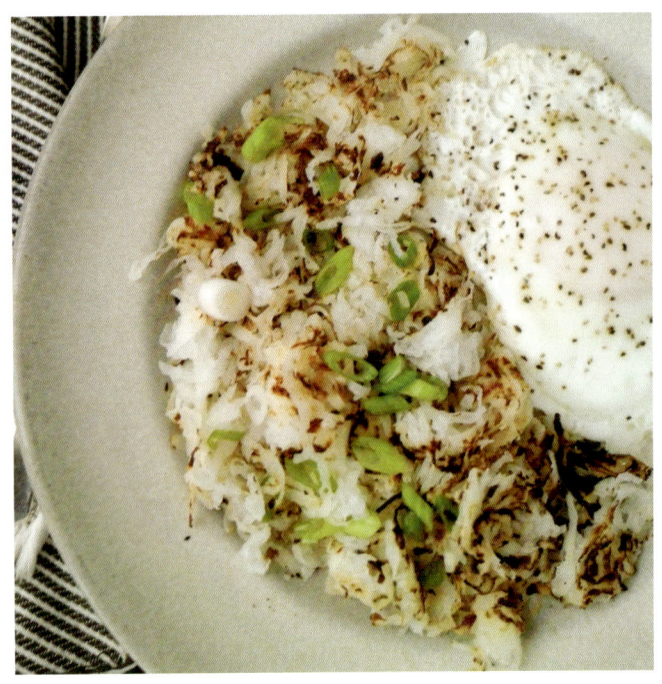

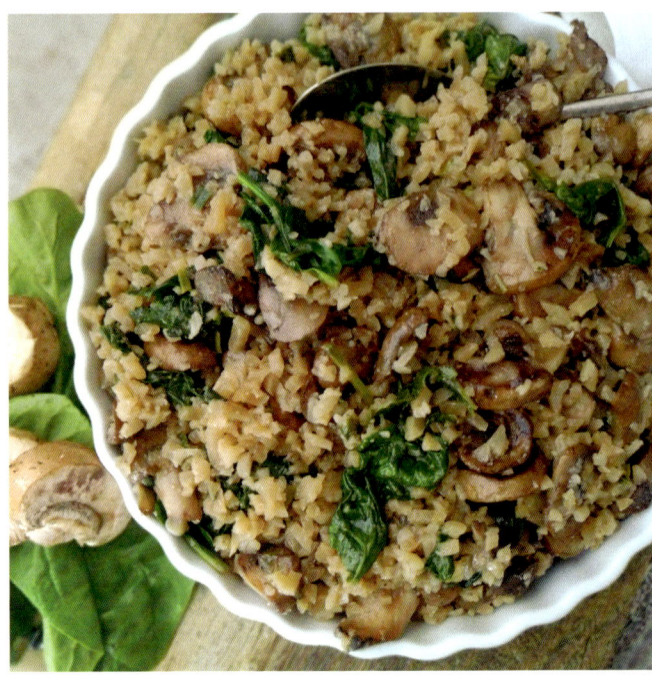

Kohlrabi Hashbrowns

INGREDIENTS
4 C. shredded kohlrabi
1 T. olive oil
½ tsp. onion powder
Salt and pepper, to taste
Chopped green onion, for topping (optional)

DIRECTIONS
1. Layer kohlrabi between several sheets of paper towels and squeeze out as much water as possible.
2. Heat oil in a large skillet over medium heat.
3. Add shredded kohlrabi; season with onion powder, salt and pepper.
4. Fry, stirring occasionally until lightly browned, about 15 minutes.
5. Top with chopped green onion, if desired.

SERVINGS
Entire recipe yield = 4 C. veggies + 1 T. oil
½ recipe yield = 2 C. veggies + 1 ½ tsp. oil

TIP: If using green onion, measure and add to veggie total.

Mushroom & Spinach Cauliflower Pilaf

INGREDIENTS
10 oz. frozen riced cauliflower
1 T. + 1 tsp. olive oil
2 ½ C. sliced baby bella mushrooms
½ C. chopped green onion
2 T. soy sauce
Garlic powder, to taste
Black pepper, to taste
2 C. fresh spinach (lightly packed), stems removed

DIRECTIONS
1. Cook riced cauliflower according to package directions. Drain if necessary; set aside.
2. Brush a large skillet with oil; heat on medium until hot. Add mushrooms and green onion; stir fry 5 minutes or until mushrooms are lightly browned.
3. Add cauliflower and stir. Drizzle with soy sauce; season with garlic powder and black pepper. Gently stir until cauliflower absorbs soy sauce.
4. Add spinach and stir fry until wilted about 1-2 minutes.

SERVINGS
Entire recipe yield = 8 C. veggies + 4 tsp. oil
¼ recipe yield = 2 C. veggies + 1 tsp. oil

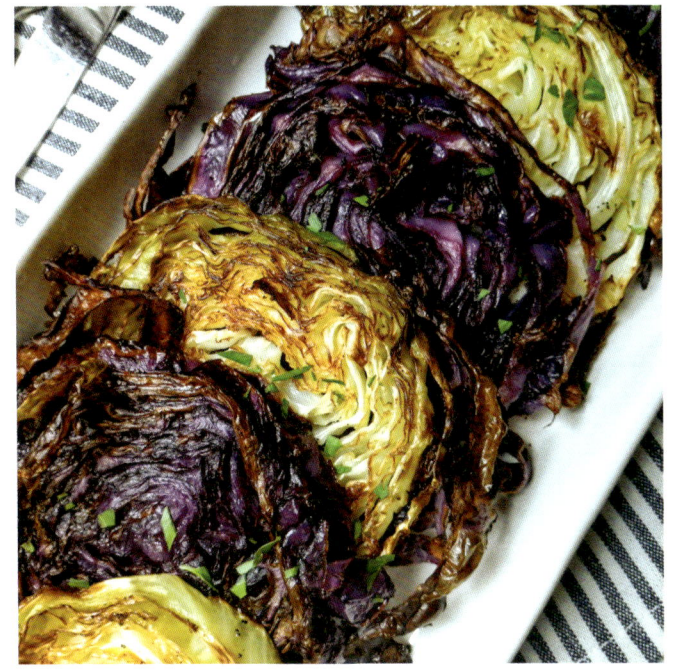

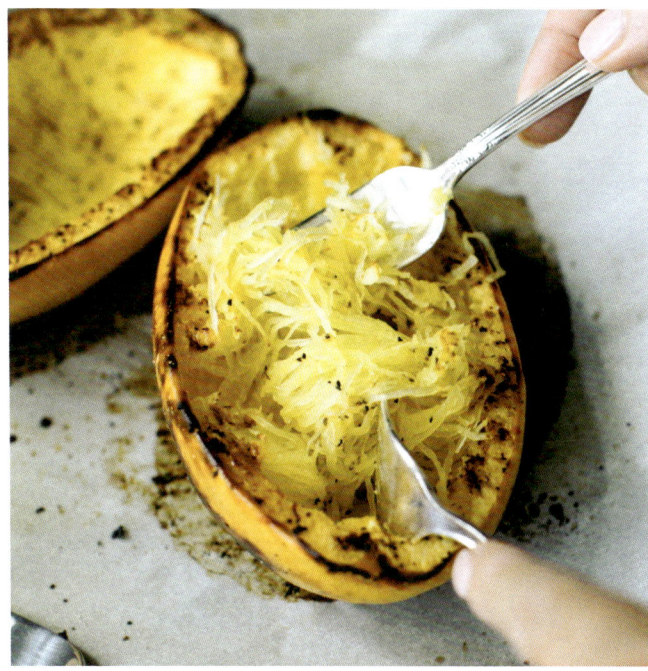

Roasted Cabbage Steaks

INGREDIENTS
1 small head red or green cabbage
4 tsp. olive oil, divided
Salt and pepper, to taste
Garlic powder, to taste

DIRECTIONS
1. Preheat oven to 425°F degrees.
2. Slice cabbage into ½" thick round discs. (For this recipe, use 4 cabbage steak slices and store remaining cabbage in fridge for another recipe.)
3. Brush steaks with ½ tsp. oil each side and place on a rimmed baking sheet; season with salt, pepper, and garlic powder.
4. Roast 30 minutes flipping steaks halfway through roasting. Steaks should be tender crisp and golden brown on both sides.

SERVINGS
Entire recipe yield (4 steaks) = 6 C. veggies + 4 tsp. oil
¼ recipe yield (1 steak) = 1 ½ C. veggies + 1 tsp. oil.

Roasted Spaghetti Squash
Aka Squoodles (spaghetti squash noodles)

INGREDIENTS
1 medium spaghetti squash
1 tsp. olive oil
Salt and pepper, to taste

DIRECTIONS
1. Preheat oven to 400°F degrees.
2. Using a large, sharp knife, slice spaghetti squash in half lengthwise. Remove seeds and stringy pulp with a spoon; discard.
3. Brush interior squash flesh with olive oil; season with salt and pepper. Roast cut side down on a rimmed, metal baking sheet 40 minutes.
4. Using a fork, remove squash from shells; discard shells. Measure amount needed (whether using as a side dish or for a recipe), then pat dry with a paper towel to remove excess moisture.
5. Season with additional salt and pepper, if desired.

SERVINGS
I loosely measure out cooked spaghetti squash by volume to get the measurement needed for a serving. For example, if 1 C. is needed, loosely measure in a 1 C. dry measuring cup. I also count ¼ tsp. oil per 1 C. serving to be included in the daily protocol count.

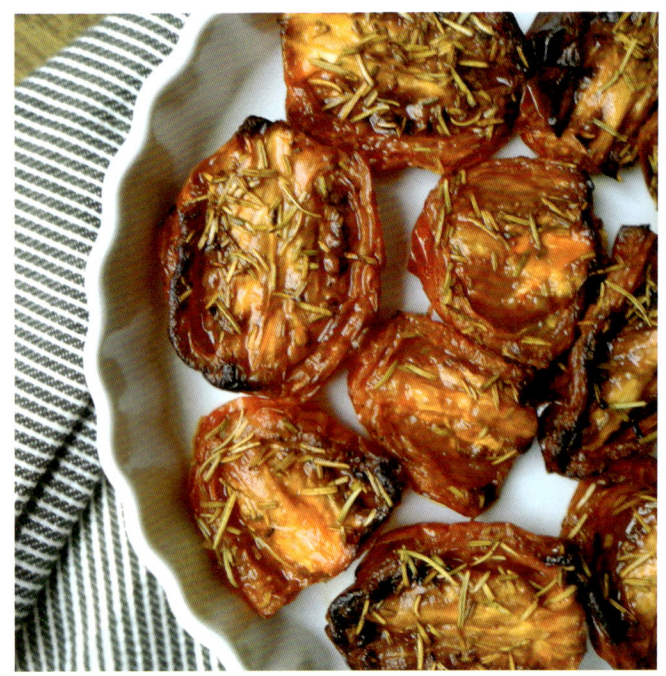
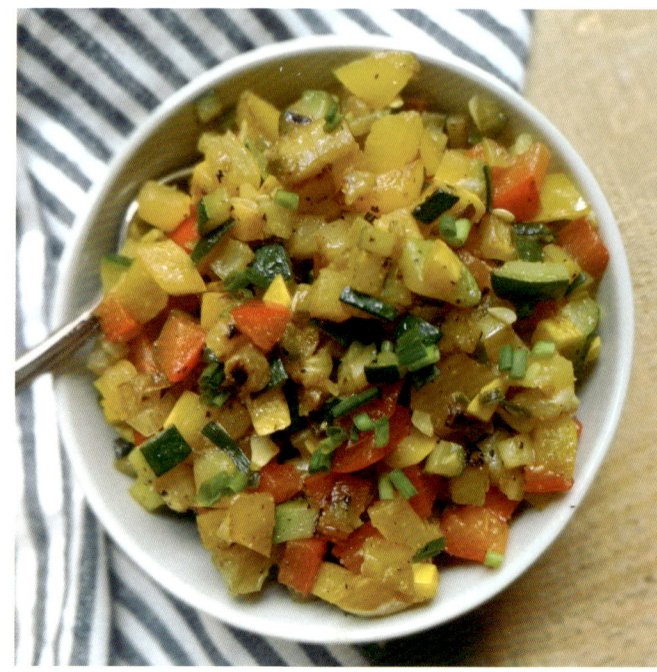

Rosemary Roasted Tomatoes
Air fryer or oven method

INGREDIENTS
2 C. (12.6 oz.) fresh Roma tomatoes
1 tsp. olive oil
1 tsp. sea salt
Dried rosemary leaves, to taste

DIRECTIONS (AIR FRYER METHOD)
1. Wash and dry tomatoes; slice in half from tip to end.
2. Brush cut side with olive oil, sprinkle with salt and a generous amount of rosemary leaves.
3. Place tomatoes in air fryer, cut side up. This may have to be done in batches depending on size of air fryer. (For standard oven roasting method, see below.)
4. Bake at 390°F degrees for 20-25 minutes.

SERVINGS
Entire recipe yield = 2 C. veggies + 1 tsp. oil

Oven Method: For standard oven roasting method, preheat oven to 425°F degrees. Place prepped tomatoes (see directions #1 and #2 above) on a parchment lined baking sheet, cut side up. Roast on lower rack of oven approximately 20 minutes or until tomatoes are lightly browned and caramelized.

Succotash

INGREDIENTS
1 T. olive oil
¼ C. + 2 T. chopped green onion
½ C. diced red bell pepper
½ C. diced yellow bell pepper
1 ¼ C. diced zucchini
1 ¼ C. diced yellow squash
2 T. diced jalapeno pepper (seeded)
1 ½ tsp. Cajun seasoning
Salt and pepper, to taste
2 tsp. lemon juice
2 tsp. chopped chives, (for topping)

DIRECTIONS
1. Heat oil in a large skillet over medium heat. Add green onion and stir fry one minute.
2. Add remaining veggies to skillet; season with Cajun seasoning, salt, and pepper. Stir fry 5 minutes or until veggies are fork tender.
3. Sprinkle succotash with lemon juice and chopped chives. Serve hot.

SERVINGS
Entire recipe yield = 4 C. veggies + 1 T. oil
½ recipe yield = 2 C. veggies + 1 ½ tsp. oil

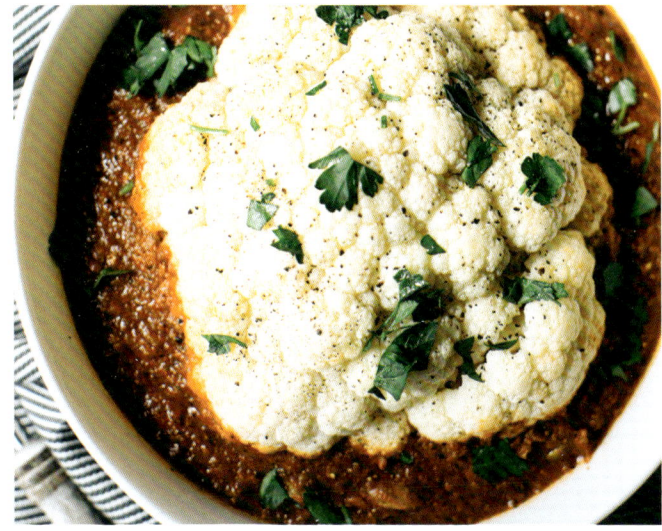

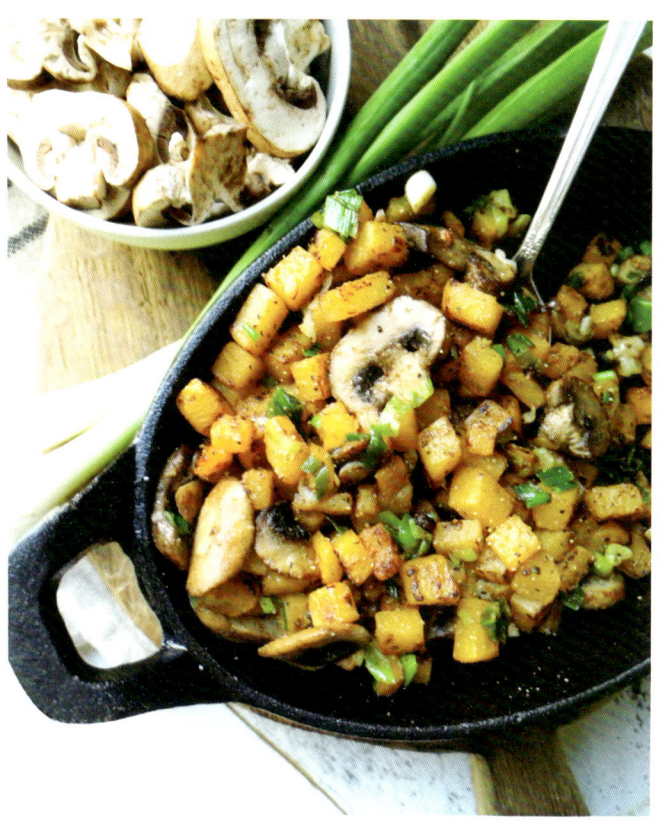

Tomato Braised Cauliflower

INGREDIENTS

1 recipe Spaghizza Sauce, pg. 148
½ C. water
1 medium head cauliflower (21 oz.), trim to remove large leaves
1 T. olive oil
Chopped fresh Italian parsley for garnish (optional)

DIRECTIONS

1. Pour the Spaghizza Sauce and water in a large saucepan; stir to mix. Bring to a low boil over medium high heat, stirring occasionally; reduce heat to medium low.
2. Place cauliflower head into center of the saucepan; push down gently. Make sure cauliflower is 1-inch from the edge of the saucepan on all sides; trim if necessary and place any trimmings into the sauce.
3. Brush the cauliflower with oil; cover saucepan and simmer 45 minutes.
4. Cauliflower will be fall-apart fork tender. To serve, slice in wedges in saucepan and scoop out with a large spoon. Plate and drizzle with Spaghizza Sauce.
5. Garnish with parsley before serving, if desired.

SERVINGS

Entire recipe yield = 10 C. veggies + 1 T. oil
⅕ recipe yield = 2 C. veggies + ½ tsp. oil

NOTE: To serve, slice a ⅕ wedge of the whole cauliflower head with immediate surrounding sauce to be as accurate to ⅕ serving size as possible.

Veggie Hash

INGREDIENTS

2 C. diced rutabaga, jicama, or celery root
1 T. + 1 tsp. olive oil
1 tsp. garlic powder
½ tsp. onion powder
1 ½ C. sliced portobella mushrooms
½ C. chopped green onion
Salt & pepper, to taste

DIRECTIONS

1. Place diced rutabaga, jicama or celery root in a large microwave proof bowl; add 1-inch water. Cover and microwave on high 5 minutes. Drain and pat dry.
2. Heat olive oil in a large skillet over medium heat. Add cooked vegetables; season with garlic powder and onion powder. Fry, stirring occasionally, until lightly browned.
3. Add mushrooms and green onion; stir fry until mushrooms are lightly browned and cooked. Season with salt and pepper.

SERVINGS

Entire recipe yield = 4 C. veggies + 4 tsp. oil
½ recipe yield = 2 C. veggies + 2 tsp. oil

Veggie Kabobs
With maple garlic soy sauce

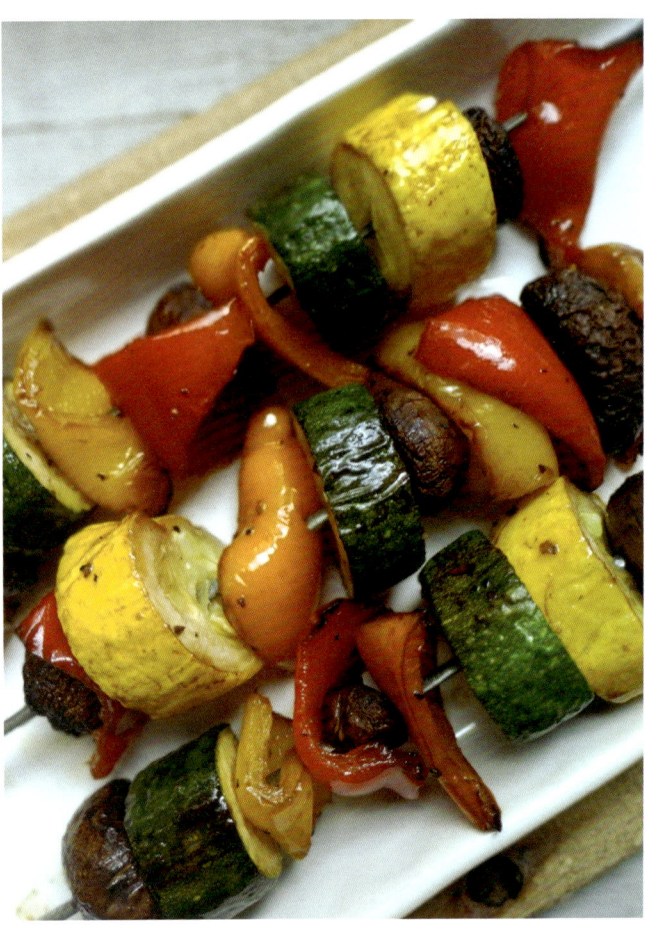

INGREDIENTS (SAUCE)
⅓ C. Ideal Protein maple syrup
⅓ C. soy sauce
¼ C. olive oil
1 tsp. minced garlic
1 tsp. apple cider vinegar
¼ tsp. black pepper

INGREDIENTS (KABOBS)
2 C. assorted bell peppers, cut in chunks
2 C. fresh whole mushrooms
2 C. (10.6 oz.) zucchini, cut in 1" slices
2 C. (8.8 oz.) yellow squash, cut in 1" slices

DIRECTIONS
1. Add sauce ingredients to a small mixing bowl; stir to combine.
2. Add kabob ingredients to a large resealable bag, pour sauce over veggies and seal bag. Turn bag several times to coat veggies; refrigerate and marinate at least 2 hours.
3. When ready to roast veggies, preheat oven to 425° F degrees.
4. Place veggies on skewers leaving at least ½" between the veggies so they cook evenly. Discard marinade.
5. Place kabobs on a baking sheet. Roast for 25 minutes flipping once during cooking.

SERVINGS
Entire recipe yield = 8 C. veggies + 4 tsp. oil (Note: most of the oil in the marinade will be discarded and not absorbed into veggies.)
¼ recipe yield = 2 C. veggies + 1 tsp. oil

TIP: These may be cooked on the grill over medium/medium high heat until lightly browned.

Zoodles
Spiralized zucchini noodles

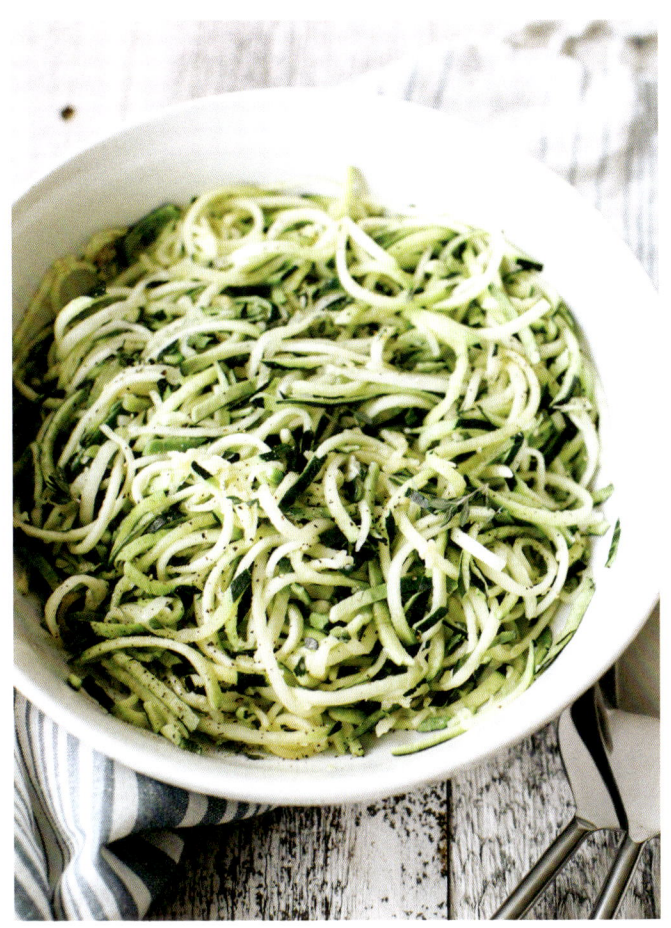

INGREDIENTS
2 medium zucchini (about 4 C. spiralized)
Sea salt
2 tsp. olive oil
½ tsp. garlic powder
Black pepper, to taste

DIRECTIONS
1. Cut ends off zucchini (no need to peel). Insert one end of zucchini into spiralizer and spiralize the zucchini into noodles.
2. Lay several sheets of paper towels on a work surface, and spread zoodles evenly onto towels. Sprinkle lightly with salt. Roll up zoodles in the paper towels and let rest 30 minutes. (This process will remove excess moisture from zoodles.)
3. Brush the bottom of a large skillet with oil and heat over medium/medium high heat.
4. Add zoodles, sprinkle with garlic powder, and sauté 2-3 minutes or until cooked al dente. Refrain from over cooking or the zoodles will turn to mush.
5. Season with black pepper, and additional salt, if desired.

SERVINGS
Entire recipe yield = 4 C. veggies + 2 tsp. oil
½ recipe yield = 2 C. veggies + 1 tsp. oil

Angel Food Cake

INGREDIENTS

2 egg whites, room temp
¼ tsp. cream of tartar
1 tsp. vanilla extract
1 Ideal Protein vanilla smoothie mix
2 T. Walden Farms strawberry syrup (for topping)

DIRECTIONS

1. Heat oven to 350°F degrees.
2. Prepare a (4 ½ x 2 ½-inch) mini angel food cake pan by lining the bottom of the pan with parchment paper. (See TIP* below.) Do not grease the sides or inner tube of the pan as the batter needs to climb up the pan.
3. Add egg whites and cream of tartar to the mixing bowl of a stand mixer.
4. Using the whisk attachment, beat egg whites on high speed until they form stiff peaks (about 2-3 minutes). Add vanilla extract in the final moments of beating.
5. Sprinkle ⅓ package of the smoothie mix over egg whites. Using a rubber spatula, gently fold in smoothie mix (doesn't have to be perfect). Refrain from over mixing or the air bubbles will be lost. Repeat process until entire smoothie mix is combined with egg whites.
6. Spoon meringue into cake pan; gently coax the batter down into pan with the spoon.
7. Bake 13-15 minutes or until top of cake turns lightly brown. Cool completely on a cooling rack in pan, right side up – no need to invert.
8. Run a knife around the center tube and inside edge of pan to loosen cake. Plate and drizzle with strawberry syrup.

SERVINGS

1 Angel Food Cake = 1 unrestricted + 2 egg whites (Consult your coach or clinic for egg white protocol counts, if any.)

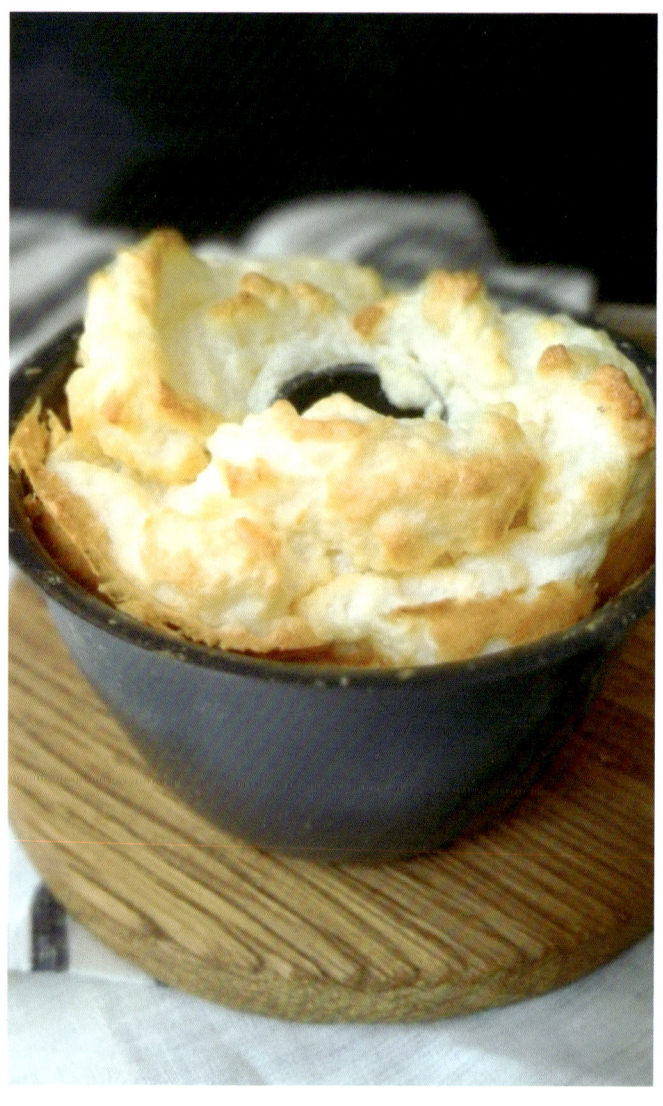

TIP: *To line the bottom of the pan, set pan on a piece of parchment paper. Trace a circle around the bottom of the pan; cut the circle out of the paper. Fold the circle in half; fold in half a second time to create a cone. Using scissors, cut enough of the tip off so that the opening fits over the center of the pan.

Apple Cobbler Cake

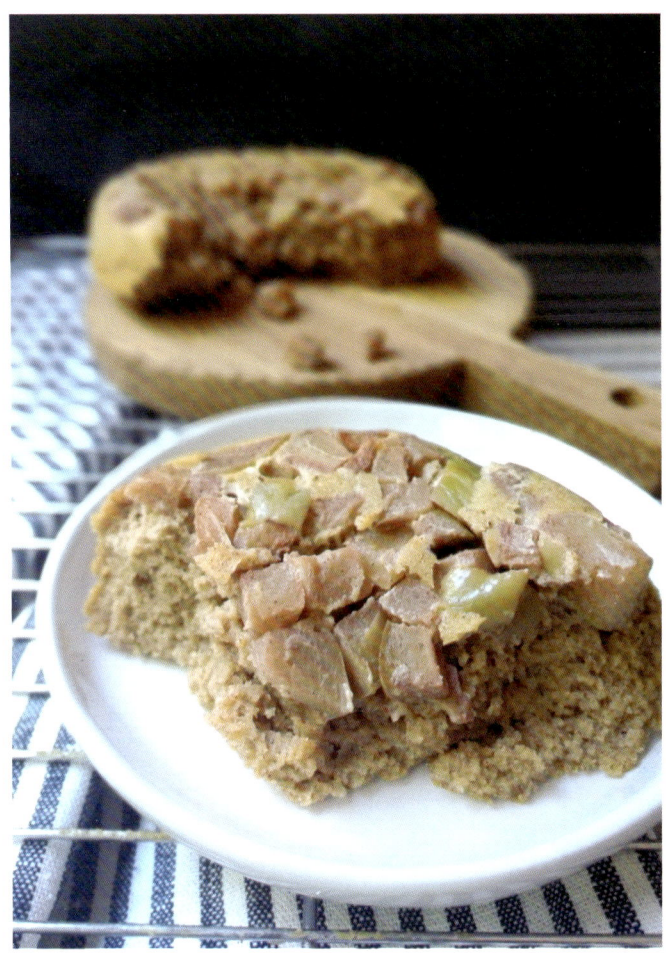

INGREDIENTS

⅔ C. Caramel Fried Apples, pg. 127
1 pkg. Ideal Protein apple cinnamon puffs
1 Ideal Protein golden pancakes mix
1 tsp. baking powder
½ tsp. cinnamon
1 large egg
1 T. water
1 T. Ideal Protein maple syrup
2 tsp. olive oil
Cooking spray

DIRECTIONS

1. Preheat oven to 350°F degrees.
2. Drain apples of any liquid and gently blot dry with paper towels. Evenly place apples on the bottom of a sprayed 5-inch round baking dish; set aside.
3. Place the dry ingredients in a bullet style blender or food processor; pulse to fine crumbs. Transfer to a mixing bowl.
4. Add liquid ingredients to a separate mixing bowl; stir to mix. Stir into dry ingredients. Batter will be stiff.
5. Evenly spread batter over apples.
6. Bake 17-19 minutes or until an inserted cake tester comes out clean.
7. Remove cake from pan and cool apple side down. For best texture, cool completely before serving. Invert cake (apple side up) for serving.

SERVINGS

Entire cake (2 servings) = 1 unrestricted + 1 restricted + 1 C. veggies (⅔ C. cooked 'apples' = 1 C. raw veggies) + 1 oz. lean protein (egg) + 2 tsp. oil
½ cake (1 serving) = ½ unrestricted + ½ restricted + ½ C. veggies (⅓ C. cooked 'apples = ½ C. raw veggies) + 0.5 oz. lean protein (egg) + 1 tsp. oil

NOTE: Because this recipe includes a restricted packet, and 1 serving (½ cake) contains ½ restricted, I count it as 1 full restricted for the day. This ensures the carb or calorie count won't exceed protocol amounts.

Blondie Cakes

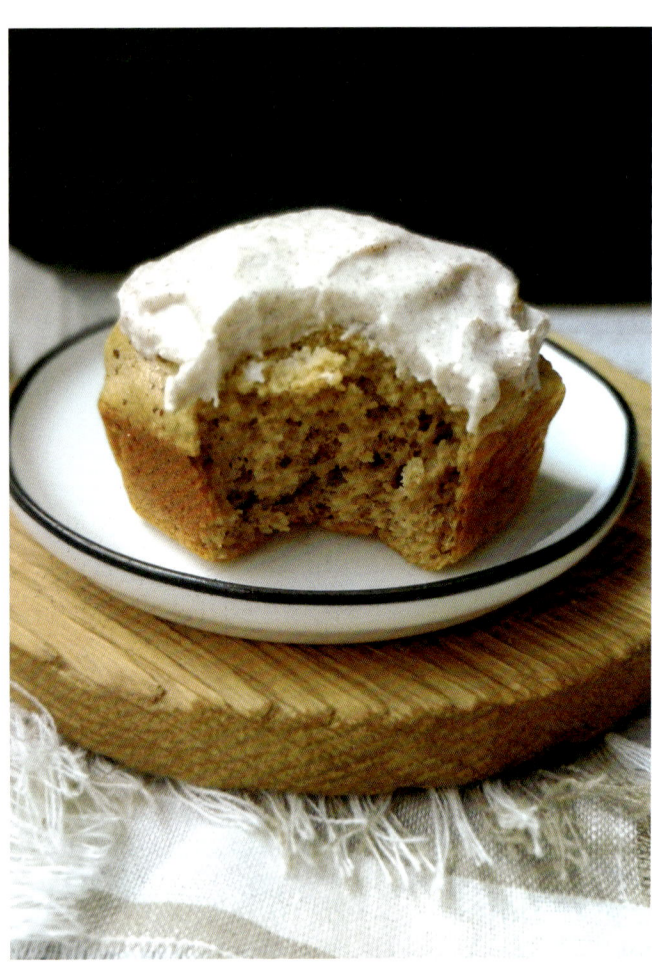

INGREDIENTS (CAKES)

1 pkg. Ideal Protein apple cinnamon puffs
1 Ideal Protein chocolate caramel mug cake mix
1 tsp. baking powder
1 large egg
2 T. water
1 T. Ideal Protein maple syrup
2 tsp. olive oil
½ tsp. vanilla extract
Cooking spray

INGREDIENTS (FROSTING, OPTIONAL)

Frosting, pg. 132
⅛ tsp. cinnamon

DIRECTIONS

1. Preheat oven to 350°F degrees.
2. Place the dry ingredients in a bullet blender or food processor; pulse to fine crumbs. Transfer to a mixing bowl.
3. Add liquid ingredients to a separate mixing bowl; stir to mix. Stir into dry ingredients.
4. Pour batter into a sprayed brownie pan (see TIP) making 4 cakes.
5. Bake 11-12 minutes or until an inserted cake tester comes out clean.
6. For best texture, remove cakes from pan and cool completely on cooling rack.
7. If desired, prepare frosting recipe adding cinnamon; stir. Frost cooled cakes.

SERVINGS

4 cakes = 1 unrestricted + 1 restricted + 1 oz. lean protein (egg) + 2 tsp. oil
2 cakes = ½ unrestricted + ½ restricted + 0.5 oz. lean protein (egg) + 1 tsp. oil

TIP: A brownie pan has square cavities (similar to a muffin tin with round cavities.)

NOTE: Because this recipe includes a restricted packet, and 1 serving (2 cakes) contains ½ restricted, I count it as 1 full restricted for the day. This ensures the carb or calorie count won't exceed protocol amounts. Serving sizes do not include frosting.

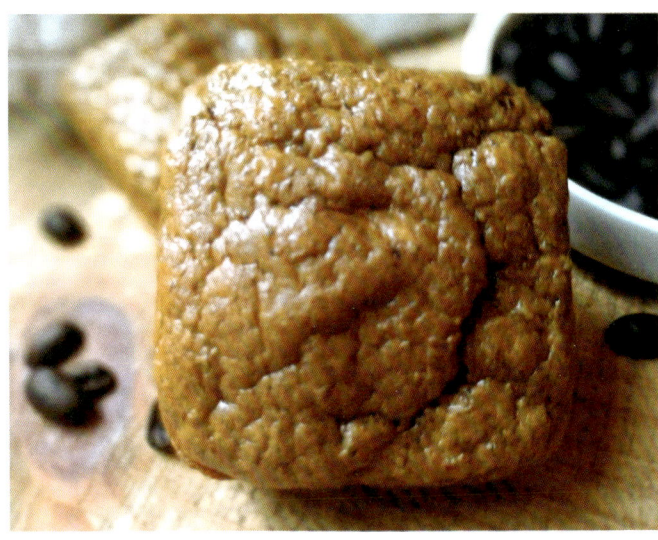

Cappuccino Cakes

INGREDIENTS

1 Ideal Protein golden or chocolate chip pancake mix
1 Ideal Protein vanilla crispy square (broken into pieces)
½ tsp. instant espresso powder
½ tsp. baking powder
1 large egg
2 T. cold coffee
2 T. water
½ tsp. vanilla extract
Cooking spray
Frosting (chocolate), pg. 132 (optional)

DIRECTIONS

1. Preheat oven to 350°F degrees.
2. Place the dry ingredients in a bullet blender or food processor; pulse to fine crumbs. Transfer to a mixing bowl.
3. Add liquid ingredients to a separate mixing bowl; stir to mix. Stir into dry ingredients.
4. Pour batter into a sprayed brownie pan (see note) making 4 cakes.
5. Bake 9-11 minutes or until an inserted cake tester comes out clean.
6. For best texture, remove cakes from pan and cool completely on a cooling rack. Frost cooled cakes, if desired.

SERVINGS

4 cakes = 2 unrestricted + 1 oz. lean protein (egg)
2 cakes = 1 unrestricted + 0.5 oz. lean protein (egg)

NOTE: A brownie pan has square cavities (similar to a muffin tin with round cavities.)

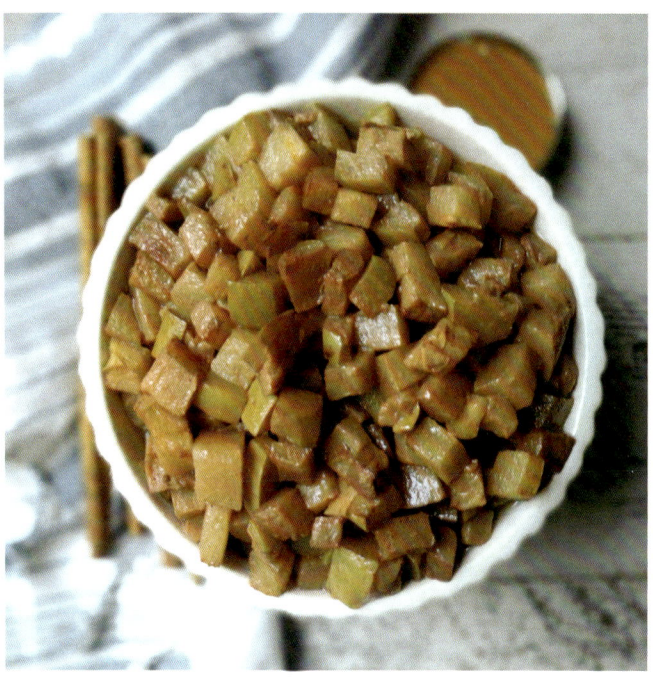

Caramel Fried Apples

Slow cooker recipe

INGREDIENTS

10 C. diced chayote squash* (peeled or unpeeled)
¼ C. apple cider vinegar
½ C. Walden Farms caramel syrup
½ C. Walden Farms pancake syrup
1 T. + 1 tsp. cinnamon
1 T. + 1 tsp. lemon juice

DIRECTIONS

1. Place diced chayote in slow cooker.
2. In a mixing bowl, whisk remaining ingredients.
3. Pour sauce mixture over chayote; stir to coat.
4. Cook on high 6 hours. Stir once halfway through cooking.

SERVINGS

Entire recipe yield = 10 C. veggies
⅕ recipe yield = 2 C. veggies

TIP: *Approximately 7-9 whole chayote squash are equivalent to 10 C. diced. Caramel Fried Apples freeze well – divide into desired serving sizes; vacuum seal or store in an airtight container.

Carrot Cake

INGREDIENTS ('CARROTS')
½ C. diced rutabaga (¼-inch cubes)
Olive oil cooking spray
¼ tsp. cinnamon
½ tsp. sugar free sweetener, granular

INGREDIENTS (CAKE)
1 Ideal Protein golden pancakes mix
1 Ideal Protein cranberry pomegranate protein bar (broken in chunks)
1 tsp. baking powder
¼ tsp. cinnamon
⅛ tsp. ground nutmeg
⅛ tsp. ground ginger
1 large egg
1 T. Walden Farms caramel syrup
1 T. water
Olive oil cooking spray
Frosting, pg. 132 (optional)

DIRECTIONS
1. Preheat oven to 425°F degrees.
2. Place rutabaga in a 5" round baking dish; lightly spray rutabaga with cooking spray. Sprinkle with cinnamon and sweetener; toss to coat.
3. Roast 20 minutes. Transfer to a work surface to cool; finely chop and set aside. Reduce oven temp to 350°F degrees.
4. Place the dry ingredients for the cake in a bullet blender or food processor; pulse to fine crumbs. Transfer to a mixing bowl.
5. Add liquid ingredients for the cake to a separate mixing bowl; stir to mix. Stir into dry ingredients. Fold in rutabaga.
6. Spray same 5" round baking dish used for cooking rutabaga; pour cake batter into baking dish.
7. Bake 16-18 minutes or until an inserted cake tester comes out clean.
8. For best texture, remove cake from pan and cool upside down on a cooling rack. Once cooled, turn right side up. Frost, if desired.

SERVINGS
Entire cake = 1 unrestricted + 1 restricted + 1 oz. lean protein (egg) + ½ C. veggies
½ cake = ½ unrestricted + ½ restricted + 0.5 oz. lean protein (egg) + ¼ C. veggies

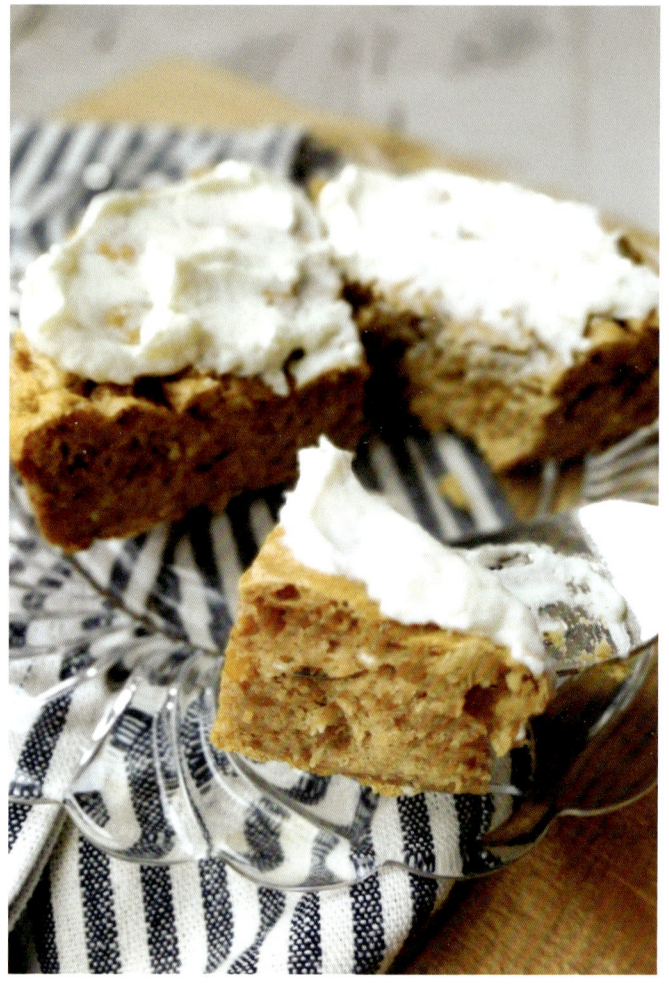

NOTE: Because this recipe includes a restricted packet, and 1 serving (½ cake) contains ½ restricted, I count it as 1 full restricted for the day. This ensures the carb or calorie count won't exceed protocol amounts.

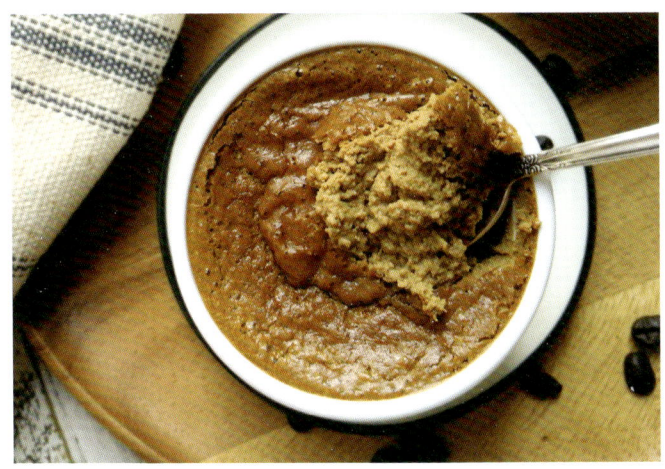

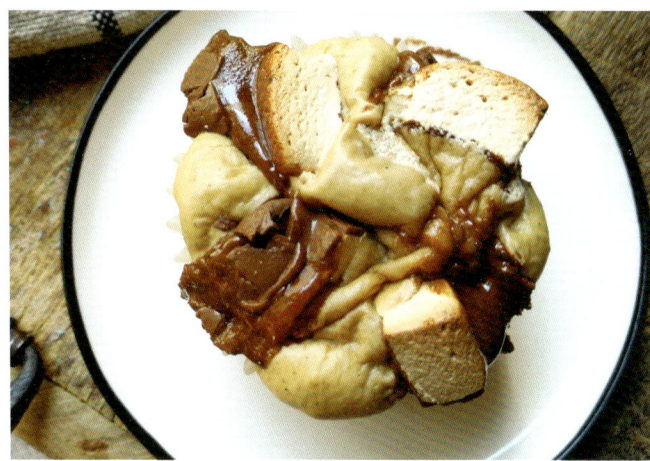

Coffee & Cream Custard

INGREDIENTS

1 large egg
1 large egg yolk
⅔ C. Caramel Fried Apples, pg. 127
¼ C. half and half cream
1 Ideal Protein cappuccino smoothie mix
1 tsp. vanilla extract

DIRECTIONS

1. Preheat oven to 300°F degrees.
2. Whisk egg and egg yolk in a mixing bowl; set aside.
3. Add remaining ingredients to a blender; blend until smooth. Stir blender mixture into eggs.
4. Place two (3 ½ x 1 ¼-inch) ramekins in a crème brûlée pan or an 8 x 8-inch baking pan, spaced apart. Evenly fill ramekins with batter.
5. Fill pan with enough hot water to bring water level halfway up sides of ramekins.
6. Bake 45 minutes. Cool on a cooling rack 1 hour, leaving ramekins in water bath.
7. Remove ramekins from pan; cover with plastic wrap and refrigerate at least 4 hours or overnight before serving.

SERVINGS

2 custards = 1 unrestricted + 1.5 oz. lean protein (egg) + 1 C. veggies (⅔ C. cooked 'apples' = 1 C. raw veggies) + 2 oz. half and half cream
1 custard = ½ unrestricted + 0.75 oz. lean protein (egg) + ½ C. veggies (⅓ C. cooked 'apples = ½ C. raw veggies) + 1 oz. half and half cream

NOTE: Only one custard should be eaten in one day due to the maximum dairy protocol.

Cookie Dough Bombs

INGREDIENTS

1 Ideal Protein chocolate caramel mug cake mix
1 Ideal Protein cookie dough swirl protein bar (cut in 8 pieces)
1 large egg
1 T. water
½ tsp. vanilla extract
Cooking spray

DIRECTIONS

1. Preheat oven to 350°F degrees.
2. Place the mug cake mix in a small mixing bowl.
3. In a separate small mixing bowl, whisk liquid ingredients to combine. Add to mug cake mix; stir to combine.
4. Pour batter into a sprayed standard size muffin tin making 2 'bombs'. Place 4 pieces of the protein bar into each bomb batter; push down so bar pieces are covered at least halfway by batter.
5. Bake 9-11 minutes or until an inserted cake tester comes out clean.
6. Remove bombs from pan -- may be served warm or cooled.

SERVINGS

2 bombs = 1 unrestricted + 1 restricted + 1 oz. lean protein (egg)
1 bomb = ½ unrestricted + ½ restricted + 0.5 oz. lean protein (egg)

NOTE: Because this recipe includes a restricted packet, and 1 serving (1 bomb) contains ½ restricted, I count it as 1 full restricted for the day. This ensures the carb or calorie count won't exceed protocol amounts.

Crustless Pumpkin Pie

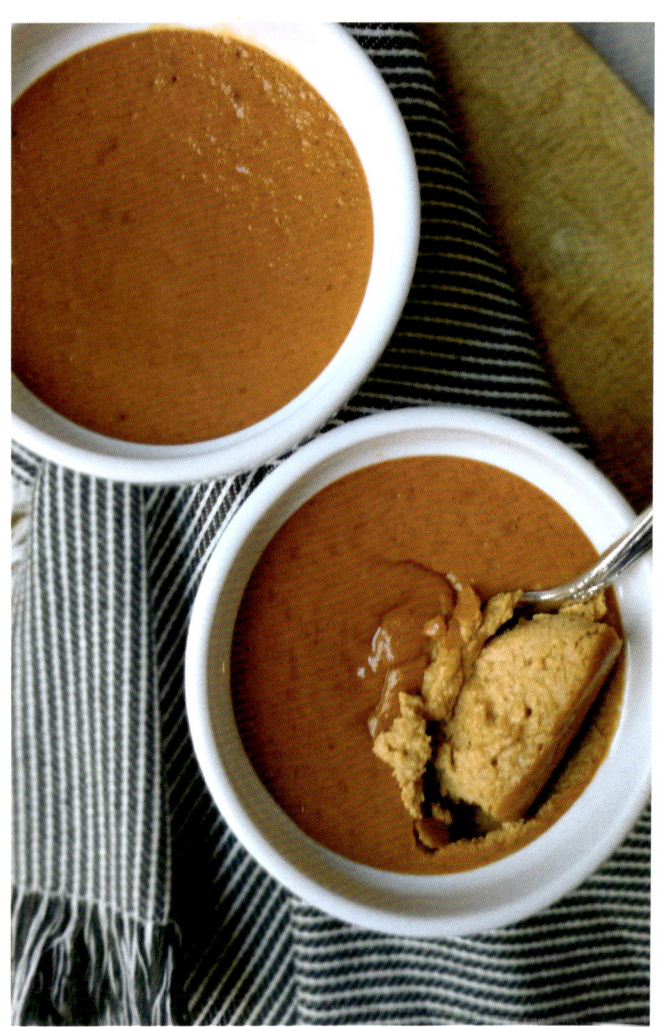

INGREDIENTS
1 large egg
1 large egg yolk
⅔ C. Caramel Fried Apples, pg. 127
¼ C. half and half cream
1 Ideal Protein vanilla smoothie mix
1 tsp. pumpkin pie flavor fountain*

DIRECTIONS
1. Preheat oven to 300°F degrees.
2. Whisk egg and egg yolk in a mixing bowl; set aside.
3. Add remaining ingredients to a blender; blend until smooth. Stir blender mixture into eggs.
4. Place two (3 ½ x 1 ¼-inch) ramekins in a crème brûlée pan or an 8 x 8-inch baking pan, spaced apart. Evenly fill ramekins with batter.
5. Fill pan with enough hot water to bring water level halfway up sides of ramekins.
6. Bake 45 minutes. Cool on a cooling rack 1 hour, leaving ramekins in water bath.
7. Remove ramekins from pan; cover with plastic wrap and refrigerate at least 4 hours or overnight before serving.

SERVINGS
2 Crustless Pumpkin Pies = 1 unrestricted + 1.5 oz. lean protein (egg) + 1 C. veggies (⅔ C. cooked 'apples' = 1 C. raw veggies) + 2 oz. half and half cream
1 Crustless Pumpkin Pie = ½ unrestricted + 0.75 oz. lean protein (egg) + ½ C. veggies (⅓ C. cooked 'apples = ½ C. raw veggies) + 1 oz. half and half cream

TIP: *Pumpkin pie flavor fountain adds color and flavor to this dish – it may be purchased online at amazon.com or olivenation.com. If it is unavailable, ¼ tsp. pumpkin pie spice may be subbed; however, the color and flavor of the pie will not be the same.

NOTE: Only one Crustless Pumpkin Pie should be eaten in one day due to the maximum dairy protocol.

Double Chocolate Caramel Cake

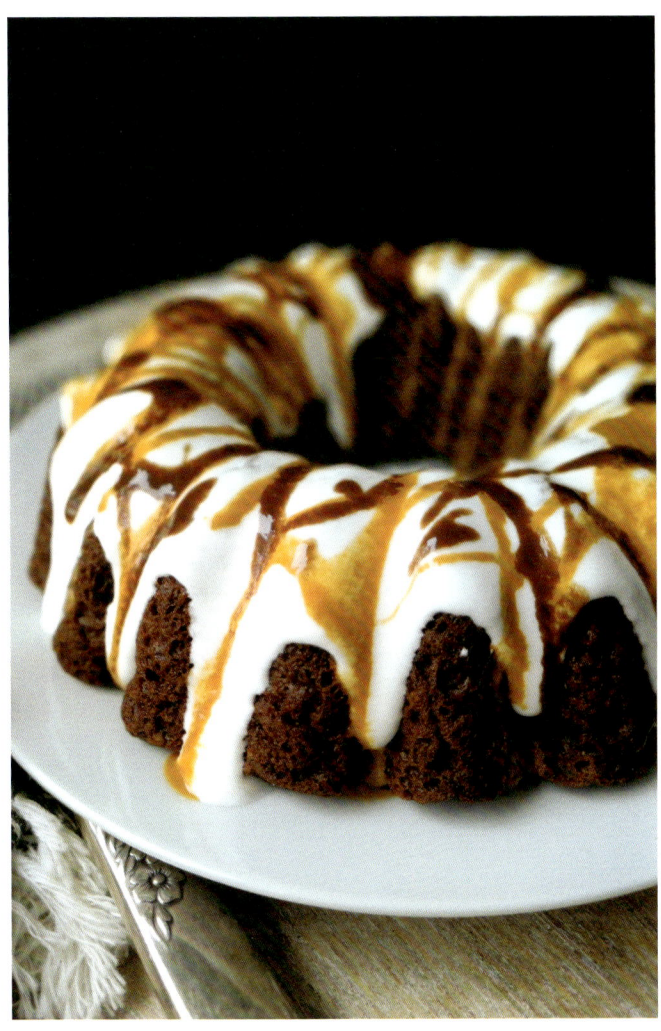

INGREDIENTS (CAKE)

2 Ideal Protein chocolate caramel mug cake mix
2 Ideal Protein chocolate smoothie mix
½ tsp. baking soda
½ tsp. baking powder
¼ C. water
¼ C. Walden Farms chocolate syrup
¼ C. half and half cream
2 large egg yolks
1 T. + 1 tsp. olive oil
2 tsp. apple cider vinegar
Cooking spray

INGREDIENTS (GLAZE)

Walden Farms marshmallow dip, to taste
Walden Farms chocolate syrup, to taste
Walden Farms caramel syrup, to taste

DIRECTIONS

1. Preheat oven to 350°F degrees.
2. Add dry ingredients to a mixing bowl; stir to mix.
3. Add liquid ingredients to a separate mixing bowl; whisk to mix. Stir into dry ingredients. Batter will be thick.
4. Spoon batter into a sprayed standard size Bundt pan. Level batter with the back of the spoon.
5. Bake 16-18 minutes or until an inserted cake tester comes out clean. Remove cake from pan and cool completely on a cooling rack before glazing.
6. To glaze, use a spoon to place marshmallow dip across the top; with the tip of the spoon, coax the dip to drip down the cake. Finish by drizzling with caramel and chocolate syrups.

SERVINGS

Entire cake = 4 unrestricted + 1 oz. lean protein (egg yolks) + 4 tsp. oil + 2 oz. half and half cream
¼ cake = 1 unrestricted + 0.25 oz. lean protein (egg yolk) + 1 tsp. oil + 0.5 oz. half and half cream

Frosting

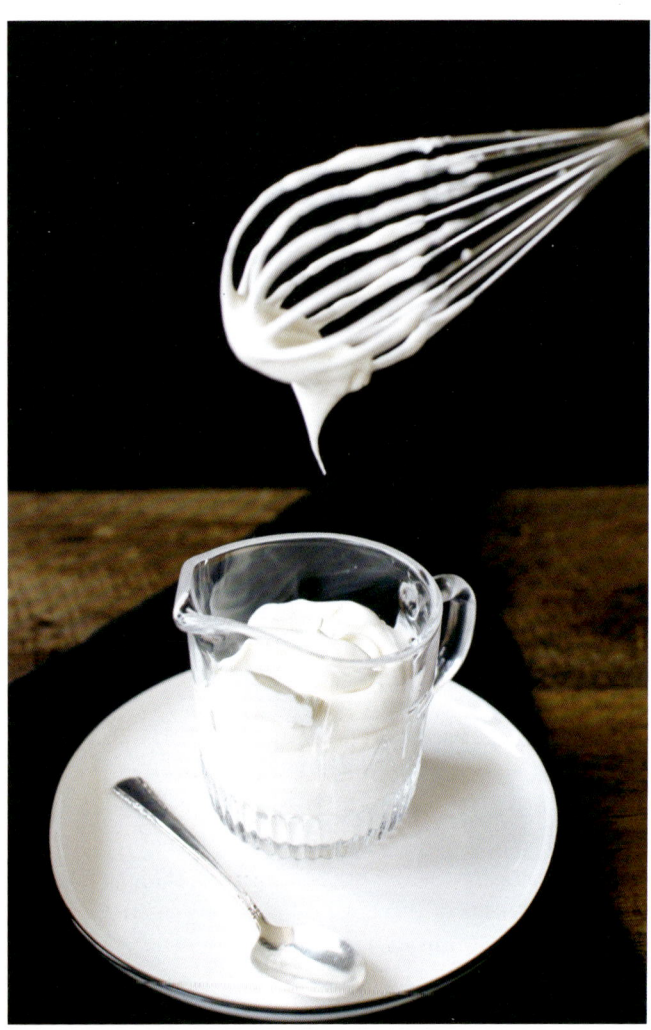

INGREDIENTS

1 T. Ideal Protein chocolate or vanilla pudding mix
2 T. Walden Farms marshmallow dip
⅛ tsp. vanilla extract

DIRECTIONS

1. Mix ingredients in a small bowl; cover and store any leftovers in fridge.

SERVINGS

Counted as 'extras' for daily protocol. Confirm 'extras' quantity with your coach or clinic.

TIP: I reserve a pudding packet for making frosting and store in fridge. Frosting flavor may be changed by adding seasonings such as cinnamon or pumpkin spice, and a variety of different flavored extracts may be used in place of the vanilla extract.

Lemon Raspberry Bundt Cake

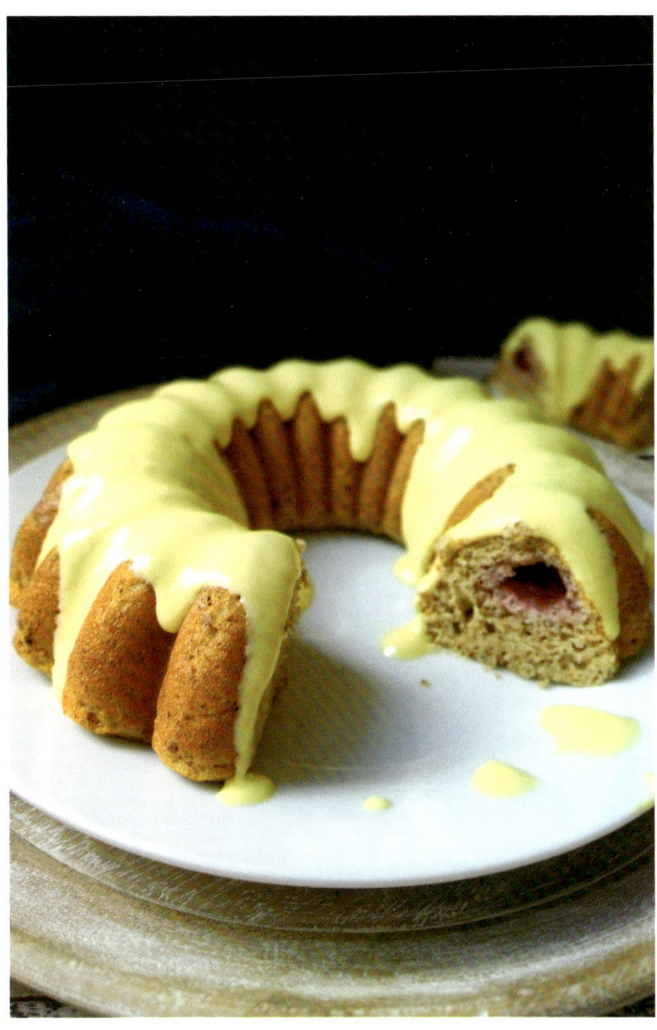

INGREDIENTS (CAKE)
2 Ideal Protein chocolate chip or golden pancakes mix
2 Ideal Protein vanilla crispy squares (broken into pieces)
1 tsp. baking powder
Zest of 1 lemon (I use a Meyer lemon*)
2 large eggs
¼ C. water
¼ C. Ideal Protein maple syrup
¼ tsp. lemon extract
3 T. Walden Farms raspberry spread
Cooking spray

INGREDIENTS (GLAZE, OPTIONAL)
3 T. Walden Farms marshmallow dip
1 T. Ideal Protein maple syrup
2-3 drops yellow food coloring, optional

DIRECTIONS
1. Preheat oven to 350°F degrees.
2. Place the dry ingredients in a bullet blender or food processor; pulse to fine crumbs. Transfer to a mixing bowl.
3. Add liquid ingredients (except raspberry spread) to a separate mixing bowl; stir to mix. Stir into dry ingredients.
4. Place ½ the batter into a sprayed standard size Bundt cake pan.
5. Evenly place the raspberry spread by the teaspoonful in a ring around center of cake batter. Pour remaining batter on top.
6. Bake 19-20 minutes or until an inserted cake tester comes out clean.
7. Remove cake from pan and cool completely on a cooling rack.
8. Combine all glaze ingredients. Spoon over cake; use spoon to coax the glaze to drip over sides.

SERVINGS
Entire cake = 4 unrestricted + 2 oz. lean protein (eggs)
¼ cake = 1 unrestricted + 0.5 oz. lean protein (eggs)

TIP: *Meyer lemons have a more fragrant rind when zested than standard lemons.

Marble Pound Cake

INGREDIENTS (CHOCOLATE BATTER)

1 Ideal Protein chocolate chip pancakes mix
1 Ideal Protein chocolate crispy square (broken into pieces)
½ tsp. baking powder
1 large egg
2 T. water
2 T. Walden Farms chocolate syrup
½ tsp. vanilla extract

INGREDIENTS (VANILLA BATTER)

1 Ideal Protein golden pancakes mix
1 Ideal Protein vanilla crispy square (broken into pieces)
½ tsp. baking powder
1 large egg
2 T. water
2 T. Ideal Protein maple syrup
½ tsp. vanilla extract
Cooking spray

DIRECTIONS

1. Preheat oven to 350°F degrees.
2. Place 4 mixing bowls on a work surface.
3. Add all chocolate batter dry ingredients to #1 bowl; stir to mix.
4. Add all chocolate batter liquid ingredients to #2 bowl; whisk to mix.
5. Add all vanilla batter dry ingredients to #3 bowl; stir to mix.
6. Add all vanilla batter liquid ingredients to #4 bowl; whisk to mix.
7. Combine chocolate batter ingredients from bowl #1 and #2; stir to mix.
8. Combine vanilla batter ingredients from bowl #3 and #4; stir to mix.
9. Coat a metal (9 x 5-inch) loaf pan with cooking spray.
10. Using an ice cream scoop, scoop chocolate batter and place in pan; repeat with vanilla batter. Randomly place batter into pan, alternating the two batters.
11. Starting at short end of pan, drag a table knife through batter making a zig zag pattern.
12. Bake 18-19 minutes or until inserted cake tester comes out clean. For best texture, remove cake from pan and cool completely on a cooling rack before serving.

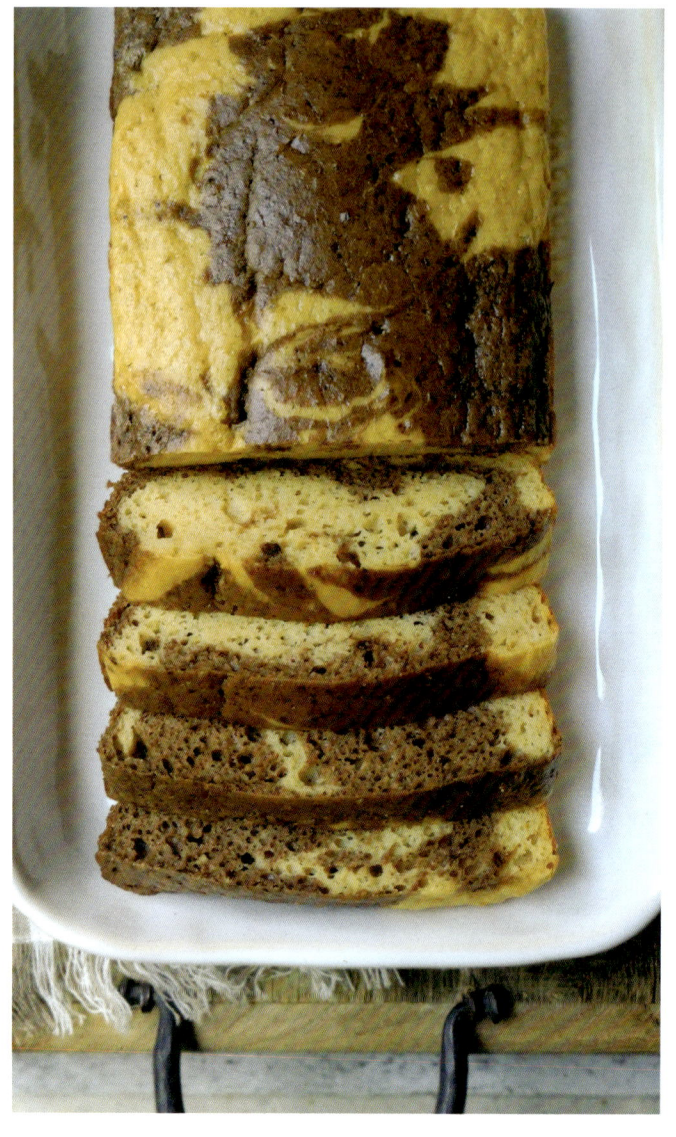

SERVINGS

Entire pound cake = 4 unrestricted + 2 oz. lean protein (eggs)
¼ pound cake = 1 unrestricted + 0.5 oz. lean protein (eggs)

Mardi Gras King Cake

INGREDIENTS (CAKE)

2 Ideal Protein golden pancakes mix
2 Ideal Protein vanilla crispy squares (broken into pieces)
1 tsp. baking powder
2 large eggs
¼ C. water
¼ C. Ideal Protein maple syrup
Cooking spray

INGREDIENTS (FILLING)

Cinnamon, to taste
3 T. Walden Farms raspberry spread

DIRECTIONS

1. Preheat oven to 350° F degrees.
2. Place the dry cake ingredients in a bullet style blender or food processor; pulse to fine crumbs. Transfer to a mixing bowl.
3. Add liquid ingredients to a separate mixing bowl; whisk to mix. Stir into dry mixture.
4. Place ½ the batter into a sprayed standard size Bundt cake pan.
5. Lightly sprinkle the top of the batter with cinnamon. Using a spoon, place teaspoon size dollops of raspberry spread in a ring around center of cake batter.
6. Pour the remaining cake batter on top of filling; level batter.
7. Bake 18-20 minutes or until an inserted cake tester comes out clean.
8. For best texture, remove cake from pan and cool completely on a cooling rack. Glaze cooled cake, if desired.

INGREDIENTS (GLAZE)

¼ C. + 2 T. Walden Farms marshmallow dip
2 T. Ideal Protein maple syrup
1 tsp. vanilla extract
2 drops green food coloring
2 drops yellow food coloring
1 drop blue + 1 drop red food coloring (making purple)

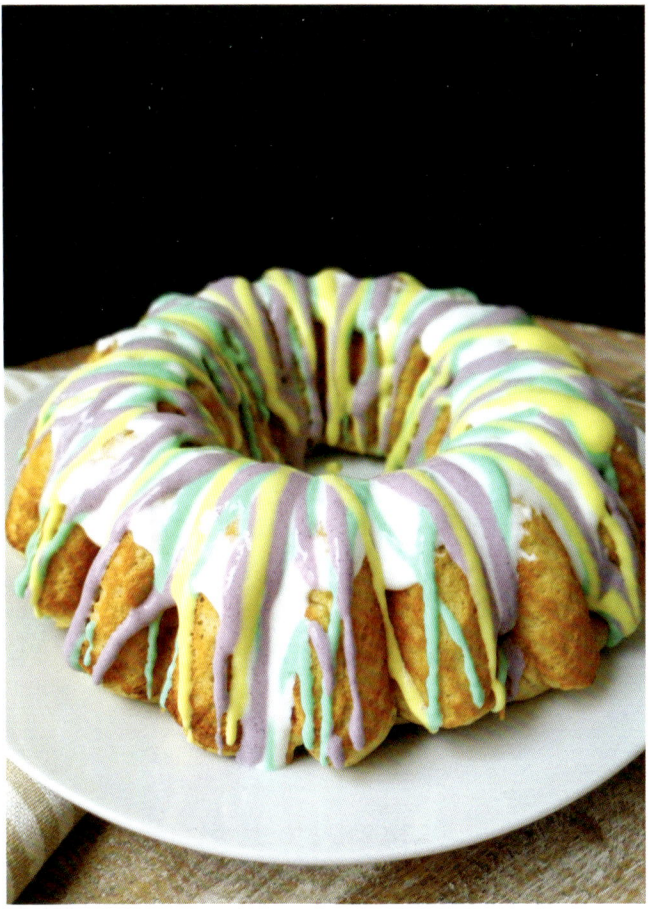

DIRECTIONS

1. Place first 3 ingredients in a small bowl; whisk until blended. Equally divide glaze into two separate bowls. Set one bowl aside.
2. Using one bowl of glaze, spoon over top of cake, coaxing glaze to drip down sides.
3. To make colored glaze, divide remaining glaze mixture into 3 small separate bowls.
4. Tint the glaze in each bowl separately using green for one, yellow for another, and the blue + red food coloring for the last.
5. Stir each one using a separate fork. Drizzle over cake.

SERVINGS

Entire cake = 4 unrestricted + 2 oz. lean protein (egg)
¼ cake = 1 unrestricted + 0.5 oz. lean protein (egg)

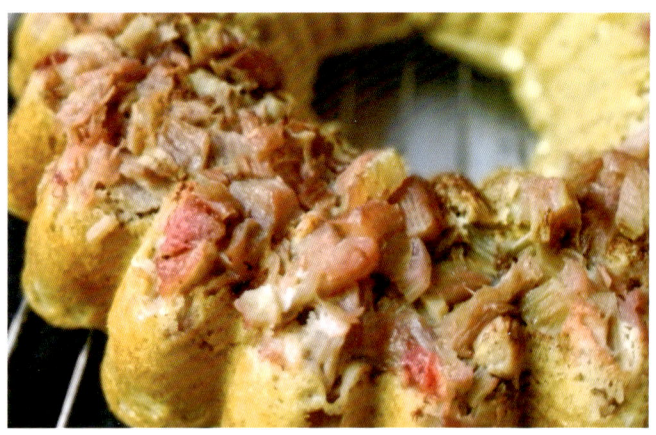
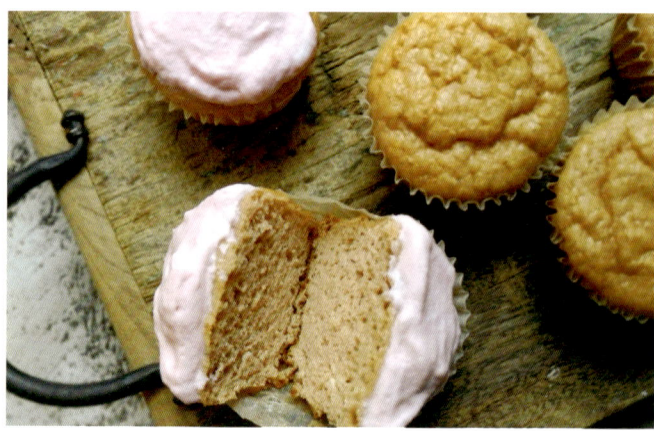

Rhubarb Dump Cake

Eggless Recipe

INGREDIENTS

1 ⅓ C. finely chopped rhubarb
1 ½ tsp. sugar free sweetener, granular
1 ½ tsp. cinnamon, divided
Cooking spray
2 Ideal Protein chocolate chip or golden pancakes mix
2 Ideal Protein maple oatmeal mix
¼ tsp. baking soda
¼ tsp. baking powder
½ C. water
2 T. Walden Farms strawberry syrup
1 tsp. vanilla extract
1 tsp. apple cider vinegar
1 T. + 1 tsp. olive oil

DIRECTIONS

1. Preheat oven to 350°F degrees.
2. In a small bowl, gently mix rhubarb with sweetener and ½ tsp. of the cinnamon. Lightly coat a standard size Bundt pan with cooking spray, and evenly spoon rhubarb into bottom of pan; set aside.
3. Add dry ingredients to a mixing bowl; stir to mix.
4. Add liquid ingredients to a separate mixing bowl; whisk to mix. Stir into dry ingredients.
5. Spoon batter into Bundt pan; level batter with the back of the spoon.
6. Bake 16-18 minutes or until an inserted cake tester comes out clean.
7. For best texture, remove cake from pan and cool completely on a cooling rack before serving.

SERVINGS

Entire cake = 4 unrestricted + 1 ⅓ C. veggies + 4 tsp. oil
¼ cake = 1 unrestricted + ⅓ C. veggies + 1 tsp. oil

Strawberry Cupcakes

INGREDIENTS

2 Ideal Protein golden pancakes mix
2 Ideal Protein vanilla crispy squares (broken into pieces)
1 tsp. baking powder
2 large eggs
¼ C. water
¼ C. Walden Farms strawberry syrup
¼ tsp. strawberry extract
Cooking spray
Frosting, pg. 132 (optional)

DIRECTIONS

1. Preheat oven to 350°F degrees.
2. Place the dry ingredients in a bullet blender or food processor; pulse to fine crumbs. Transfer to a mixing bowl.
3. Add liquid ingredients to a separate mixing bowl; whisk to mix. Stir into dry ingredients.
4. Pour batter into a sprayed standard size cupcake tin making 8 cupcakes.
5. Bake 12-13 minutes or until an inserted cake tester comes out clean.
6. For best texture, remove cupcakes from pan and cool completely on a cooling rack. Frost, if desired.

SERVINGS

8 cupcakes = 4 unrestricted + 2 oz. lean protein (egg)
2 cupcakes = 1 unrestricted + 0.5 oz. lean protein (egg)

TIP: A few drops of red food coloring in the batter and the frosting help to make this cupcake achieve a strawberry-like color.

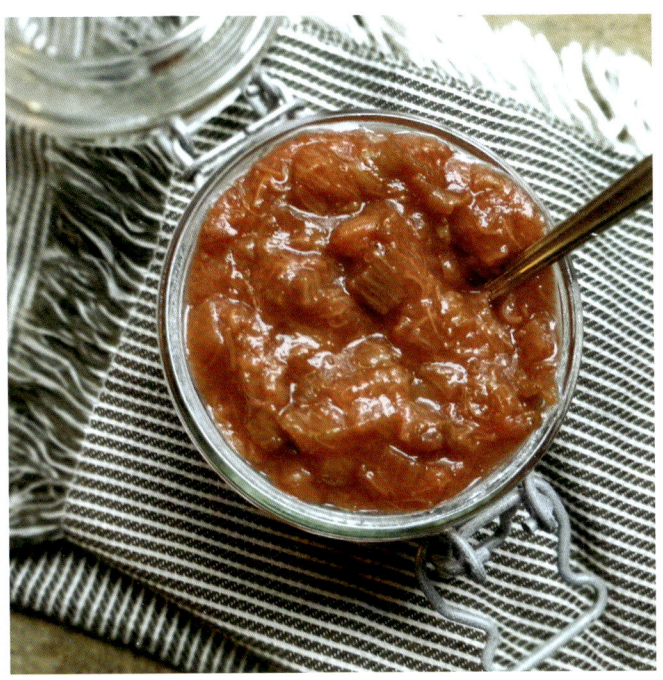

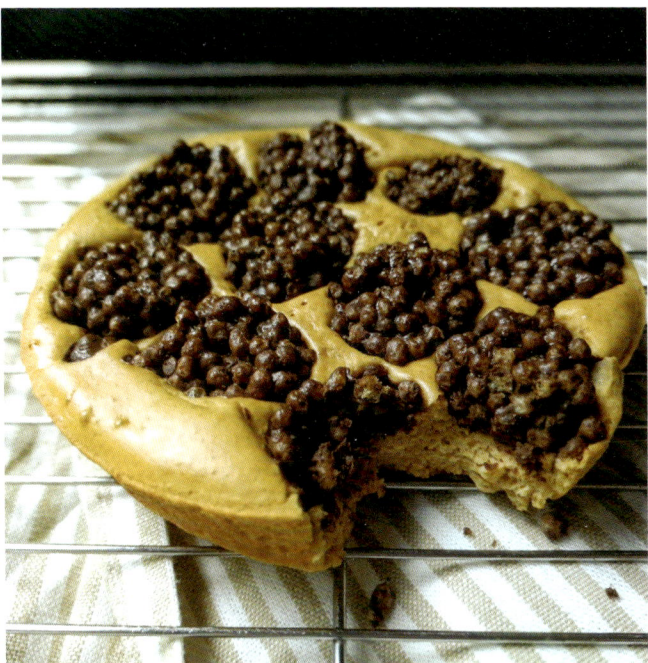

Strawberry Rhubarb Compote

INGREDIENTS

3 C. fresh or frozen rhubarb (cut in 1-inch chunks)
2 T. Walden Farms strawberry syrup
1 T. Ideal Protein maple syrup
1 tsp. lemon juice
½ tsp. vanilla extract
¼ tsp. cinnamon

DIRECTIONS

1. Place all ingredients in a medium saucepan; stir to mix. Bring to a low boil over medium heat.
2. Reduce heat to medium low. Simmer 10 minutes or until rhubarb is stewed, stirring often.
3. Store covered in fridge.

SERVINGS

Entire recipe yield = 3 C. veggies
⅓ recipe yield = 1 C. veggies

TIP: Add compote to smoothies and shakes, top pancakes, waffles or oatmeal, or layer with pudding making a parfait.

Turtle Crunch Cake

INGREDIENTS

1 large egg
2 T. water
1 T. Walden Farms caramel syrup
1 Ideal Protein chocolate caramel mug cake mix
1 pkg. Ideal Protein salted caramel chocolate clusters
Cooking spray

DIRECTIONS

1. Preheat oven to 350°F degrees.
2. Add liquid ingredients to a small mixing bowl; whisk to mix. Add mug cake mix; stir to combine.
3. Pour batter into a sprayed 5-inch round baking dish. Place clusters on top of batter in a single layer.
4. Bake 18-20 minutes or until an inserted cake tester comes out clean.
5. Remove cake from pan and cool completely on a cooling rack.

SERVINGS

Entire cake = 2 unrestricted + 1 oz. lean protein (egg)
½ cake = 1 unrestricted + 0.5 oz. lean protein (egg)

condiments

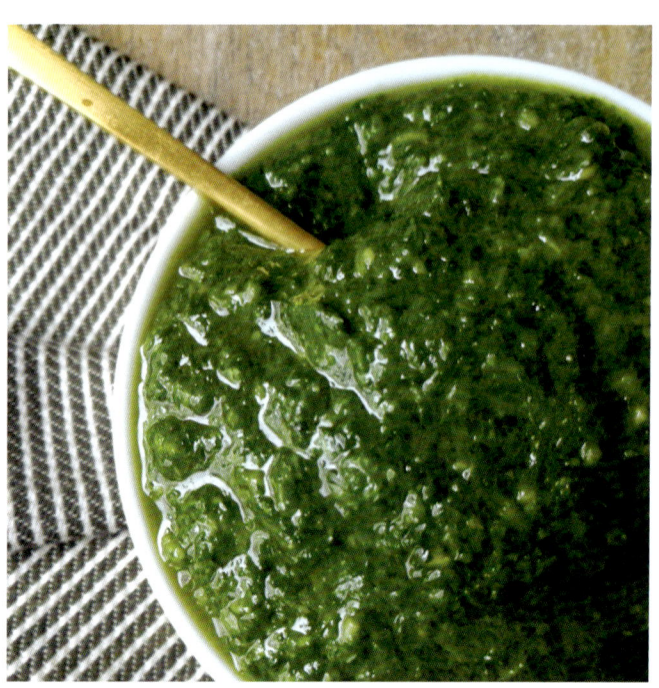

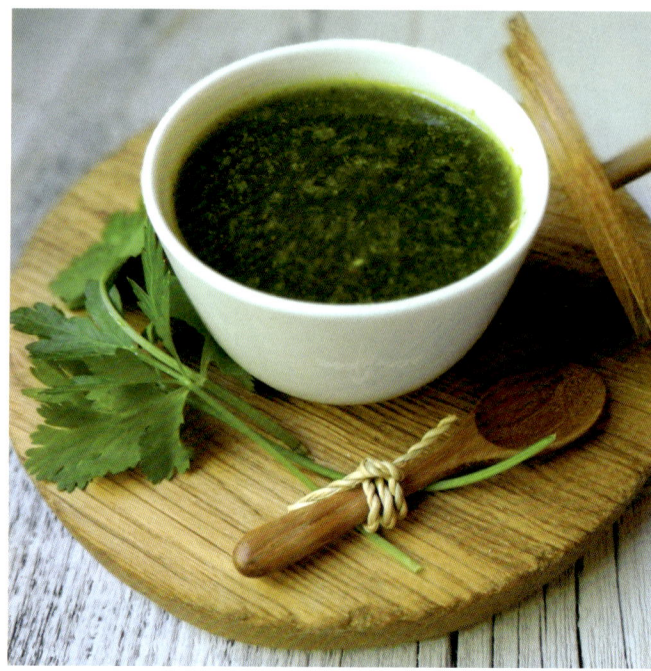

Basil Pesto

INGREDIENTS
1 C. fresh basil leaves, stems removed
(moderately packed)
1 C. fresh spinach leaves, stems removed
(moderately packed)
¼ C. mild olive oil
1 T. minced garlic
1 ½ tsp. lemon juice
¼ tsp. sea salt

DIRECTIONS
1. Place all ingredients in a food processor; blend on high until emulsified to desired texture.
2. Store in an airtight container in the fridge. Before putting lid on container, lay a piece of plastic wrap directly on top of pesto to seal out air. This will allow the pesto to remain a bright green color longer.

SERVINGS
1 T. Pesto = ⅛ tsp. oil

Chimichurri Sauce

INGREDIENTS
1 C. fresh Italian parsley, firmly packed
1 C. fresh cilantro, firmly packed
4 garlic cloves
2 tsp. dried oregano
½ C. olive oil
2 T. apple cider vinegar
1 tsp. sea salt
¼ tsp. freshly ground black pepper
¼ tsp. crushed red pepper flakes

DIRECTIONS
1. Place all ingredients in a blender or food processor and pulse just until blended; no need to puree unless that is the preferred consistency.
2. Keep refrigerated; before serving, let sauce come to room temperature.

SERVINGS
1 T. Sauce = 1½ tsp. oil

TIP: Serve as a condiment with lean cooked meats; exceptionally good served with flank steak.

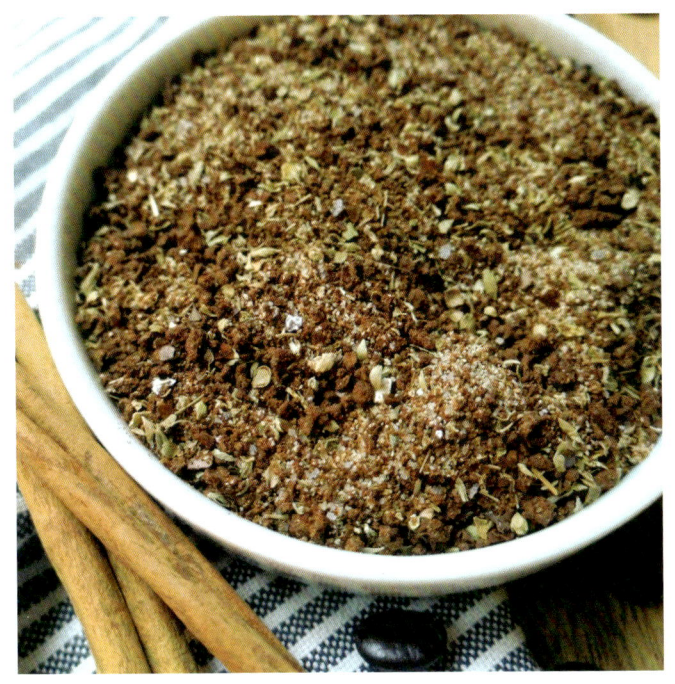
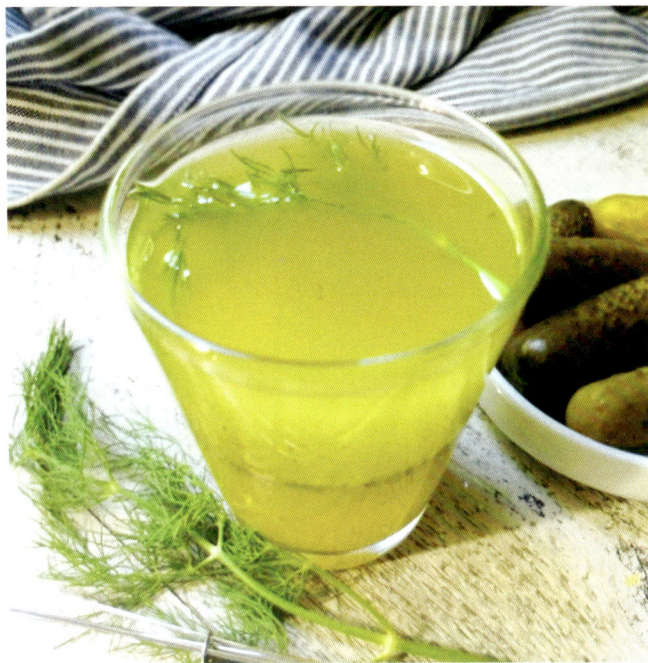

Coffee Spice Rub

INGREDIENTS
2 T. instant espresso coffee granules
2 tsp. ground cumin
2 tsp. dried oregano leaves
1 ½ tsp. garlic powder
1 ½ tsp. sea salt
1 tsp. unsweetened cocoa powder
½ tsp. smoked paprika
¼ tsp. cinnamon

DIRECTIONS
1. Add ingredients to a bowl and stir to combine.
2. Store in an airtight container.

SERVINGS
Varies

TIP: Use as a rub for large cuts of meat such as beef and pork roasts.

Dill Pickle Vinaigrette

INGREDIENTS
½ C. mild olive oil
½ C. dill pickle juice (from pickle jar)
¾ tsp. Dijon mustard
⅛ tsp. garlic powder
1 tsp. chopped fresh dill

DIRECTIONS
1. Place all ingredients in a small mixing bowl. Whisk with a fork to blend.
2. Cover and store refrigerated; whisk before serving.

SERVINGS
1 T. Vinaigrette = 1 ½ tsp. oil

NOTE: Dill pickles/juice must not have added sugar; check ingredients label on jar.

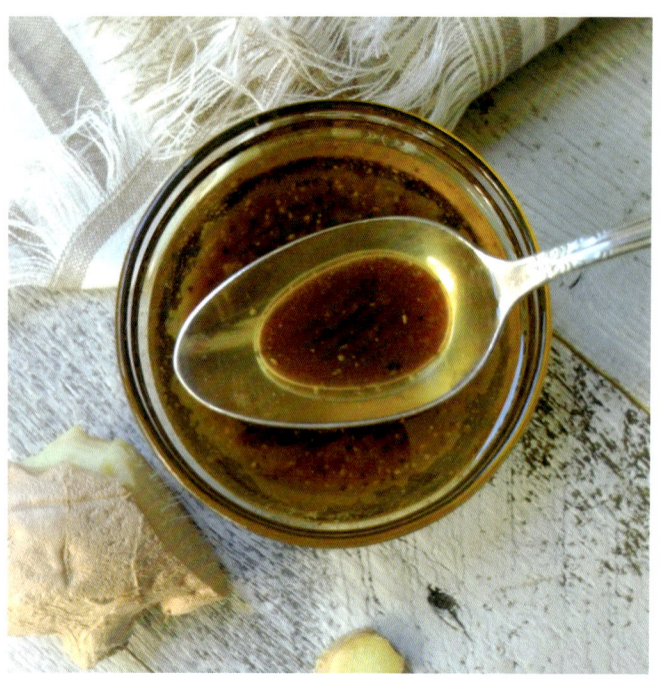
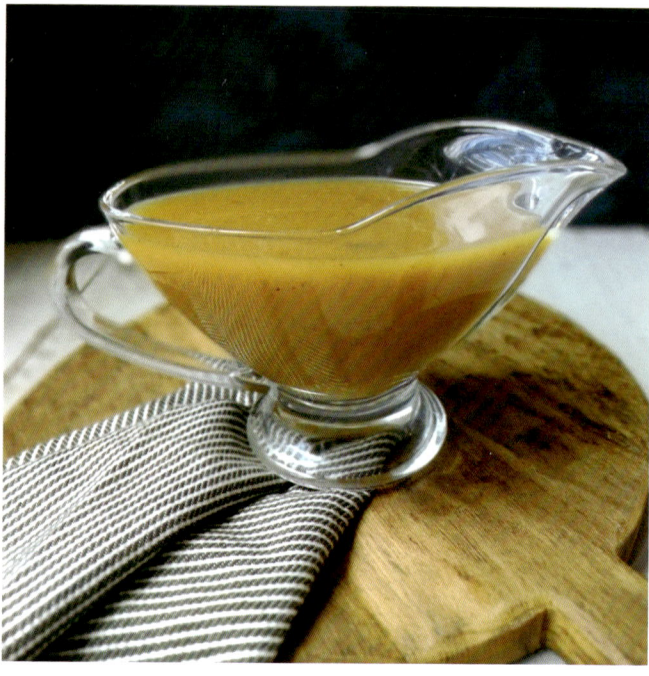

Ginger Soy Vinaigrette

INGREDIENTS
2 T. apple cider vinegar
¼ tsp. ground ginger
1 T. soy sauce
¼ tsp. sugar free sweetener, granular
¼ tsp. Ideal Protein salt
¼ tsp. black pepper
¼ tsp. hot sauce
⅓ C. olive oil

DIRECTIONS
1. In a medium bowl, stir all ingredients to combine (except oil); whisk in oil.
2. Cover and store refrigerated; whisk before serving.

SERVINGS
1 T. Vinaigrette = 2 tsp. oil

Gravy

INGREDIENTS
2 C. turkey, chicken, or beef broth
1 tsp. konjac powder*
1 tsp. soy sauce
½ tsp. onion powder
Black pepper, to taste

DIRECTIONS
1. Add all ingredients to a small saucepan; whisk to mix.
2. Heat over medium/medium high heat while stirring. Bring gravy to a low boil; continue to stir 1 minute or until thickened. Serve hot.

SERVINGS
Consult your clinic or coach for protocol counts for this recipe as part of any 'extras' for the day.

TIP: *Konjac powder (or glucomannan powder) is a natural thickener made from the root of a konjac plant and may easily be found online at amazon.com or other online nutritional ecommerce sites.

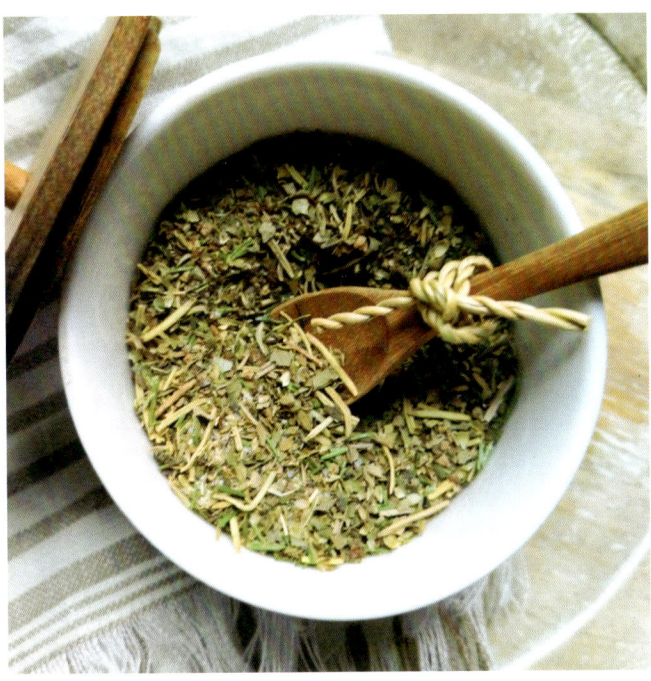

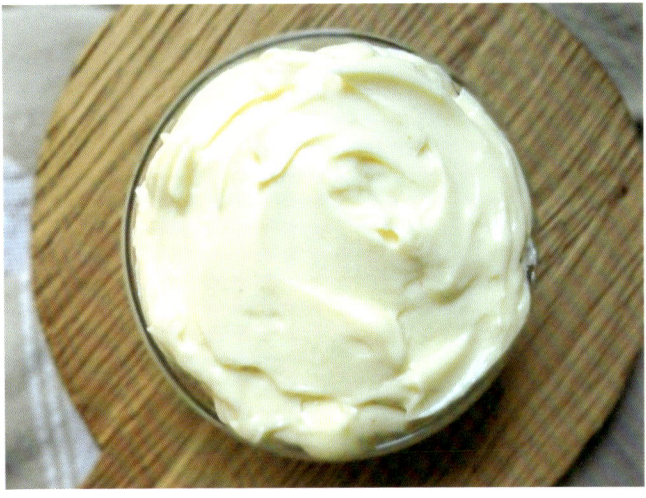

Greek Seasoning

INGREDIENTS
2 tsp. salt
2 tsp. dried basil
2 tsp. dried oregano
½ tsp. dried thyme
2 tsp. garlic powder
1 tsp. dried dill weed
1 tsp. marjoram
1 tsp. black pepper
1 tsp. parsley flakes
1 tsp. rosemary
½ tsp. cinnamon
½ tsp. nutmeg

DIRECTIONS
1. Add ingredients to a bowl and stir to combine.
2. Store in an airtight container.

SERVINGS
n/a

Janeva's Mayonnaise

This recipe is easier than it looks—read entire recipe before making mayonnaise!

INGREDIENTS
2 large egg yolks (room temp)
1 T. Dijon mustard
1 pinch sea salt
1 C. mild olive oil (I use Bertolli® organic)
1 tsp. apple cider vinegar

DIRECTIONS
1. In order listed, place ingredients in a large, tall container. (Container should be 3" inches or less in diameter, but wide enough to accommodate a stick blender.)
2. Place a stick immersion blender into container, hold straight and be sure the blender rests on container bottom.
3. Hold blender stationary on the bottom of the container while blending on high for 8-10 seconds, until the oil mixture starts to emulsify into white mayonnaise. Continue to blend by *very slowly* drawing blender straight up the container to finish emulsifying the mayonnaise.
4. If the mayonnaise doesn't completely emulsify, slowly plunge blender down into mayonnaise to the bottom. Holding the blender at a slight angle, pull up slowly. Repeat these steps as necessary to emulsify oil completely until mayonnaise is creamy.
5. Vigorously stir mayonnaise with a butter knife after final blend with the stick blender. Store refrigerated up to one week.

SERVINGS
1 T. Mayonnaise = 2 tsp. oil

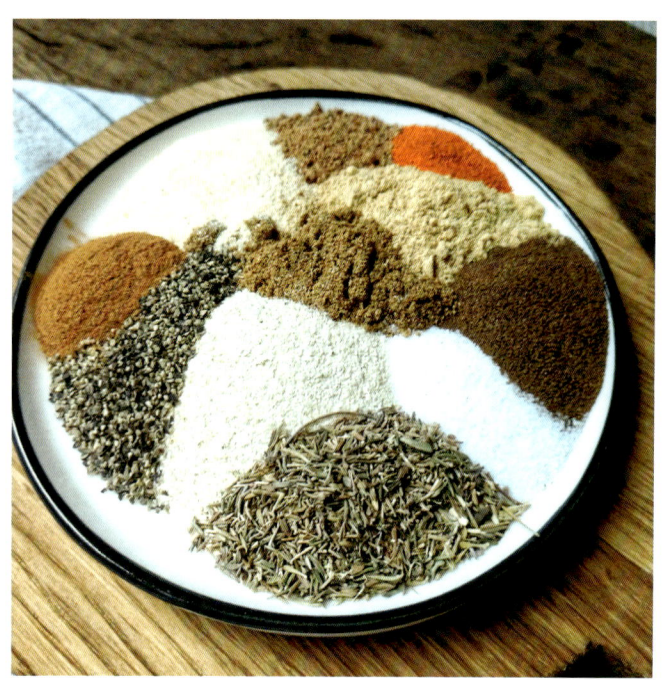

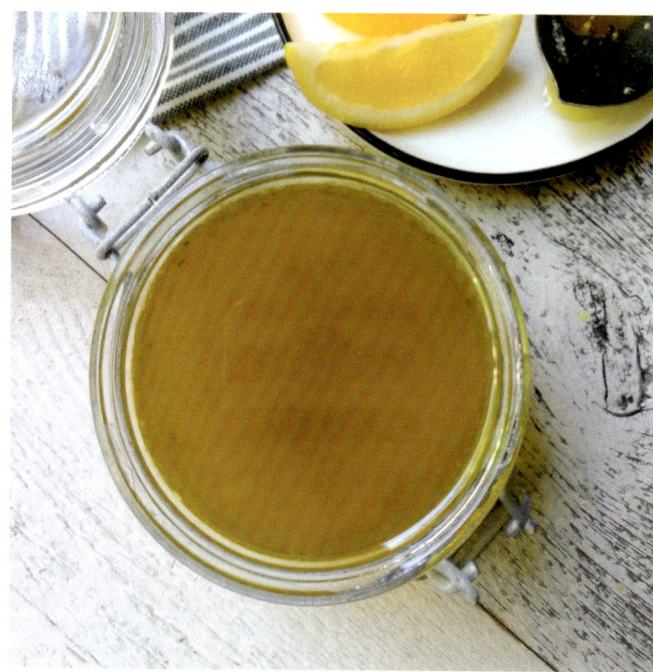

Jerk Seasoning

INGREDIENTS
1 T. ground coriander
2 tsp. garlic powder
2 tsp. ground ginger
2 tsp. onion powder
1 tsp. salt
1 tsp. pepper
1 tsp. dried thyme
¾ tsp. ground nutmeg
¾ tsp. ground allspice
½ tsp. ground cinnamon
¼ tsp. cayenne pepper

DIRECTIONS
1. Add ingredients to a bowl and stir to combine.
2. Store in an airtight container.

SERVINGS
Varies

Lebanese Garlic Lemon Dressing

INGREDIENTS
½ C. fresh lemon juice
½ C. extra virgin olive oil
3 cloves garlic, minced
1 tsp. kosher or sea salt
⅛ tsp. black pepper

DIRECTIONS
1. Place all ingredients in a small mixing bowl. Whisk with a fork to blend.
2. Cover and store refrigerated; whisk before serving.

SERVINGS
1 T. Dressing = 1 ½ tsp. oil

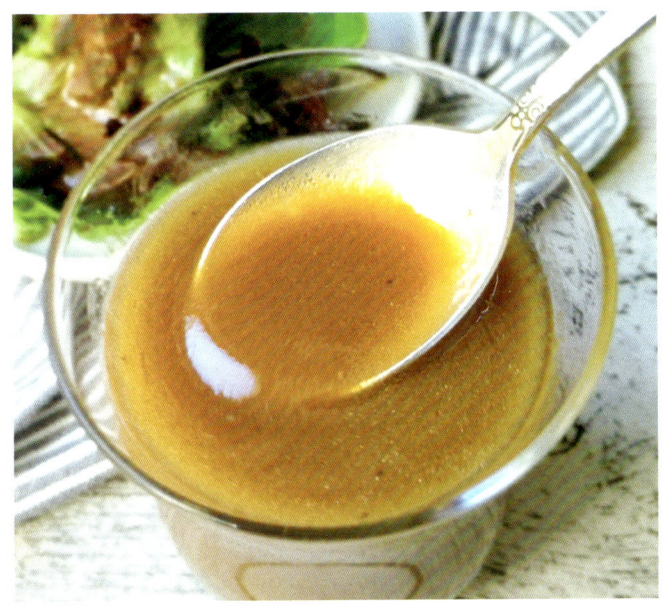

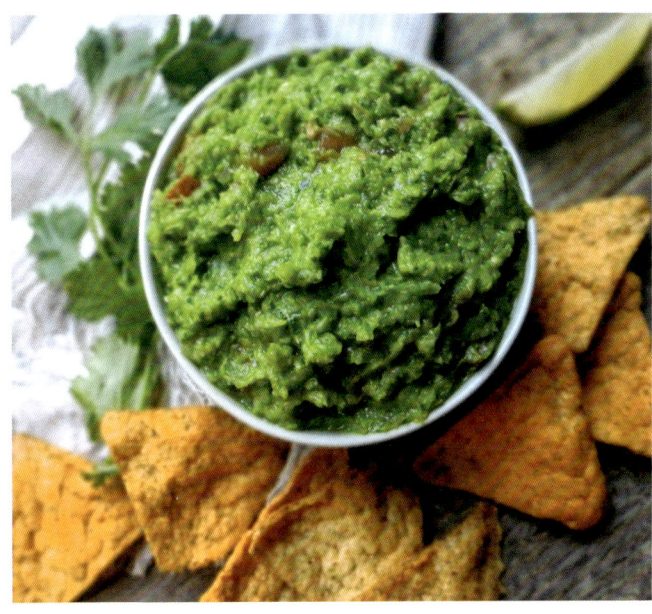

Maple Soy Vinaigrette

INGREDIENTS
½ C. soy sauce
½ C. apple cider vinegar
½ C. Ideal Protein maple syrup
2 T. sugar free sweetener, granular
2 T. Dijon mustard
1 small clove garlic, finely chopped
½ tsp. ground ginger
¼ tsp. Ideal Protein salt
¼ tsp. black pepper
½ C. olive oil

DIRECTIONS
1. In a medium bowl, stir all ingredients to combine (except oil); whisk in oil.
2. Cover and store refrigerated; whisk before serving.

SERVINGS
1 T. Vinaigrette = ½ tsp. oil

Mockamole
A guacamole-style condiment made with asparagus

INGREDIENTS
1 ¾ C. asparagus, cut in 1" pieces (discard woody ends)
1 large bowl ice water
1 T. lime juice
¼ C. chopped fresh cilantro
¼ C. chopped green onion
½ jalapeno pepper, seeded and minced
1 tsp. minced garlic
Salt and pepper, to taste
3 T. Pico de Gallo, pg. 145

DIRECTIONS
1. Place a steamer basket in a large saucepan or Dutch oven. Add 1 inch water and heat to a low boil. Add asparagus to basket, cover, and steam asparagus over medium heat 10 minutes.
2. Immediately transfer asparagus into ice water; cool 2 minutes, drain, and transfer asparagus to a food processor. Add remaining ingredients (except Pico de Gallo.) Puree.
3. Place asparagus puree in a medium bowl; fold in Pico de Gallo.
4. Store in refrigerator; serve chilled.

SERVINGS
Measure amount being used and count that amount toward the daily veggie protocol. For example, ½ C. Mockamole = ½ C. veggies.

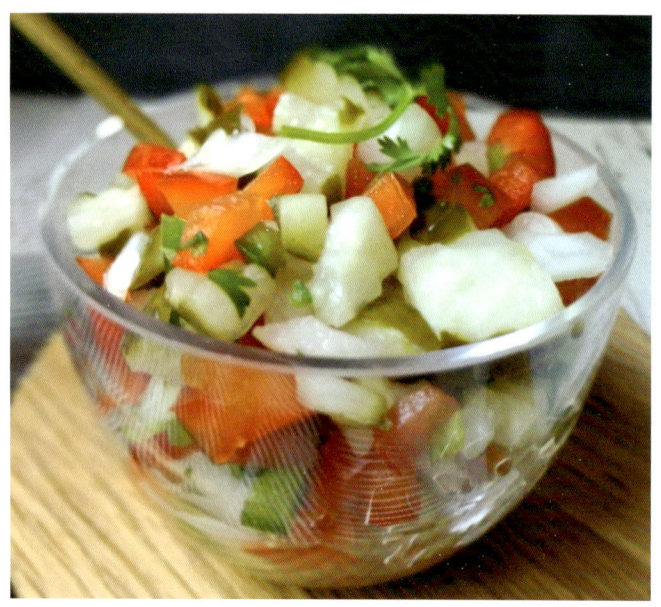
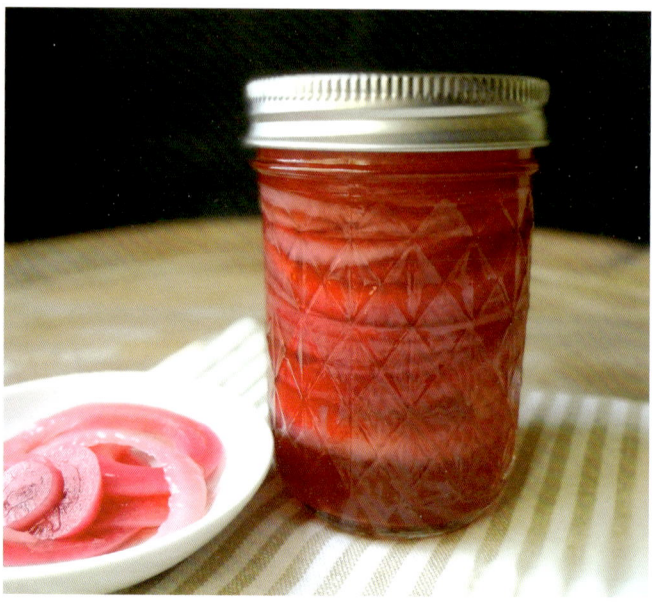

Pickle De Gallo

A rift of the classic Pico de Gallo made with pickles as the surprise ingredient!

INGREDIENTS

1 ½ C. diced kosher pickles
1 C. diced red bell pepper
½ C. diced yellow onion
1 jalapeno pepper, seeded and minced
2 T. chopped fresh cilantro
2 T. jarred pickle juice
½ tsp. sugar free sweetener, granular

DIRECTIONS

1. Place all ingredients in a medium mixing bowl. Toss gently to mix; store covered in fridge up to one week.

SERVINGS

Measure amount being used and count that amount toward the daily veggie protocol. For example, ½ C. Pickle de Gallo = ½ C. veggies.

TIP: Pickle de Gallo is excellent served with Ideal Protein chips, added to salads, or served over burgers and other proteins for added flavor.

Pickled Red Onions

INGREDIENTS

1 medium red onion
½ C. water
¼ C. apple cider vinegar
¼ C. white vinegar
3 T. Ideal Protein maple syrup
1 ½ tsp. fine sea salt
¼ tsp. red pepper flakes

DIRECTIONS

1. Cut ends off onion and remove skin; slice onion into ⅛" slices. Set aside.
2. Add all remaining ingredients to a microwave proof bowl (I use a 2 C. glass measuring cup as this makes it easy to fill jars later in recipe); whisk ingredients to blend.
3. Heat pickling mixture in the microwave 1 minute on high. Stir to mix and let cool to room temperature.
4. Place onion slices in a canning jar(s). Pour pickling liquid over onions, covering completely; seal jar with lid. Let sit at room temp 6 hours; then store in fridge 24 hours before consuming.
5. Store refrigerated.

SERVINGS

Measure amount being used and count that amount toward the daily veggie protocol. For example, ¼ C. Pickled Red Onions = ¼ C. veggies.

TIP: Use as a condiment served on meats, salads, or any other dish requiring extra flavor.

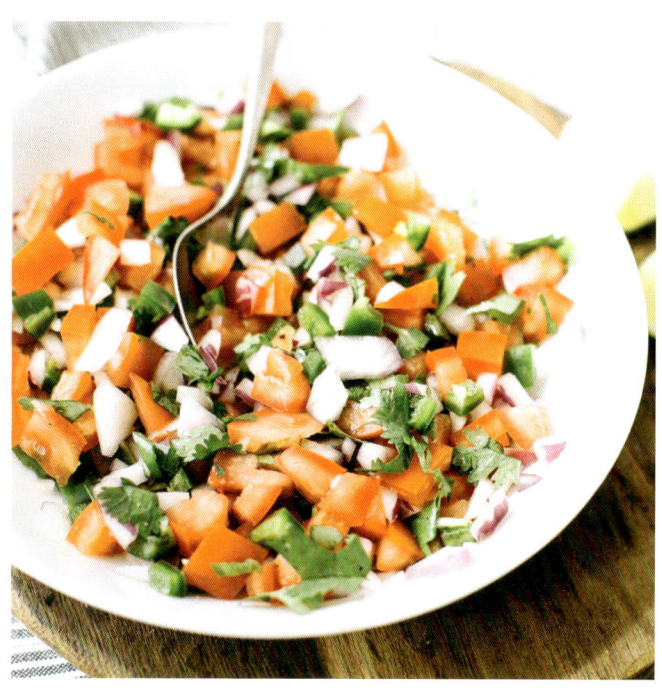

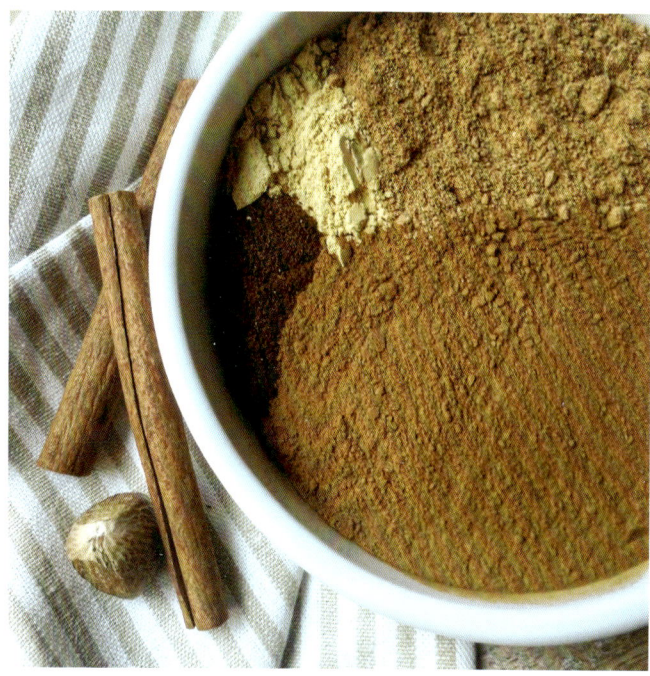

Pico de Gallo

Mexican-style salsa

INGREDIENTS

1½ C. diced fresh Roma tomatoes
1 C. diced red or yellow onion
⅔ C. chopped fresh cilantro
1 - 2 jalapeno peppers, seeded and finely chopped
Juice of ½ lime, or to taste
Sea salt, to taste

DIRECTIONS

1. In a medium bowl, gently fold all ingredients to combine.
2. Store in a covered container in refrigerator.

SERVINGS

Measure amount being used and count that amount toward the daily veggie protocol. For example, ½ C. Pico de Gallo = ½ C. veggies.

Pumpkin Pie Spice

INGREDIENTS

¼ C. ground cinnamon
1 T. + 1 tsp. ground nutmeg
1 tsp. ground ginger
1 tsp. ground cloves

DIRECTIONS

1. Add ingredients to a bowl and stir to combine.
2. Store in an airtight container.

SERVINGS

Varies

TIP: Add to coffee, smoothies, oatmeal, pancake batter or baked goods.

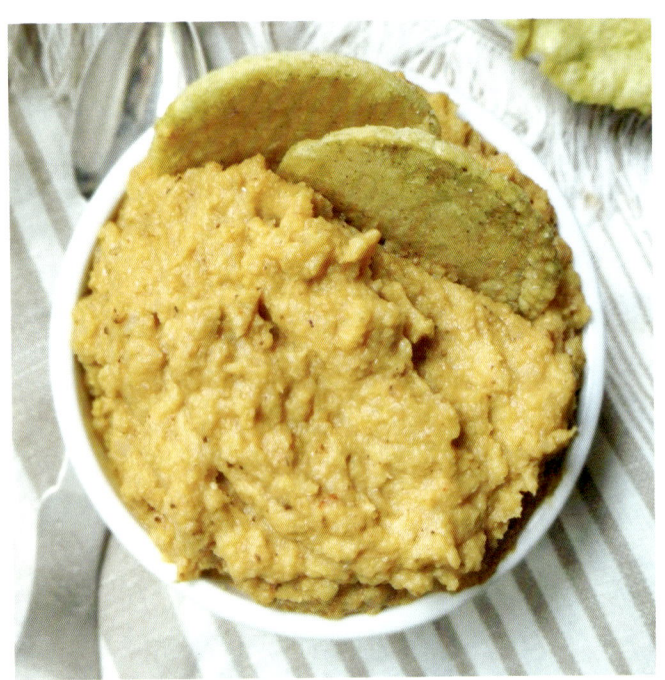

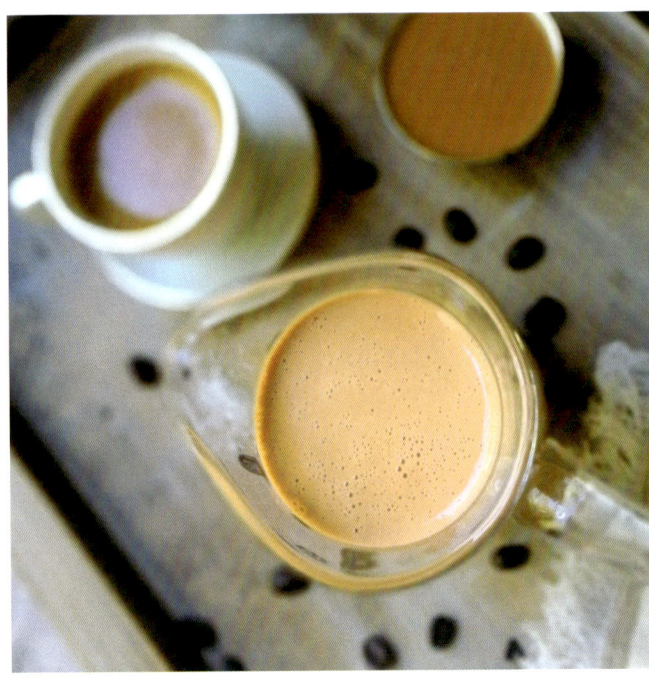

Roasted Cauliflower Hummus

INGREDIENTS

4 C. (14 oz.) cauliflower florets, cut in bite size pieces
1 T. + 1 tsp. extra virgin olive oil
1 tsp. smoked paprika
½ tsp. garlic powder
1 tsp. kosher salt
½ tsp. ground cumin
¼ tsp. red pepper flakes
1 T. lemon juice
⅓ C. chicken broth, fat free

DIRECTIONS

1. Preheat oven to 425°F degrees. Place cauliflower florets, olive oil and dry seasonings in a resealable bag. Shake to coat florets.
2. Spread florets onto a baking sheet. Roast 20-23 minutes, flipping once during roasting.
3. Place roasted florets and remaining ingredients in a blender or food processor; blend until creamy. You may add more chicken broth if necessary for desired texture.

SERVINGS

Entire recip yield = 4 C. veggies + 4 tsp. oil
½ recipe yield = 2 C. veggies + 2 tsp. oil

TIP: Serve with vegetables or Ideal Protein chips.

Salted Caramel Coffee Creamer

INGREDIENTS

½ C. half and half cream
½ C. Ideal Protein vanilla shake (ready-to-drink)
½ C. Walden Farms caramel syrup
Pinch of sea salt

DIRECTIONS

1. In a medium bowl, mix all ingredients together – transfer to a covered storage container with a pour spout. I like to use my Ideal Protein shaker cup.
2. Keep refrigerated.

SERVINGS

Entire recipe yield = 1 ½ C. creamer
6 T. = 1 oz. half and half cream + 2 extras (shake + syrup)
3 T. = 0.5 oz. half and half cream + 1 extra (shake + syrup)

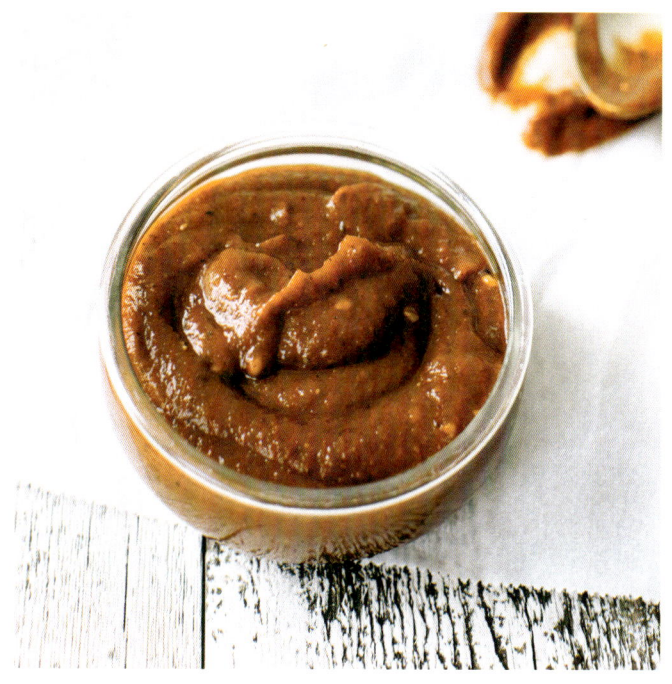

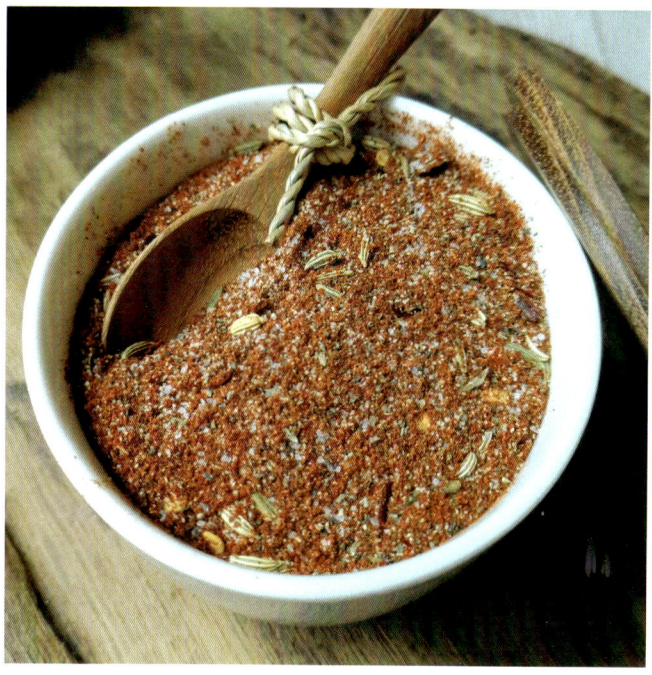

Sassy BBQ Sauce

INGREDIENTS
1 C. Heinz No Added Sugar Ketchup*
1 T. olive oil
1 T. liquid smoke
1 T. apple cider vinegar
1 T. lemon juice
1 T. sugar free sweetener, granular
1 T. onion powder
1 tsp. minced garlic
1 tsp. chili powder
½ tsp. salt
½ tsp. black pepper

DIRECTIONS
1. Add all ingredients to a small saucepan; stir to mix.
2. Cover and simmer 20 minutes, stirring occasionally. Remove cover and simmer an additional 5 minutes, stirring occasionally.
3. Store BBQ sauce in refrigerator.

SERVINGS
Entire recipe yield = 2 C. veggies (1 C. ketchup equivalent to 2 C. tomatoes) + 1 T. oil
2 T. BBQ sauce = ¼ C. veggies + (oil is a trace amount per serving)

TIP: *Walden Farms ketchup may be substituted for the Heinz brand ketchup. If using Walden Farms brand, eliminate the veggie count in the servings.

Sausage Seasoning

INGREDIENTS
3 ½ tsp. paprika
1 ½ tsp. sea salt
¾ tsp. garlic powder
1 tsp. fennel seed
1 tsp. black pepper
¼ tsp. crushed red pepper flakes, optional

DIRECTIONS
1. Add ingredients to a bowl and stir to combine.
2. Store in an airtight container.

SERVINGS
Varies

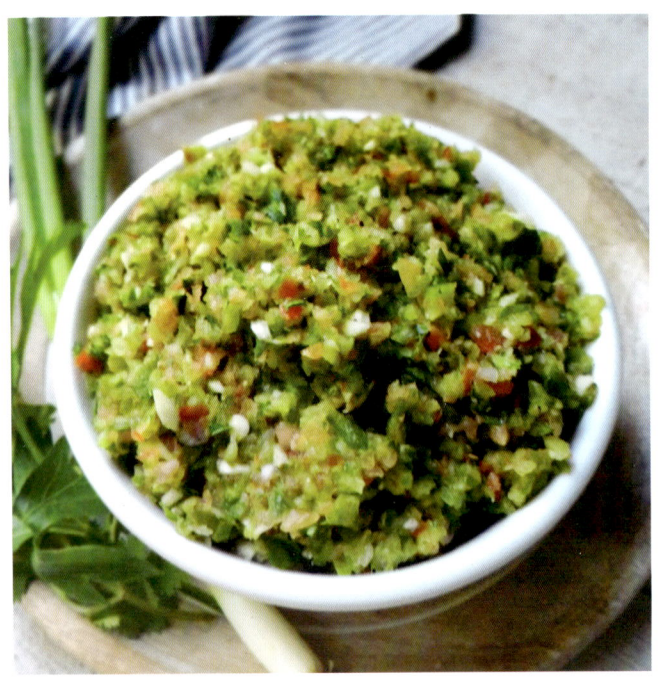

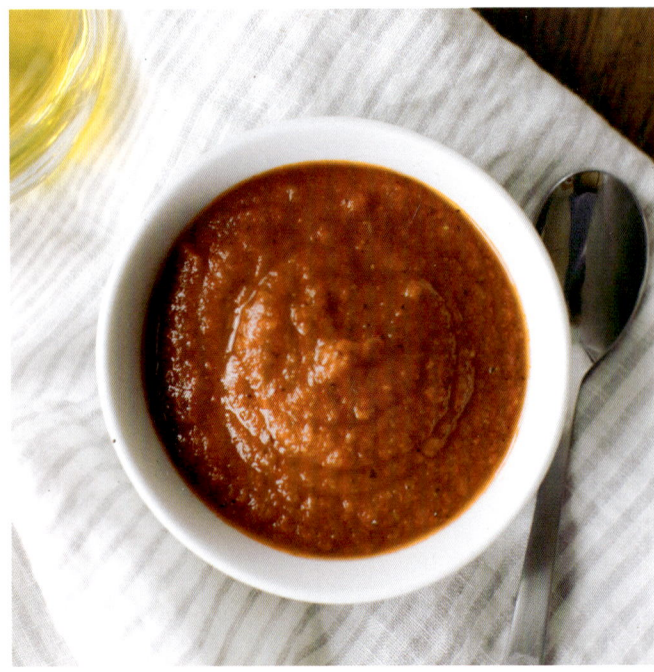

Sofrito

For uses, see tip below

INGREDIENTS

2 C. green bell pepper, cut in chunks
1 C. red bell pepper, cut in chunks
2 C. chopped fresh tomato
1 C. (3.5 oz.) green onion
10 garlic cloves, peeled
1 C. fresh cilantro, firmly packed
½ C. fresh Italian parsley, firmly packed
1 tsp. kosher salt
½ tsp. black pepper

DIRECTIONS

1. Place all ingredients in a food processor; blend to the consistency of a pesto.
2. Drain in a mesh strainer; store covered in fridge.

SERVINGS

Measure amount being used and count that amount toward the daily veggie protocol. For example, ½ C. Sofrito = ½ C. veggies.

TIP: There are several uses for this Latin inspired condiment that adds extra flavor to any dish. Add to soups, stews or egg dishes. Top casseroles, cauliflower rice, cooked lean meats, fish or seafood with Sofrito. Makes a great dip for chips and crackers.

Spaghizza Sauce

Perfect for recipes requiring a tomato-based sauce

INGREDIENTS

28 oz. can crushed tomatoes
2 T. tomato paste
¼ tsp. black pepper
½ tsp. crushed red pepper flakes
1 tsp. onion powder
1 tsp. garlic powder
1 T. dried Italian seasoning
1 tsp. salt
2 T. apple cider vinegar
2 T. extra virgin olive oil

DIRECTIONS

1. Place all ingredients in a blender; blend until tomatoes are pureed.
2. Pour mixture into a medium saucepan and bring to a low boil. Reduce to low heat; simmer for 25-30 minutes, stirring occasionally.
3. Refrigerate sauce until use.

SERVINGS

Entire recipe yield = 5 C. veggies + 2 T. oil
⅕ recipe yield = 1 C. veggies + 1 ¼ tsp. oil

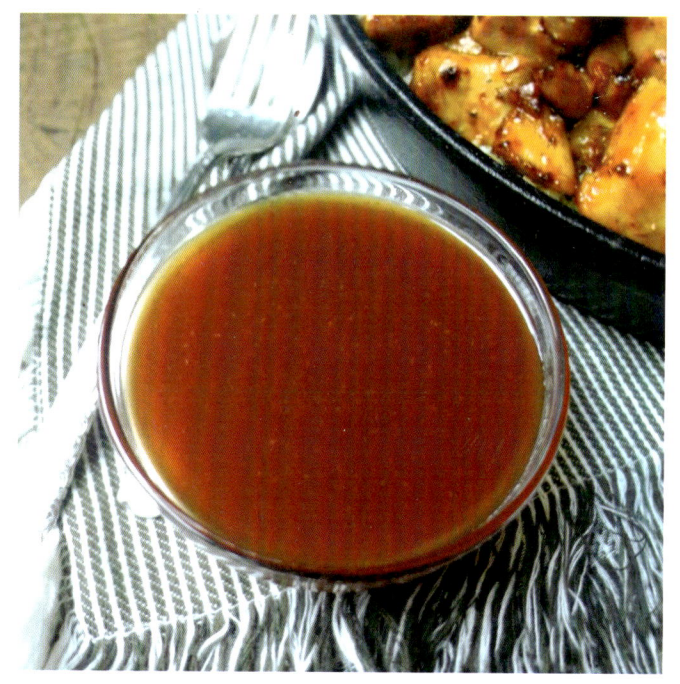

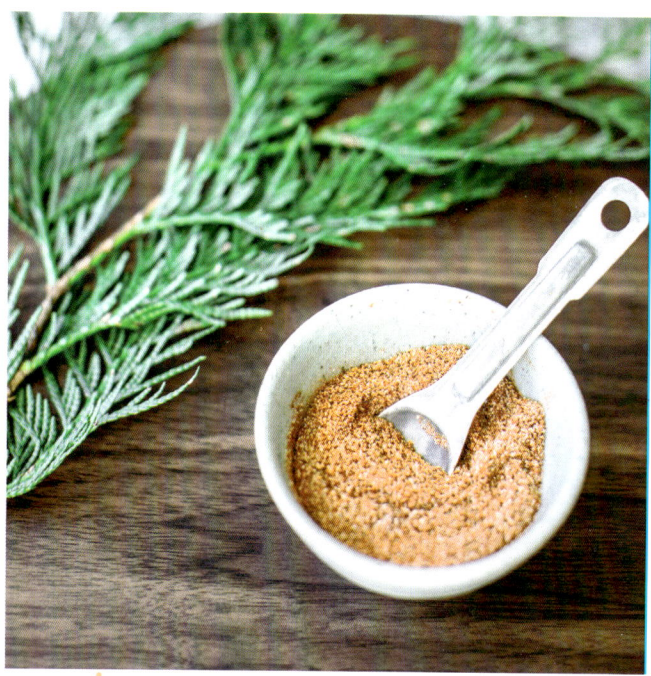

Sweet & Sour Sauce

INGREDIENTS
½ C. sugar free sweetener, granular
⅓ C. apple cider vinegar
2 T. Heinz No Added Sugar Ketchup
2 T. tomato paste
1 T. Ideal Protein maple syrup
1 T. soy sauce
½ tsp. garlic powder

DIRECTIONS
1. In a medium mixing bowl, whisk all ingredients together until thoroughly mixed.
2. Store refrigerated.

SERVINGS
2 T. sauce = 1/4 C. veggies (approximately)

TIP: Excellent for use with pork or chicken stir fry, meatballs, etc.

Taco Seasoning

INGREDIENTS
1 ½ T. chili powder
2 T. cumin
1 ½ T. paprika
1 ½ T. onion powder
1 T. garlic powder
⅛ to ½ tsp. cayenne, or to taste

DIRECTIONS
1. Add ingredients to a bowl and stir to combine.
2. Store in an airtight container.

SERVINGS
Varies

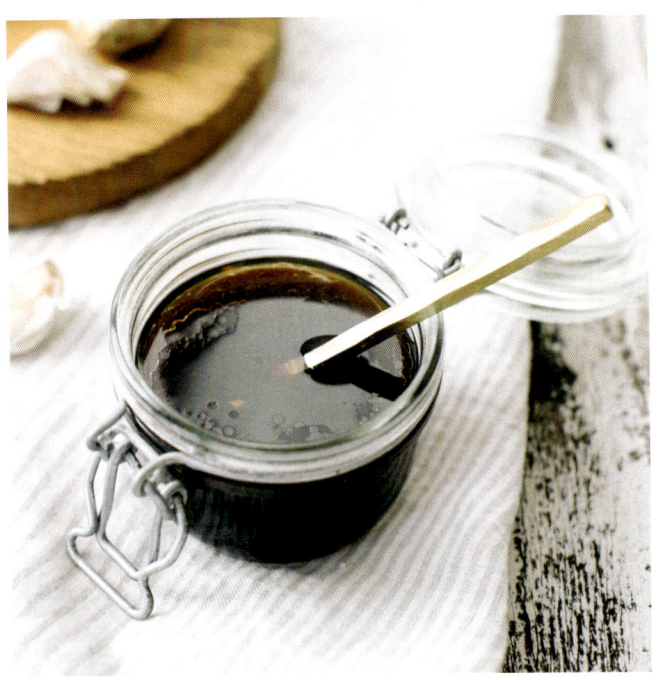

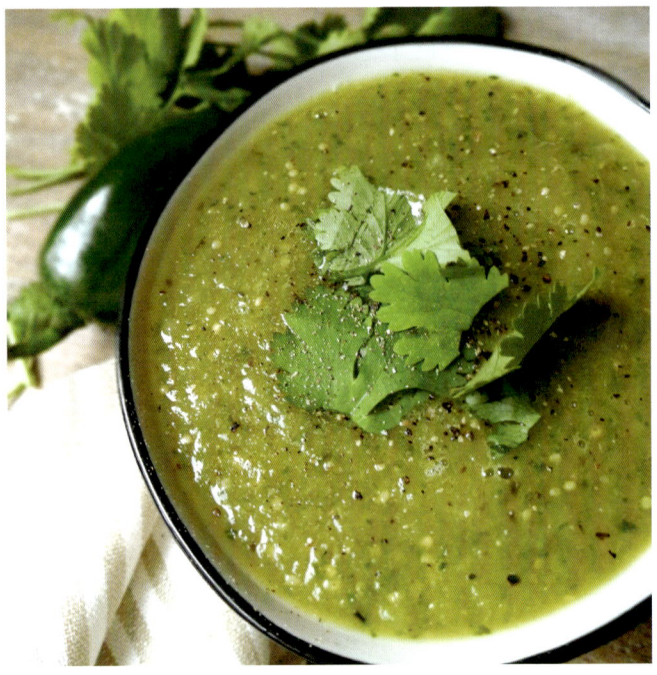

Teriyaki Sauce

INGREDIENTS
½ C. low sodium soy sauce
¼ C. toasted sesame oil
2 T. Ideal Protein maple syrup
1 T. minced ginger
1 tsp. minced garlic

DIRECTIONS
1. Add all ingredients to a small saucepan; stir to mix.
2. Heat to a low boil on medium; reduce heat and simmer about 10 minutes or until mixture slightly thickens.
3. Store refrigerated in an airtight container.

SERVINGS
1 T. Teriyaki Sauce = 1 tsp. oil

Tomatillo Salsa Verde

INGREDIENTS
6 medium tomatillos
2 medium jalapenos
½ medium yellow onion
2 garlic cloves
½ C. fresh cilantro
1 T. lime juice
½ tsp. sea salt

DIRECTIONS
1. Move oven rack to top rung and turn on broiler.
2. Remove husks from tomatillos, slice in half. Place cut side down on a foil lined baking sheet.
3. Slice jalapenos in half, remove pulp and seeds; discard. Place cut side down on same baking sheet as tomatillos.
4. Broil tomatillos and jalapenos about 2 minutes until the skin is blistered and blackened. Cool.
5. Add cooled tomatillos and jalapenos to a blender with remaining ingredients; pulse or blend until smooth (or desired texture.)
6. Taste and adjust lime juice and salt, if necessary.

SERVINGS
Measure amount being used and count that amount toward the daily veggie protocol. For example, ½ C. Tomatillo Salsa Verde = ½ C. veggies.

TIP: Use the salsa to top Ideal Protein Dorados, eggs, casseroles, salads, or meats.

Zucchini Salsa

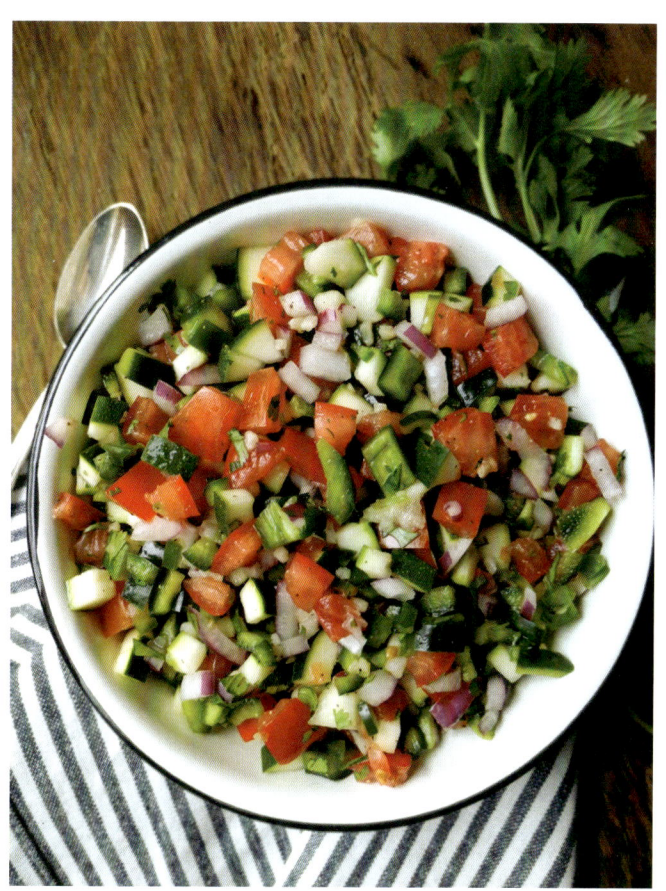

INGREDIENTS

1 C. chopped Roma tomatoes (seeds and pulp removed)
1 ½ C. chopped zucchini
½ C. chopped poblano pepper (seeded)
½ C. chopped red or yellow onion
1 jalapeno pepper, seeded and diced
2 T. finely chopped fresh cilantro
1 tsp. minced garlic
3 T. lime juice
½ tsp. sea salt
¼ tsp. black pepper

DIRECTIONS

1. In order listed, add all ingredients to a medium mixing bowl. Toss to coat.
2. Store refrigerated.

SERVINGS

Measure amount being used and count that amount toward the daily veggie protocol. For example, ½ C. Zucchini Salsa = ½ C. veggies.

TIP: Use this salsa the same way you would use a Mexican-style salsa – add to eggs, casseroles or meats; use as a condiment with Ideal Protein chips.

snacks & miscellaneous

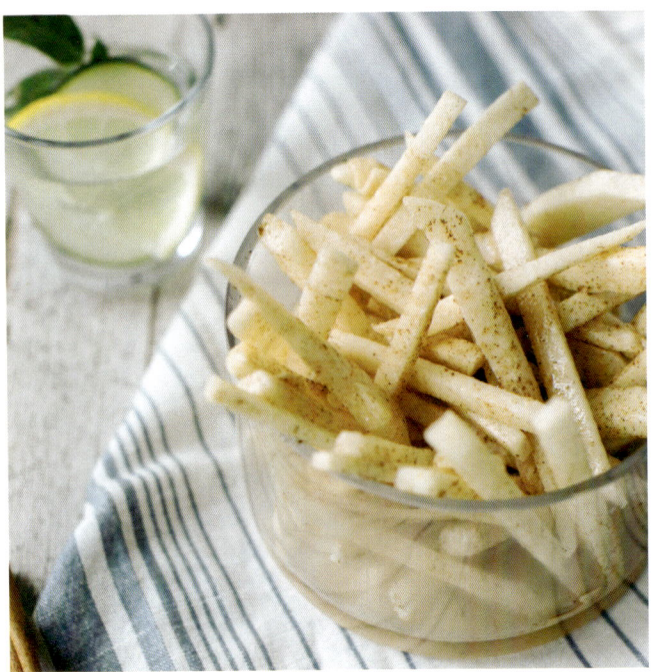

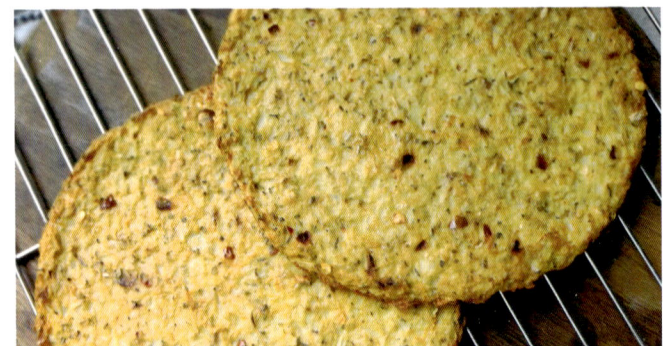

CaULIflower Pizza Crusts

INGREDIENTS
14 oz. frozen riced cauliflower
½ tsp. Italian seasoning
½ tsp. garlic powder
½ tsp. crushed red pepper
1 large egg

DIRECTIONS
1. Preheat oven to 400°F degrees.
2. Cook riced cauliflower according to package directions; drain and cool.
3. Add remaining ingredients to a small bowl. Whisk to blend; set aside.
4. Place cooled cauliflower rice in the center of a clean, thin dish towel. Using the towel, wring the cauliflower by squeezing out as much water as possible until the rice is 'dry' and no water drains from the towel. (Do not rush this step or the crust won't cook properly and will be too soggy; this procedure may take 3-4 minutes to squeeze out all the water.)
5. Place the cauliflower rice and egg mixture in a large bowl and mix until well blended.
6. Line a baking sheet with parchment paper. Evenly divide crust mixture in half; spread mixture in two 6-inch circles on baking sheet.
7. Bake 30 minutes; flip crusts and bake another 10 minutes. Cool on cooling rack.
8. Top with your favorite pizza toppings.

SERVINGS
2 cauliflower crusts = 4 C. veggies + 1 oz. lean protein (egg)
1 cauliflower crust = 2 C. veggies + 0.5 oz. lean protein (egg)

Caramel Apple Jicama Stix

INGREDIENTS
3 C. (13.8 oz.) jicama stix (cut jicama the size of fries)
2 T. Walden Farms caramel syrup
1 T. + 2 tsp. apple cider vinegar
1 T. Ideal Protein maple syrup
1 T. olive oil
1 tsp. cinnamon
Pinch of sea salt

DIRECTIONS
1. Place jicama stix in a large resealable bag; set aside.
2. In a medium bowl, whisk the remaining ingredients.
3. Pour the caramel mixture over the stix; seal bag and toss to coat.
4. Marinate in fridge 2-4 hours for best flavor; toss to coat before serving.

SERVINGS
Entire recipe yield = 3 C. veggies +1 T. oil
⅓ recipe yield = 1 C. veggies + 1 tsp. oil

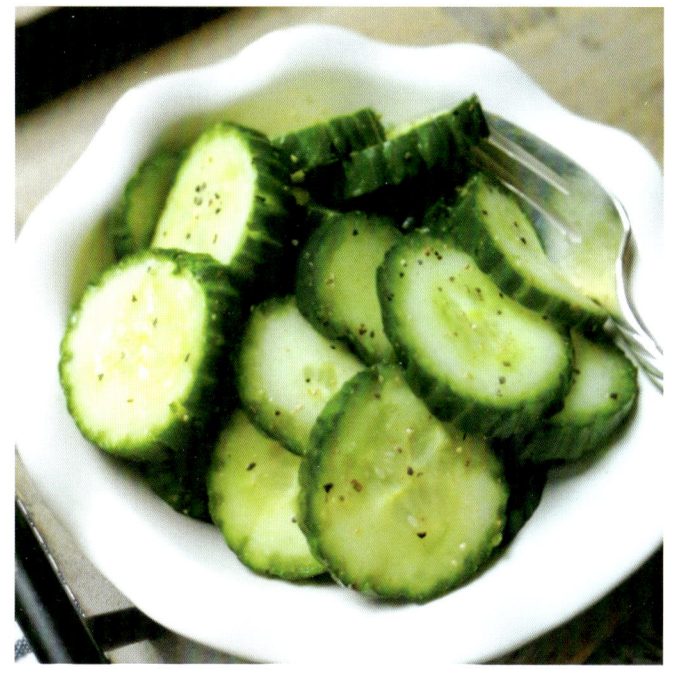

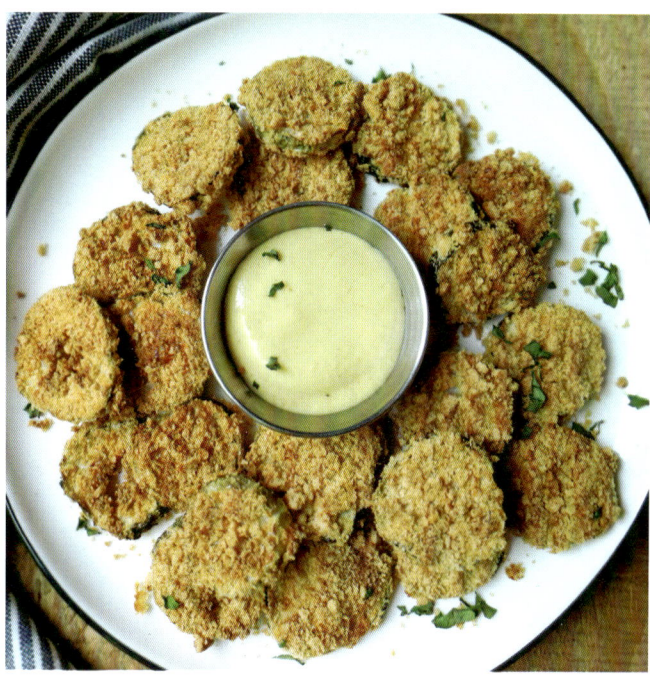

Cucumber Coins

A tangy, salty-sweet portable snack

INGREDIENTS

1 English cucumber, unpeeled
2 T. sugar free sweetener, granular
1 ½ tsp. ground coriander
1 tsp. kosher salt
¼ tsp. black pepper
¼ tsp. onion powder
3 T. apple cider vinegar
2 T. cold water

DIRECTIONS

1. Slice cucumber into ¼" coins; set aside.
2. In a small bowl, whisk remaining ingredients.
3. Place cucumber in a large resealable plastic bag and pour dressing mixture over the top of cucumbers. Seal bag and toss to coat.
4. Store in refrigerator.

SERVINGS

Measure amount being used and count that amount toward the daily veggie protocol. For example, ½ C. cucumbers = ½ C. veggies.

Fried Pickles

Air fryer recipe

INGREDIENTS

1 pkg. Ideal Protein dill pickle zippers (crushed to fine crumbs)
3 T. liquid egg whites (more if needed)
1 C. dill pickle slices
Olive oil cooking spray

DIRECTIONS

1. Spread crushed dill pickle zipper crumbs on a small plate.
2. On a separate small plate, add liquid egg whites.
3. Dredge pickle slices in egg whites and press into crumbs, covering both sides.
4. In one layer, add pickle slices to air fryer. Lightly coat both sides with olive oil cooking spray.
5. Air fry 15 minutes at 350˚ F degrees flipping once during cooking.

SERVINGS

Entire recipe yield = 1 C. veggies + 1 restricted

TIP: To make Fried Pickles using oven method, preheat oven to 400˚F degrees; follow directions 1-4. Place pickles on a parchment lined baking sheet and bake 20 minutes flipping once during baking.

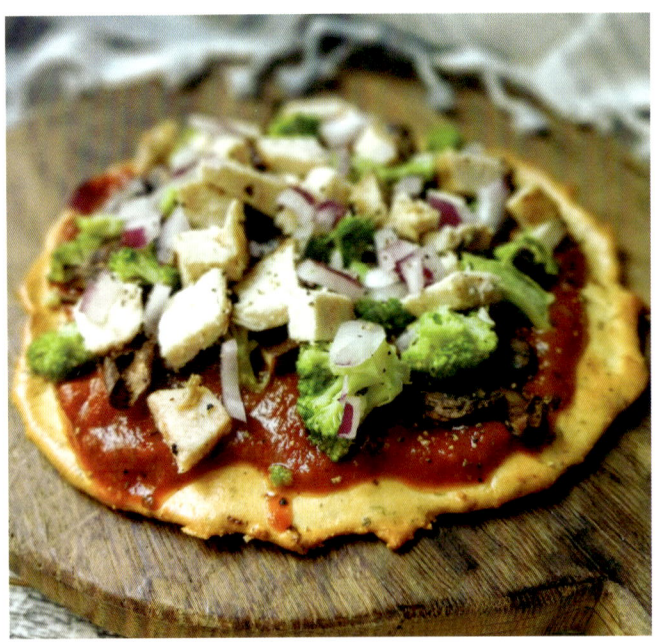

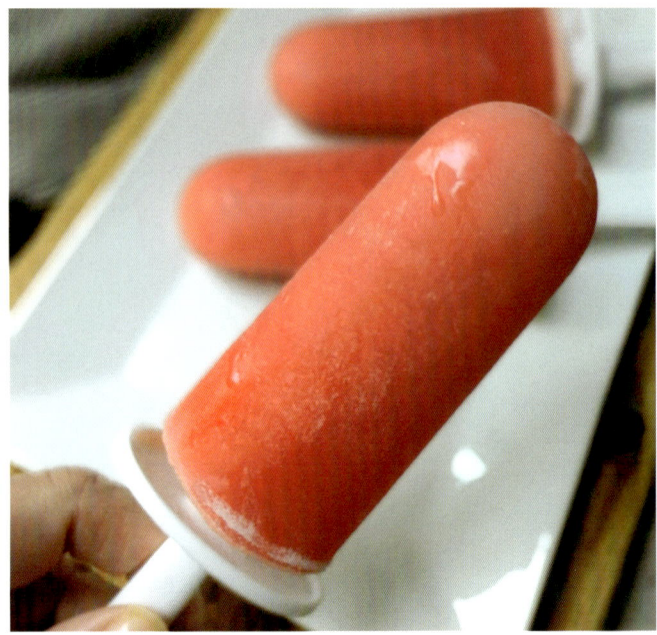

Perfect Pizza Crust

INGREDIENTS
1 Ideal Protein mashed potatoes mix
½ tsp. garlic powder
¼ tsp. salt
¼ tsp. Italian seasoning
¼ tsp. onion powder
¼ tsp. crushed red pepper flakes
1 tsp. olive oil
3 T. water
Cooking spray

DIRECTIONS
1. Preheat oven to 350° F degrees.
2. In a medium bowl, mix the dry ingredients.
3. Add liquid ingredients; stir to mix.
4. Line a rimmed baking sheet with parchment paper. Evenly spread batter in a 7-inch circle with a spatula or back of spoon sprayed with cooking spray.
5. Bake 10 minutes. Remove from oven and poke several holes in the crust with a fork; flip crust over. Bake an additional 10 minutes.
6. Cool completely; this will allow the crust to become crispier.

SERVINGS
Entire recipe yield = 1 unrestricted + 1 tsp. oil

TIP: As a serving suggestion, top with Spaghizza Sauce (pg. 148), roasted veggies, and lean protein of choice, if desired.

Raspberry Mango Popsicles

INGREDIENTS
1 Ideal Protein raspberry gelatin mix
½ C. boiling water
1 Ideal Protein mango shake (ready-to-drink)

DIRECTIONS
1. Combine raspberry gelatin and boiling water in a medium mixing bowl; stir until gelatin is dissolved.
2. Add mango shake to gelatin mixture; stir to combine.
3. Fill popsicle molds and freeze.

SERVINGS
Entire recipe yield = 1 unrestricted
(Total amount of popsicles will vary based on popsicle mold size; eat all of them no matter the size, and count as 1 unrestricted.)

NOTE: Gelatin mix is not counted in recipe yield – it is allowed as an extra (4th packet) every other day.

TIP: Vanilla or Chocolate Ideal Protein ready-to-drink shake flavors will also work in place of the mango shake.

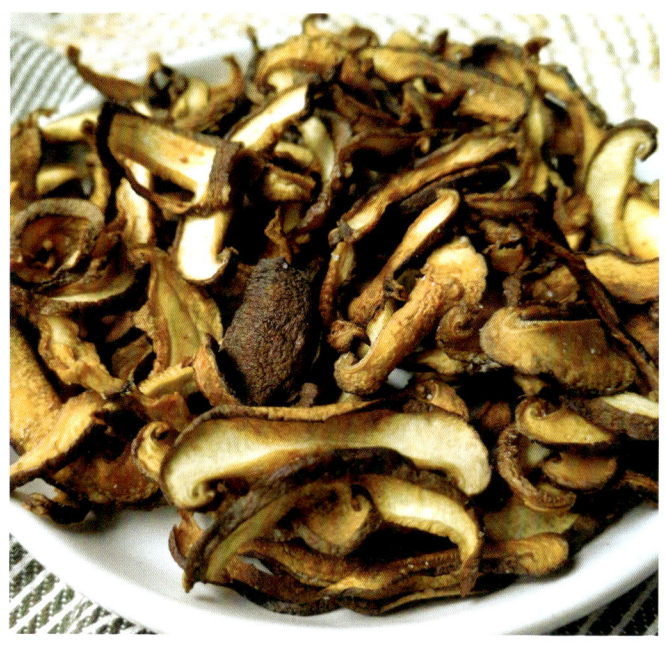

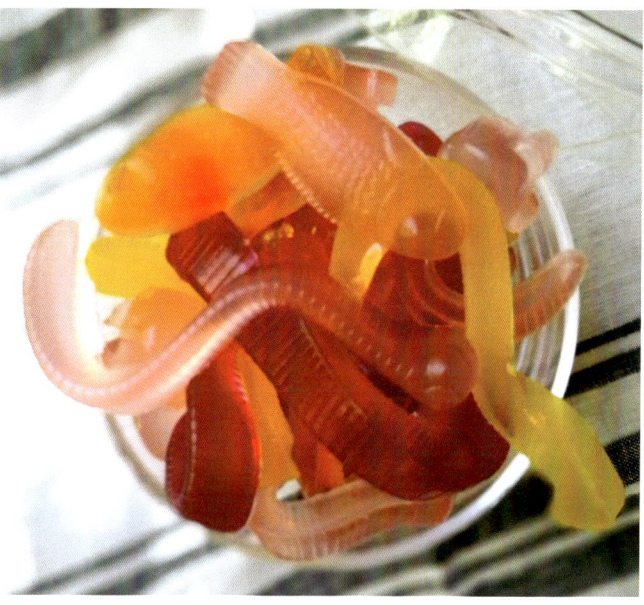

Shiitake Bacon

Tastes like crispy bacon pieces!

INGREDIENTS

2 C. thinly sliced shiitake mushrooms
Olive oil cooking spray
Sea salt, to taste

DIRECTIONS

1. Preheat oven to 375°F degrees.
2. Coat a rimmed baking sheet with cooking spray.
3. Spread mushroom slices in one layer on baking sheet, spacing apart. Lightly spray mushrooms with cooking spray to coat; season lightly with salt.
4. Bake 20-30 minutes, turning with a spatula once during baking (baking time varies based on thickness of slices and water content in mushrooms). Bake mushrooms until they are dark brown and crispy but not burned.
5. During baking, remove mushroom slices that bake earlier than others. Serve immediately or bacon will lose its crispy texture.

SERVINGS

Entire recipe yield = 2 C. veggies + ½ tsp. oil (approximately)

TIPS: Baking time will vary depending on the thickness of the mushrooms; watch closely toward end of bake time or they will burn quickly.

Sour Gummies

INGREDIENTS

1 packet Ideal Protein water enhancer (any flavor)
1 packet Knox® unflavored gelatin
3 T. boiling water
2 T. cold water

DIRECTIONS

1. Add water enhancer and gelatin powder to a vessel with a spout (I use a glass liquid measuring cup).
2. Stir in boiling water until gelatin is dissolved; add cold water and stir to mix.
3. Place gummy molds on a baking sheet (this will help stabilize the silicone molds when moving from work surface to fridge). Pour gelatin mixture into silicone gummy molds.
4. Refrigerate 1 hour; remove gummies from molds. For storing, place gummies in an airtight container and store refrigerated.

SERVINGS

This recipe will make approximately 8 pieces depending on the shape and size of the mold. Essentially the water enhancers are unlimited when mixed with water; however, the gelatin packet has some calories and will need to be counted toward daily protocol. Consult your coach or clinic for protocol serving size.

TIP: For a sweeter, less intense sour taste, use ½ packet Ideal Protein water enhancer powder in place of the full packet.

Zesty Italian Parmesan Crackers

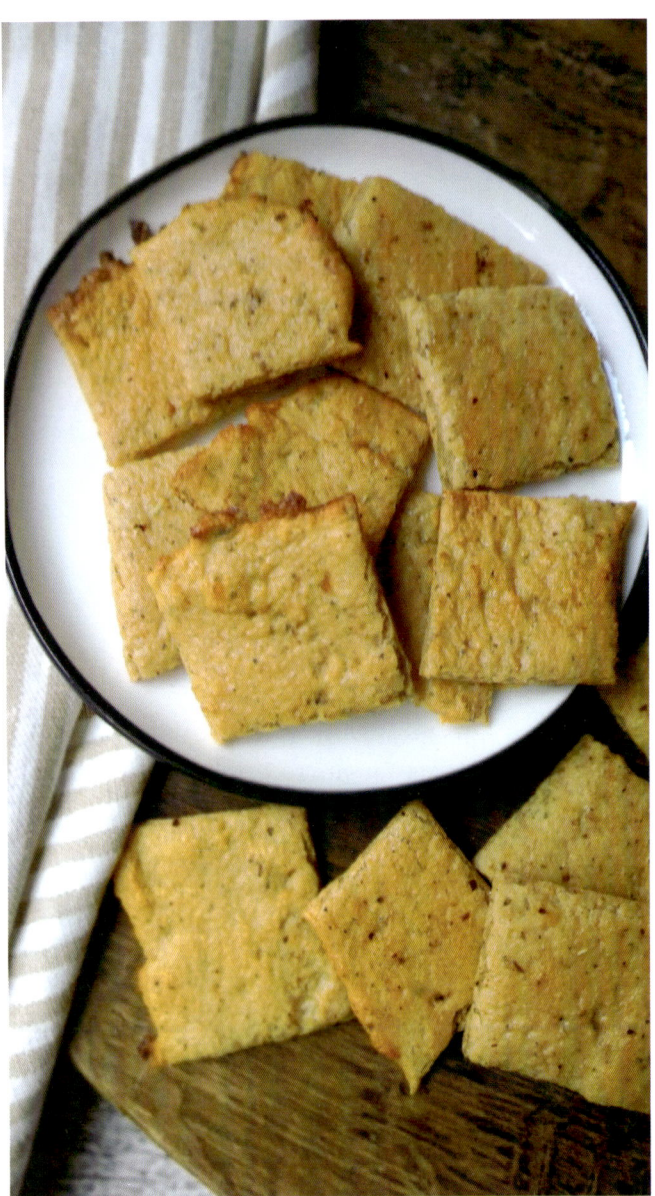

INGREDIENTS

1 Ideal Protein crispy cereal mix
1 Ideal Protein garlic parmesan croutons
¼ tsp garlic powder
¼ tsp. Ideal Protein salt
¼ tsp. Italian seasoning
Pinch of crushed red pepper flakes
3 T. water
1 tsp. olive oil

DIRECTIONS

1. Preheat oven to 350˚F degrees.
2. Place dry ingredients in a bullet blender or food processor; pulse to fine crumbs. Transfer to a mixing bowl; stir in liquid ingredients.
3. Line a rimmed baking sheet with parchment paper; spread batter in a cracker-thin square with a rubber spatula. (Spraying spatula with cooking spray helps to prevent sticking.)
4. Bake 15 minutes. Using a pizza cutter, cut into cracker size pieces and flip pieces over. Bake an additional 5 minutes.
5. Watch the crackers closely toward the end of bake time as they will brown quickly.
6. Cool crackers on pan 20 minutes. Crackers will crisp as they cool.

SERVINGS

Entire recipe yield = 1 unrestricted + 1 tsp. oil

NOTE: One Ideal Protein crouton packet is allowed per day as an 'extra' but is not counted toward the 3 required Ideal Protein food packets. Therefore, it is not counted in the servings.

category index

ideal protein packet index